Bovine Respiratory Disease

Guest Editors

VICKIE L. COOPER, DVM, MS, PhD
BRUCE W. BRODERSEN, DVM, MS, PhD

VETERINARY CLINICS OF NORTH AMERICA: FOOD ANIMAL PRACTICE

www.vetfood.theclinics.com

Consulting Editor
ROBERT A. SMITH, DVM, MS

July 2010 • Volume 26 • Number 2

SAUNDERS an imprint of ELSEVIER, Inc.

W.B. SAUNDERS COMPANY
A Division of Elsevier Inc.

1600 John F. Kennedy Boulevard • Suite 1800 • Philadelphia, PA 19103-2899

http://www.vetfood.theclinics.com

VETERINARY CLINICS OF NORTH AMERICA: FOOD ANIMAL PRACTICE Volume 26, Number 2
July 2010 ISSN 0749-0720, ISBN-13: 978-1-4377-2504-9

Editor: John Vassallo; j.vassallo@elsevier.com

Veterinary Clinics of North America: Food Animal Practice (ISSN 0749-0720) is published in March, July, and November by Elsevier Inc., 360 Park Avenue South, New York, NY 10010-1710. Subscription prices are $179.00 per year (domestic individuals), $265.00 per year (domestic institutions), $89.00 per year (domestic students/residents), $208.00 per year (Canadian individuals), $346.00 per year (Canadian institutions), $263.00 per year (international individuals), $346.00 per year (international institutions), and $135.00 per year (international and Canadian students/residents). To receive student/resident rate, orders must be accompanied by name of affiliated institution, date of term, and the signature of program/residency coordinator on institution letterhead. *Clinics* subscription prices. All prices are subject to change without notice. **POSTMASTER:** Send address changes to *Veterinary Clinics of North America: Food Animal Practice*, Elsevier Health Sciences Division, Subscription Customer Service, 3251 Riverport Lane, Maryland Heights, MO 63043. Customer Service (orders, claims, online, change of address): Elsevier Health Sciences Division, Subscription Customer Service, 3251 Riverport Lane, Maryland Heights, MO 63043. Tel: 1-800-654-2452 (U.S. and Canada); 314-447-8871 (ouside U.S. and Canada). Fax: 314-447-8029. E-mail: journalscustomerservice-usa@elsevier.com (for print support); journalsonlinesupport-usa@elsevier.com (for online support).

Reprints. For copies of 100 or more, of articles in this publication, please contact the Commercial Reprints Department, Elsevier Inc., 360 Park Avenue South, New York, NY 10010-1710. Tel.: 212-633-3812; Fax: 212-462-1935; E-mail: reprints@elsevier.com.

Veterinary Clinics of North America: Food Animal Practice is covered in *Current Contents/Agriculture, Biology and Environmental Sciences, MEDLINE/PubMed (Index Medicus), and Excerpta Medica.*

Printed and bound by CPI Group (UK) Ltd, Croydon, CR0 4YY
Transferred to Digital Print 2011

Contributors

CONSULTING EDITOR

ROBERT A. SMITH, DVM, MS
Diplomate, American Board of Veterinary Practitioners; Veterinary Research and
Consulting Services, LLC, Greeley, Colorado

GUEST EDITORS

VICKIE L. COOPER, DVM, MS, PhD
Senior Clinician, Department of Veterinary Diagnostic and Production Animal Medicine,
College of Veterinary Medicine, Iowa State University, Ames, Iowa

BRUCE W. BRODERSEN, DVM, MS, PhD
Assistant Professor, Veterinary Diagnostic Center, School of Veterinary Medicine and
Biomedical Sciences, University of Nebraska—Lincoln, Lincoln, Nebraska

AUTHORS

MARK R. ACKERMANN, DVM, PhD
Diplomate, American College of Veterinary Pathologists; Professor, Department of
Veterinary Pathology, College of Veterinary Medicine, Iowa State University, Ames, Iowa

KEN G. BATEMAN, DVM, MSc
Associate Professor, Department of Population Medicine, University of Guelph, Guelph,
Ontario, Canada

BRUCE W. BRODERSEN, DVM, MS, PhD
Assistant Professor, Veterinary Diagnostic Center, School of Veterinary Medicine and
Biomedical Sciences, University of Nebraska—Lincoln, Lincoln, Nebraska

HUGH Y. CAI, DVM, MSc, DVSc
Veterinary Microbiologist, Animal Health Laboratory, Laboratory Services Division,
University of Guelph, Guelph, Ontario, Canada

FERNANDA CASTILLO-ALCALA, DVM, DVSc
Associate Professor, Ross University School of Veterinary Medicine, Basseterre, St Kitts,
West Indies

JEFF L. CASWELL, DVM, DVSc, PhD
Diplomate, American College of Veterinary Pathologists; Professor, Department of
Pathobiology, University of Guelph, Guelph, Ontario, Canada

M.M. CHENGAPPA, DVM, PhD
Diplomate, American College of Veterinary Microbiologists; Professor, Department of
Diagnostic Medicine and Pathobiology, Kansas State University College of Veterinary
Medicine, Manhattan, Kansas

SHAFIQUL CHOWDHURY, DVM, PhD
Professor, Department of Pathobiological Sciences, School of Veterinary Medicine, Louisiana State University, Baton Rouge, Louisiana

ANTHONY W. CONFER, DVM, PhD
Diplomate, American College of Veterinary Pathologists; Regents Professor and Sitlington Endowed Chair, Department of Veterinary Pathobiology, College of Veterinary Medicine, Oklahoma State University, Stillwater, Oklahoma

VICKIE L. COOPER, DVM, MS, PhD
Senior Clinician, Department of Veterinary Diagnostic and Production Animal Medicine, College of Veterinary Medicine, Iowa State University, Ames, Iowa

RACHEL DERSCHEID, DVM
College of Veterinary Medicine, Iowa State University, Ames, Iowa

ALAN R. DOSTER, DVM, PhD
Diplomate, American College of Veterinary Pathologists; Professor, Veterinary Diagnostic Center, School of Veterinary Medicine and Biomedical Sciences, University of Nebraska—Lincoln, Lincoln, Nebraska

T.A. EDWARDS, DVM
Midwest Feedlot Services, Inc, Kearney, Nebraska

PATRICK J. GORDEN, DVM
Diplomate, American Board of Veterinary Practitioners; Senior Clinician, Food Supply Veterinary Medicine, College of Veterinary Medicine, Iowa State University, Ames, Iowa

DEE GRIFFIN, DVM, MS
Great Plains Veterinary Educational Center, School of Veterinary Medicine and Biomedical Sciences, University of Nebraska—Lincoln, Clay Center, Nebraska

CLINTON JONES, PhD
School of Veterinary and Biomedical Sciences, Nebraska Center for Virology, University of Nebraska—Lincoln, Lincoln, Nebraska

JENNIFER KUSZAK, BS, MS
Nebraska Veterinary Diagnostic Center, School of Veterinary Medicine and Biomedical Sciences, University of Nebraska—Lincoln, Lincoln, Nebraska

D. SCOTT MCVEY, DVM, PhD
Nebraska Veterinary Diagnostic Center, School of Veterinary Medicine and Biomedical Sciences, University of Nebraska—Lincoln, Lincoln, Nebraska

MICHAEL D. NICHOLS, DVM
Senior Veterinarian, US Beef Veterinary Operations, Pfizer Animal Health, Vega, Texas

JASON S. NICKELL, DVM
Department of Diagnostic Medicine/Pathobiology, Kansas State University, Manhattan; Bayer Animal Health, Shawnee Mission, Kansas

ROGER J. PANCIERA, DVM, PhD
Diplomate, American College of Veterinary Pathologists; Professor Emeritus
of Pathobiology, Department of Veterinary Pathobiology, Oklahoma State University,
Stillwater, Oklahoma

PAUL PLUMMER, DVM, PhD
Diplomate, American College of Veterinary Internal Medicine; Assistant Professor,
Food Supply Veterinary Medicine, College of Veterinary Medicine, Iowa State University,
Ames, Iowa

JULIA RIDPATH, PhD
Ruminant Diseases and Immunology Research Unit, United States Department of
Agriculture, Agricultural Research Service, National Animal Disease Center, Ames, Iowa

JAMES A. ROTH, DVM, PhD
Diplomate, American College of Veterinary Microbiologists; Professor, Veterinary
Microbiology and Preventative Medicine, College of Veterinary Medicine, Iowa State
University, Ames, Iowa

LINDA J. SAIF, MS, PhD
Distinguished University Professor, Department of Veterinary Preventive Medicine, Food
Animal Health Research Program, Ohio Agricultural Research and Development Center,
College of Veterinary Medicine, The Ohio State University, Wooster, Ohio

GERALD L. STOKKA, DVM, MS
Pfizer Animal Health, Cooperstown, North Dakota

SHAUN H. SWEIGER, DVM, MS
Beef Production Medicine Faculty Member, Veterinary Diagnostic and Production Animal
Medicine Department, Iowa State University College of Veterinary Medicine, Lloyd Vet
Med Center, Ames, Iowa; Owner/Operator, Sweiger Enterprises, LLC; President, CATTLE
STATS, LLC, Oklahoma City, Oklahoma

BRAD J. WHITE, DVM, MS
Associate Professor, Department of Clinical Sciences, Kansas State University,
Manhattan, Kansas

Contents

Pneumonia is a major cause of death and economic losses to the cattle industry. Recognizing the patterns of pneumonic lesions and understanding the pathogenesis of the various types of pneumonia are important for correct diagnosis and interpretation of the lesions. Bacterial pneumonias consist of bronchopneumonia, fibrinous pneumonia, and pleuropneumonia as well as caseonecrotic, aspiration, and tuberculous pneumonias. Two major patterns of interstitial pneumonia are recognized in cattle, and verminous pneumonia is associated with *Dictyocaulus viviparus* infection.

There are a variety of factors and conditions that predispose cattle to pneumonia. Cattle have anatomic and cellular differences from humans and other species and are managed in groups/herds, all of which can increase susceptibility to microbial pathogens. This article highlights the basic innate immune response of the respiratory tract and newer developments in the understanding of adaptive immune responses of the bovine respiratory tract, placing special emphasis on features unique to cattle.

Respiratory disease in nursing calves is a common, yet sporadic herd event. In herds that experience respiratory disease, this can be a frustrating experience. Beef cow operations have an expectation of losses during the calving season. Losses because of respiratory disease in calves, that are at least 1 month up to weaning age, is not a normal expectation. Veterinarians providing services and advice to these operations must be able to present scientific and logical recommendations to manage these events. A strong working knowledge of the risk factors contributing to clinical disease is necessary to developing prevention strategies.

Incidence rates for bovine respiratory disease (BRD) in dairy cattle have remained essentially unchanged over the last 20 years. Dairy calves are more commonly affected than adult animals, with BRD being the principal cause of death in weaned dairy calves. The lack of progress in controlling respiratory disease demonstrates that there continues to be significant room for improvement in controlling this multifactorial syndrome, and that dairy producers need assistance in applying evolving husbandry practices to improve the health of dairy cattle. Therefore, it seems prudent to focus the management strategies on preventing disease through sound management of the transition period, along with sound vaccination and biosecurity programs.

The authors provide a review of the foundations of a sound preconditioning or backgrounding health program for stocker cattle. A systematic approach to a health program for high-risk stocker calves has been used, with discussion of purchasing and arrival considerations; nutritional management; cattle movement management; prevention, control, and treatment of bovine respiratory disease (BRD); and the use of information management in the control of BRD.

Vaccines and antibiotics are still relied upon as the standard methods of bovine respiratory disease (BRD) prevention, control, and therapy. Success in building disease resistance begins with genetic selection and continues with colostrum management and reducing pathogen exposure. Purchasing single-source cattle with a history of pre- and post-weaning procedures will minimize pathogen exposure and enhance immunity. Using cattle-handling techniques and facilities that promote low stress will allow host immune defenses to remain effective against bacterial and viral colonization. Lastly, controlling BRD must be managed through a comprehensive herd health immunization and management program that effectively addresses disease challenges common to the operation.

This article provides an overview of implementing metaphylactic antimicrobial protocols to certain classes of cattle on arrival to stocker and feedlot production systems. The goal of this management practice is to reduce the negative health and performance effects induced by bovine respiratory disease (BRD). This article emphasizes the multiple factors that influence the decision for mass medication, including weight (age) of the cattle, distance traveled, environmental conditions, previous health history, visual inspection of the cattle at arrival, and prediction of the risk of disease. Current data suggest that metaphylactic programs significantly reduce negative health effects and improve feed performance that can be observed in cattle stricken with BRD.

BHV-1 is an important pathogen of cattle. Because of its ability to induce immune suppression, BHV-1 is an important agent in the multifactorial disorder, bovine respiratory disease complex (BRDC). BHV-1 encodes several proteins that inhibit various arms of the immune system suggesting that these proteins are important in the development of BRDC.

Bovine respiratory syncytial virus (BRSV) is a major cause of respiratory disease and a major contributor to the bovine respiratory disease (BRD) complex. BRSV infects the upper and lower respiratory tract and is shed in nasal secretions. The close relatedness of BRSV to human respiratory syncytial virus (HRSV) has allowed researchers to use BRSV and HRSV to elucidate the mechanisms by which these viruses induce disease. Attempted vaccine production using formalin-inactivated vaccine resulted in exacerbated disease when infants became exposed to HRSV. Cattle vaccinated with formalin-inactivated virus had enhanced disease when inoculated with BRSV. This article discusses various aspects of BRSV, its epidemiology, pathogenesis, diagnostic tests, immunity, and vaccination.

The contribution of bovine viral diarrhea viruses (BVDV) to the development of bovine respiratory disease is the sum of several different factors. These factors include the contribution of acute uncomplicated BVDV infections, the high incidence of respiratory disease in animals persistently infected with BVDV, the immunosuppression that accompanies acute BVDV infections and predisposes animals to secondary infections, and the synergy resulting in increased virulence occurring in coinfections of BVDV with other pathogens. Immunosuppression, which is associated with infection with all BVDV, may have the greatest impact of these factors. Control of BVDV infections rests on reducing exposure by removing BVDV persistently infected animals, increasing herd resistance by vaccination, and instituting biocontrol methods that limit the opportunity for introduction of BVDV into herds and management units.

Bovine coronaviruses (BCoVs) cause respiratory and enteric infections in cattle and wild ruminants. BCoV is a pneumoenteric virus that infects the upper and lower respiratory tract and intestine. It is shed in feces and nasal secretions and also infects the lung. BCoV is the cause of 3 distinct clinical syndromes in cattle: (1) calf diarrhea, (2) winter dysentery with hemorrhagic diarrhea in adults, and (3) respiratory infections in cattle of various ages including the bovine respiratory disease complex or shipping fever of feedlot cattle. No consistent antigenic or genetic markers have been identified to discriminate BCoVs from the different clinical syndromes. At present, there are no BCoV vaccines to prevent respiratory BCoV infections in cattle, and the correlates of immunity to respiratory BCoV infections are unknown. This article focuses on respiratory BCoV infections including viral characteristics; epidemiology and interspecies transmission; diagnosis, pathogenesis, and clinical signs; and immunity and vaccines.

Mycoplasma bovis has recently emerged as an important cause of chronic caseonecrotic bronchopneumonia, arthritis, and tenosynovitis in beef cattle. *Mycoplasma bovis* can act as a primary pathogen, yet many cases are coinfected with other bacteria or viruses, and evidence suggests that *M. bovis* colonizes and perpetuates lung lesions that were initiated by other bacteria, such as *M. haemolytica*. *Mycoplasma bovis* elicits a robust humoral immune response, but the resulting antibodies are not protective because of the variable surface proteins, and vaccines have not yet been shown to prevent disease. *Mycoplasma bovis* infections are responsible for a high proportion of the chronic disease occurring in feedlots, and the welfare of such animals is an important aspect of feedlot health management.

Pneumonia caused by the bacterial pathogens discussed in this article is the most significant cause of morbidity and mortality of the BRDC. Most of these infectious bacteria are not capable of inducing significant disease without the presence of other predisposing environmental factors, physiologic stressors, or concurrent infections. *Mannheimia haemolytica* is the most common and serious of these bacterial agents and is therefore also the most highly characterized. There are other important bacterial pathogens of BRD, such as *Pasteurella multocida*, *Histophulus somni*, and *Mycoplasma bovis*. Mixed infections with these organisms do occur. These pathogens have unique and common virulence factors but the resulting pneumonic lesions may be similar. Although the amount and quality of research associated with BRD has increased, vaccination and therapeutic practices are not fully successful. A greater understanding of the virulence mechanisms of the infecting bacteria and pathogenesis of pneumonia, as well as the characteristics of the organisms that allow tissue persistence, may lead to improved management, therapeutics, and vaccines.

THE CLINICS ARE NOW AVAILABLE ONLINE!

Access your subscription at:
www.theclinics.com

Preface

Bovine Respiratory Disease

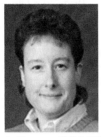 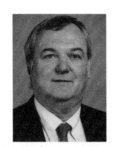

Vickie L. Cooper, DVM, MS, PhD   Bruce W. Brodersen, DVM, MS, PhD
Guest Editors

The cattle industry today faces many of the same challenges they have over the past several decades. Fortunately, disease emergence has been relatively static other than recognition of new strains of old viruses. The industry may seemingly be unchanged, but in reality, many new challenges have arisen in terms of environmental issues and continued awareness of biosecurity issues in cattle management. It has been 13 years since the last update on respiratory disease in *Veterinary Clinics of North America: Food Animal Practice* was published. Disease detection relative to respiratory disease has improved greatly. Control of bovine viral diarrhea virus (BVDV) has taken quantum leaps forward with the advent of immunohistochemistry and application of molecular biology technologies toward testing for cattle persistently infected with BVDV. In some situations, this has reduced the incidence of respiratory disease and has paid premiums to producers. Similarly, tests to detect other diseases have improved. Improvement in identification of disease will help producers respond to disease outbreaks in a more timely fashion. It is our hope this issue will update readers on contributing factors and management of the bovine respiratory disease complex.

We would like to thank each of the authors for contributing their articles to this issue. Without them, this would not have been possible. We would also like to thank John Vassallo, Editor at the Saunders/Elsevier Company, for his patience and guidance with this issue. Our coworkers have been supportive through this endeavor and we

Vet Clin Food Anim 26 (2010) xiii–xiv
doi:10.1016/j.cvfa.2010.04.011

thank them for their support. Lastly, we would like to thank our families for their love and support.

Vickie L. Cooper, DVM, MS, PhD
Department of Veterinary Diagnostic and Production Animal Medicine
Iowa State University
1600 South 16th Street
Ames, IA 50011, USA

Bruce W. Brodersen, DVM, MS, PhD
Veterinary Diagnostic Center
School of Veterinary Medicine and Biomedical Sciences
University of Nebraska—Lincoln
1900 North 42nd Street
Lincoln, NE 68506-0907, USA

E-mail addresses:
vcooper@iastate.edu (V.L. Cooper)
bbrodersen1@unl.edu (B.W. Brodersen)

Pathogenesis and Pathology of Bovine Pneumonia

Roger J. Panciera, DVM, PhD[a], Anthony W. Confer, DVM, PhD[b],*

KEYWORDS

- Bronchopneumonia • Fibrinous pneumonia • Pleuropneumonia
- Aspiration pneumonia • Caseonecrotic pneumonia
- Interstitial pneumonia • Embolic pneumonia
- Verminous pneumoniae

Despite availability and use of many bovine respiratory pathogen vaccines and new antimicrobial drugs as well as greater understanding of the pathogenesis of bovine respiratory disease (BRD), pneumonia, ranging from subclinical to fatal, remains a major cause of morbidity, mortality, and economic loss to the beef and dairy cattle industries.[1,2] When cattle are subjected to stresses, such as weaning, shipment, and commingling with animals from other sources, transmission of various infectious agents and proliferation of endogenous—yet potentially pathogenic—microbes occur often, resulting in damage to the respiratory tract with subsequent upper or lower respiratory disease.[3] Most fatal forms of BRD and often the outcome of this stress/infectious agent scenario are severe bacterial (including mycoplasmal) pneumonias. In addition, other forms of severe respiratory disease and pneumonia, such as acute interstitial pneumonia (AIP), exist whose pathogenesis are less well established. Finally, incidental and less frequent causes of bovine pneumonia include embolic, verminous, and aspiration pneumonias.

This article focuses on pathogenesis and pathologic characteristics of selected types of bovine pneumonia with emphasis on gross pathologic changes. Readers are referred to several recent articles and textbooks for more complete histopathologic descriptions.[3–5] Emphasis is on bacterial and AIP, major causes of losses primarily in feedlot and stocker cattle. Bacterial pneumonia usually occurs within the first 6 to 10 days after stress, such as shipping or commingling, with interstitial pneumonias often occurring 70 or more days later.[6] Bacterial pneumonia is second to diarrheal disease as a cause of illness and losses in dairy calves. In addition, several

[a] Department of Veterinary Pathobiology, Oklahoma State University, 212 McElroy Hall, Stillwater, OK 74078-2007, USA
[b] Department of Veterinary Pathobiology, Oklahoma State University, 224 McElroy Hall, Stillwater, OK 74078-2007, USA
* Corresponding author.
E-mail address: anthony.confer@okstate.edu

Vet Clin Food Anim 26 (2010) 191–214
doi:10.1016/j.cvfa.2010.04.001
0749-0720/10/$ – see front matter © 2010 Elsevier Inc. All rights reserved.

of the minor pneumonias of cattle are discussed on a lesion recognition and differential diagnosis basis.

BOVINE BACTERIAL PNEUMONIA

The role of bovine respiratory viruses in precipitating severe BRD and bacterial pneumonias has long been known. Bovine herpesvirus-1 (BHV-1) (infectious bovine rhinotracheitis virus); parainfluenza virus-3 (PI-3); and bovine respiratory syncytial virus (BRSV) are recognized as primary respiratory pathogens.[5,7] During the past 25 years, the roles of other viruses have been speculated on and investigated; several, including bovine rhinoviruses and adenoviruses, have been dismissed as minimal pathogens at best and bovine viral diarrhea virus (BVDV) has been recognized as a major pathogenic partner in BRD.[8] A pathogenic role for bovine respiratory coronavirus has been postulated, but if such a role exists, it is still under investigation.[9] BHV-1, PI-3, BRSV, and BVDV can cause some degree of acute respiratory disease. BHV-1 is well recognized as a cause of severe upper respiratory lesions, ranging from hemorrhage to diphtheritic membranes.[4] With the exception of certain instances of BRSV, fatality is usually not associated with those infections alone. Instead, their roles are primarily to assist in establishing a respiratory environment that is favorable to colonization and replication by several pathogenic bacteria resulting in pneu-monia.[10–14] This is done through two major mechanisms. The first is by alteration in mucosal surfaces such that adhesion of bacteria to virus-infected cells is enhanced; further colonization occurs more readily in areas of virus-induced mucosal erosion than in intact mucosa.[15–17] The second is modification of the innate and adaptive immune systems through altered alveolar macrophage function, suppression of lymphocyte proliferation and induced apoptosis, and modified cytokine and other inflammatory mediator release.[17]

In an overview of the pathogenesis of pneumonia in feedlot cattle in a 1983 sympo-sium on BRD, Thomson[18] described only *Mannheimia haemolytica* (formerly *Pasteur-ella haemolytica*) and *Pasteurella multocida* as bacterial pathogens in the BRD complex. Since that time, *Histophilus somni* (formerly *Haemophilus somnus*), *Arcano-bacterium pyogenes*, *Mycoplasma bovis*, and, most recently, *Bibersteinia trehalosi* (formerly *Pasteurella trehalosi*) have also been recognized as additional bacterial agents associated with severe bovine bacterial pneumonia (**Table 1**).[19,20] These bacteria are ubiquitous in the cattle population as normal nasopharyngeal commen-sals and, after stress or viral infection, can proliferate and be inhaled into the lungs. Each has its own cadre of virulence factors, including biofilm, capsules, adhesins, toxins, and enzymes, that enhance its ability to colonize the lower airway, evade the immune system, resist antimicrobial treatment, cause tissue destruction, and incite an intense inflammatory response.[10]

Differences in various virulence factors possessed by each bacterial species are responsible for the relative pathogenicity and lesions indicative of that particular infec-tion (see **Table 1**). *M haemolytica* virulence factors include protein adhesins, capsular polysaccharide, lipopolysaccharide (LPS), iron-binding proteins, secreted enzymes, and a ruminant-specific RTX toxin—leukotoxin (LKT).[14] LPS and LKT are the two factors responsible for most of the destructive lesions of *M haemolytica* infection. Specific adhesins include a glycoprotein, N-acetyl-D-glucosamine, that mediates adherence to tracheal epithelial cells and activates the oxidative burst of bovine neutrophils. Heat-modifiable outer membrane protein A (OmpA) and the surface lipo-protein 1 mediate *M haemolytica* binding to bronchial epithelial cells. In addition, the *M haemolytica* capsule may function as an adhesin in addition to its antiphagocytic

Table 1
Major BRD pathogenic bacteria and their virulence factors

Bacterium	Capsule	Endotoxin	Exotoxins	Adhesin Proteins	Secreted Enzymes	Other Factors
Mannheimia haemolytica	Yes	LPS	LKT	• OmpA • Lipoprotein I • N-acetyl-D-glucosamine • Fibrinogen-binding proteins	• Neuraminidase • Sialoglycoprotease	• Biofilm
Pasteurella multocida	Yes	LPS	*P multocida* Toxin—rarely in BRD isolates	• OmpA • Type IV fimbriae • FHA	• Neuraminidase	• Biofilm
Histophilus somni	No	LOS	None			• Biofilm • IgBPs • Histamine
Mycoplasma bovis	No	No	Polysaccharide toxin (?)	• VSPs		• Biofilm • Hydrogen peroxide
Arcanobacterium pyogenes	No	No	Pyolysin	• Collagen-binding protein	• Proteases • DNAase	• Biofilm
Bibersteinia trehalosi	Yes	Yes	LKT ± (strain dependent)	• Two OmpA • Fibrinogen-binding proteins	• Novel protease • Superoxide dismutase	

properties. Fibrinogen-binding proteins have been identified.[21] Neuraminidase and sialoglycoprotease modify cell surfaces and may enhance bacterial adhesion. *M haemolytica* LPS has typical endotoxic and proinflammatory properties, causes vasculitis, and complexes with LKT enhancing LKT receptor production and augmenting LKT activity. LKT induces dose-related changes in bovine leukocytes, ranging from osmotic swelling, membrane pore formation, and necrosis to apoptosis or release of proinflammatory cytokines, oxygen-free radicals, and cellular protease.[14,22-24] Evidence of biofilm formation with reduced antimicrobial susceptibility has been demonstrated.[25]

P multocida virulence factors are less numerous than those identified in *M haemolytica*. Several adhesins, a thick polysaccharide capsule, and LPS are the major factors responsible for bacterial colonization, evasion of host defense, tissue destruction, and inflammation.[13] Adhesins are responsible for bacterial adherence to and colonization of cell surfaces. These include type IV fimbriae, OmpA, neuraminidase, and filamentous hemagglutinin (FHA). In addition, OmpA and various iron-binding proteins, such as hemoglobin-binding protein A and transferrin-binding protein A, bind fibronectin; and other extracellular matrix proteins may aid in invasion. The importance of capsule as a virulence determinant in the pathogenesis of *P multocida* infection is due to its antiphagocytic properties. *P multocida* LPS is a potent stimulator of inflammatory cytokines and a predominant inciter of pulmonary inflammation.[13] Evidence of biofilm formation with reduced antimicrobial susceptibility has been demonstrated.[25]

H somni are nonencapsulated, and the virulence factors include lipooligosaccharide (LOS) and various outer membrane proteins, especially transferrin-binding proteins and immunoglobulin-binding proteins (IgBPs).[12] LOS can mediate endothelial cell apoptosis and, through antigenic phase variation, can assist the bacterium to escape the host immune response. LOS is the primary factor responsible for lesion formation by causing thrombosis, inflammation, and tissue destruction. IgBPs assist the bacterium to evade host defenses. They are surface-exposed fibrillar protein networks that bind the Fc domain of bovine IgG2 and are responsible for virulent strains that are resistant to phagocytosis and complement-mediated serum killing.[26] *H somni* produces histamine, which in conjunction with anti–major outer membrane protein IgE, may account for early respiratory lesions.[12,27,28] Recently, biofilm production by *H somni* within the host was documented, which allows the bacterial colonies to evade host defense and resist antimicrobial drugs. FHA proteins may be involved in that process.[29]

M bovis virulence factors include variable surface proteins (VSPs) that function as adhesins allowing the bacterium to colonize bronchioles. VSPs are responsible for phenotypic variation among *M bovis* strains and, through antigenic phase variations, allow for evasion of host immune responses.[30,31] A polysaccharide toxin has been described; however, the role or even existence of that toxin remains controversial. *M bovis* strains may produce hydrogen peroxide, which forms oxygen-free radicals and causes host lipid peroxidation. The formation of biofilm has been associated with many *M bovis* strains, and that trait enhances immune and antimicrobial resistance and colonization.[32]

A pyogenes produces a collagen-binding protein (CbpA) that allows it to bind collagen and promotes adhesion to host cells.[33] A cholesterol-dependent cytolysin (pyolysin) that is a pore-forming cytolysin/hemolysin has been characterized.[34,35] Adhesion may also be mediated by type II fimbriae and by two neuraminidases that cleave sialic acids and expose cell receptors. Several extracellular matrix-binding proteins that bind to collagen or fibronectin and exoenzymes (DNase and proteases) assist in invasion of tissue and degradation of proteins and nucleic acids. In addition, *A pyogenes* can evade host defenses by invasion of epithelium by intracellular survival in macrophages and by formation of biofilm.[36]

Virulence factors of *B trehalosi* are not as well understood as those of many of the other BRD bacterial pathogens; however, there are many similarities with *M haemolytica*. Strains are encapsulated, and some strains are positive for LKT whereas others are not.[37] It is not clear whether or not strains that are LKT deficient are pathogenic. A novel protease has been demonstrated in *B trehalosi* isolated from bighorn sheep, and high antibodies to it were found in healthy sheep.[38] Fibrinogen-binding proteins have been identified.[21] Adhesion to epithelial surfaces could be mediated by the two OmpA molecules expressed in *B trehalosi*.[39]

Identification of pathogenic bacteria at necropsy depends on many factors, including type and number of antimicrobial treatments, extent of tissue decomposition, sample collection, holding, and shipping methods, transit time to laboratory, and method of bacterial detection. Traditional culture, immunohistochemistry, in situ hybridization, and polymerase chain reaction (PCR) techniques are available in various laboratories across North America. Technique sensitivity and specificity differ among these tests, and results may vary depending on the test applied. For example, *H somni* was cultured from only 10 of 65 cases of pneumonia, yet the bacterium was demonstrated by immunohistochemistry, in situ hybridization, and PCR in 17, 19, and 29 of the cases, respectively.[40] In feedlots in particular, there is strong correlation between the time of onset of pneumonia, acuteness of the lesion, and the etiologic agents that can be isolated from that lesion. For example, Booker and colleagues[41] using immunohistochemistry demonstrated that in lungs from cattle dying of peracute to subacute pneumonia, *M haemolytica*, *H somni*, and *M bovis* were demonstrated in approximately more than 80%, less than 20%, and 50% to 60% of the lungs, respectively. In contrast, the incidences of *M haemolytica*, *H somni*, and *M bovis* were approximately 40%, 30%, and 90%, respectively, in chronic pneumonia; lungs were not examined for *P multocida*. Using bacteriologic culture, Fulton and colleagues[42] demonstrated that when *M haemolytica* was isolated from lungs of cattle dying of pneumonia the mean onset of fatal disease was approximately 19 days in the feedlot. In contrast, when *M haemolytica* was not isolated from the lungs, the mean day at onset was approximately 33 days on feed. The opposite was true for *Mycoplasma* sp isolation, whereas onset of disease was approximately 70 days for positive lungs and 29 days for negative lungs. To complicate matters further, multiple pathogenic bacteria are often isolated from individual cases of bovine pneumonia at necropsy resulting in an inability to identify the primary pathogen or pathogens. In several studies, more than 60% of the lungs from cattle dying of bacterial pneumonia contained more than one potentially pathogenic bacterial species.[41–43] Therefore, reliance on microbiologic techniques applied to lungs at necropsy, using culture or another means, such as PCR or immunohistochemistry, is likely not providing a clear representation of the role of specific pathogens in initiating the lesion. Finally, the characteristics and type of pneumonic lesion present at necropsy are determined by the inciting causative bacteria and concurrent or predisposing pathogens as well as the effectiveness or ineffectiveness of host defense mechanisms. In addition, lesion characteristics are highly dependent on acuteness or chronicity of the lesion as well as the types, numbers, and length of treatments received.[5]

Inhaled bacterial pathogens first colonize the bronchoalveolar junction, overcome host defenses, incite inflammation at that site, and spread through contiguous airways or through adjacent components of lung tissue to produce three general types or patterns of pneumonia. These are suppurative bronchopneumonia (also called lobular bronchopneumonia), fibrinous pneumonia or pleuropneumonia (also called lobar pneumonia or fibrinous bronchopneumonia), and caseonecrotic pneumonia (also called mycoplasmal pneumonia).[4,44] These various types of bronchopneumonia are classified based on the type of exudation present, initial site of bacterial localization in the airway, influence of various bacterial virulence factors, host resistance, and rapidity and method of spread of the infection within the lung. In addition, specific bronchopneumonia subclassifications are more commonly associated with specific bacteria.

Suppurative Bronchopneumonia (Lobular Bronchopneumonia)

This form of pneumonia is the most common form seen in BRD of young dairy calves and most often associated with P multocida infection, although other respiratory bacteria may also produce the lesion.[3,4,13] Suppurative bronchopneumonia occurs when bronchial colonization of moderately virulent bacteria initiates a suppurative bronchitis with progressive spread along airways resulting in an obviously bronchiole-centered lesion within each lung lobule. The pneumonia is bilateral, cranioventrally distributed, and moderately firm (**Fig. 1**). In acute lesions, affected lobes are fairly uniform in color varying from pink, pink-gray, dark red, red-gray, or gray with minimal to mild interlobular septal edema (**Fig. 2**). Pleuritis is usually not present; however, if present, it consists of small foci of pleural dullness to small clusters of fibrin strands. On cut surface within lobules, there are variable-sized, partially discreet tan to gray foci indicative of a pattern of bronchiolar and peribronchiolar inflammation (**Fig. 3**). Remaining areas of lobules are pink to dark red representing various amounts of inflammation, congestion, and atelectasis. Intrabronchial purulent to mucopurulent exudate may be grossly obvious or in more subtle cases require a gentle squeeze to express exudate.

As bronchopneumonia becomes more chronic, palpation reveals a more lumpy distribution of consolidation with more obvious purulent bronchitis, bronchiectasis, and abscess formation. Inter- and intralobular fibrosis is present. Affected bronchioles may be prominent due to peribronchial fibrosis with dilated, mucoid to purulent, exudate-filled lumens. Shrunken, obscured lumens due to bronchiolitis obliterans become prominent histopathologically, but those changes are not readily grossly recognized. Focal fibrinous to fibrous adhesions may develop between parietal and visceral pleura especially over underlying abscesses. In chronic cases, A pyogenes is usually cultured particularly from bronchiectatic airways and abscesses, whereas other parts of the lung may yield multiple bacterial species.

Fibrinous Pneumonia or Fibrinous Pleuropneumonia (Fibrinous Bronchopneumonia, Lobar Pneumonia)

This form of pneumonia is typical of that produced by M haemolytica and to a lesser extent H somni and is the most common form of acute pneumonia in weaned, stressed beef cattle (shipping fever).[3,4] Fibrinous pneumonia occurs when there is overwhelming centrifugal spread of the inflammatory process from the primary locus of colonization in the bronchioles via extension from lobules into adjacent lobules within the cranioventral lobes. The rapid intra- and interlobular spread of M haemolytica is thought due to the effects of LPS on vascular integrity, severe cytolytic effects of LKT on resident and responding leukocytes, and the tissue destructive effects of released enzymes, oxygen radicals, and inflammatory mediators during that process.[14,45]

Fibrinous pneumonia is a bilateral, cranioventrally distributed, very firm, minimally compressible lung consolidation (**Fig. 4**). Fibrinous pneumonia is characterized by wide distension of interlobular septa with yellow gelatinous edema or coagulated

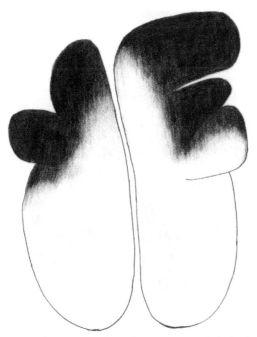

Fig. 1. Bronchopneumonia (suppurative bronchopneumonia, lobular bronchopneumonia).

fibrin. Fibrin thrombi may be visible in distended interlobular lymphatics. Consolidated lobes have a marbled appearance, a descriptive term indicating that each lobule is reasonably uniform in color with a multicolor patchwork or marbled pattern of lobules ranging from pink, pink-tan, dark red, to red-gray (**Fig. 5**). Large, irregular foci of pink-tan coagulation necrosis are frequently within lobules and may involve entire lobules. These necrotic foci are usually outlined by a discrete pale line representing intense accumulations of inflammatory cells and result from intralesional vasculitis and thrombosis that develop. Bronchi contain fibrinous coagulum but not frank pus.

Fibrinous pleuropneumonia (fibrinonecrotic pneumonia and pleuropneumonia) is likewise a bilateral, cranioventral, marbled pneumonia in which a fibrinous pleuritis

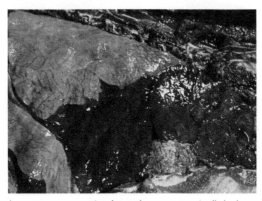

Fig. 2. Cranioventral, acute, suppurative bronchopneumonia (lobular pneumonia).

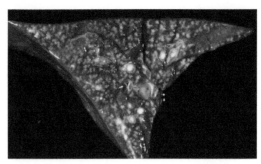

Fig. 3. Acute suppurative bronchopneumonia demonstrating bronchiolar and peribronchiolar pattern of inflammation with pus-filled airways.

of varying intensity is present (**Fig. 6**). The presence of pleuritis is an indication of the aggressiveness of the lung infection such that there is extension of infection and inflammation from alveoli to subpleural connective tissue and onto the visceral pleural surface. In early stages, pleural granularity, dullness, and fine fibrinous strands are present. Later, more intense broad sheets of yellow fibrin may obscure the appearance of the underlying lung. Fibrinous adhesions are likely present between parietal and visceral pleura. Fibrin-rich, yellow fluid within the pleural cavity is highly variable in quantity. In contrast to *M haemolytica*–associated pneumonia, *H somni*–associated fibrinous pneumonia may have accompanying lesions of myocarditis, myocardial infarction, and fibrinous synovitis.

Chronic pneumonic changes similar to those seen in bronchopneumonia occur in cattle that survive acute fibrinous pneumonia or pleuropneumonia.

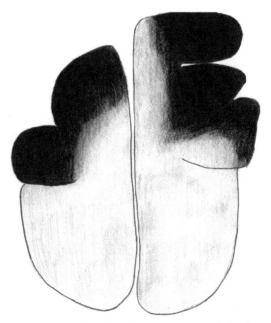

Fig. 4. Fibrinous pneumonia and fibrinous pleuropneumonia (lobar bronchopneumonia).

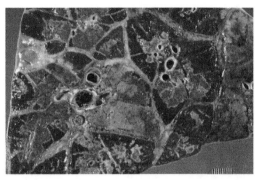

Fig. 5. Fibrinous pneumonia (lobar pneumonia) demonstrating marbled appearance due to pale areas of coagulation necrosis and dark areas of acute pneumonia. Interlobular septa are distended with fibrin-rich exudate.

Caseonecrotic Bronchopneumonia (Mycoplasmal Pneumonia)

In recent years in North America, this type of pneumonia has been recognized as characteristic of chronic *Mycoplasma* infection, especially *M bovis*, which is more virulent than other bovine Mycoplasma spp.[32,46] In many studies of BRD, *Mycoplasma* spp can be demonstrated in more than 70% of pneumonia cases usually in combination with other bacteria. Sole *Mycoplasma* spp isolation occurs in less than 20% of BRD cases.[41,43]

Mycoplasma spp colonize the ciliated epithelium of the respiratory tract producing a mild mucopurulent bronchitis and bronchiolitis and, through persistent infection, pulmonary lesions may develop.[31] In mild, subacute cases, the main lesion is large peribronchial lymphocytic cuffs. Systemic spread of *M bovis* may lead to serofibrinous synovitis and otitis media.[47] Gross examination of the lung at this stage likely reveals no obvious changes or small patchy red to red-gray areas of cranioventral atelectasis.

With *M bovis* infection, however, many calves develop chronic, multifocal, caseous necrosis within the cranial lung lobes (caseonecrotic bronchopneumonia). Although the pathogenesis of this lesion is still under investigation, bacterial antigen is demonstrated surrounding necrotic foci suggestive of a cause and effect relationship.[48–50] *M bovis* virulence factors responsible for this lesion are not currently understood. At necropsy, the cranioventral lobes are expanded with firm consolidation, which is often

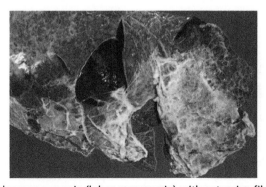

Fig. 6. Fibrinous pleuropneumonia (lobar pneumonia) with extensive fibrinous exudate.

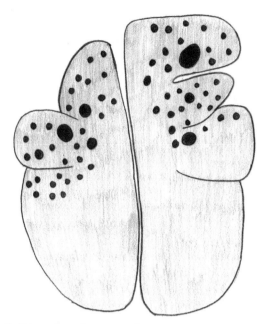

Fig. 7. Caseonecrotic (*Mycoplasma*) pneumonia.

visibly and palpably nodular (**Fig. 7**). Clusters of discrete yellow foci of caseous necrosis are present within lobules, and these foci often range from 1 to 10 mm in diameter (**Fig. 8**). The surrounding lobular tissue is often mottled to uniformly gray to dark red. In more severe lesions, necrotic foci coalesce and can involve an entire lobule. When the lung is squeezed, the necrotic material falls out as a single mass or multiple pieces. Sequestra may be seen. Expressed bronchial exudate may be mucoid to mucopurulent; the character of the exudate is likely determined by the presence or absence of other bacteria. A caseous to caseofibrinous synovitis or otitis may accompany the pneumonia.

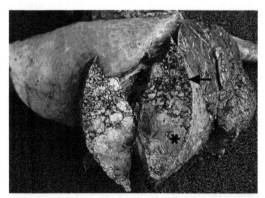

Fig. 8. Caseonecrotic bronchopneumonia typical of *M bovis* infection. Small (*arrow*) to large (*asterisk*) areas of coalescing foci of necrosis are present. (*Courtesy of* Dr Jeff Caswell, University of Guelph, Guelph, Ontario, Canada.)

INTERSTITIAL PNEUMONIA

The term, *interstitial pneumonia*, designates a lesion rather than a disease. The lesion may be acquired by delivery of causative factors through pulmonary circulation or by airways. Whatever the route of exposure, primary damage occurs to structures in alveolar septa (ie, alveolar type I pneumocytes or vascular endothelial cells) and to bronchiolar Clara cells. Subsequently, the fibrin-rich plasma exudation phase occurs creating severe edema and intraalveolar hyaline membranes.[3,5] This exudative phase is followed by type II pneumocyte proliferation, and, with time, alveolar septal fibrosis. Type II pneumocyte hyperplasia can be extensive resulting in alveoli lined by cuboidal epithelium in an acinar or gland-like appearance (sometimes referred to as pulmonary fetalization or adenomatosis).

There are many established causes of interstitial pneumonia, which include, but are not limited to, various chemical compounds, such as 3-methylindole (3MI); viruses, such as BRSV; migrating parasite larvae; immune mechanisms; toxic gases; and perhaps environmental conditions.[3,51,52] In many instances, however, the causative factor is not known. Interstitial pneumonia occurs in various patterns of lung involvement. The best characterized pathologically is diffuse AIP (**Fig. 9**), whereas less well characterized is secondary interstitial pneumonia, which is distinguished by coexisting, probably preceding, cranioventral bronchopneumonia with extensive interstitial pneumonia in caudal areas of lungs (**Fig. 10**). A third, less well-characterized pattern, involves various areas of lung, predominantly caudal, dorsal with intervening areas of more normal, but prominently pale, overinflated lobules or groups of lobules, forming a so-called checkerboard pattern (**Fig. 11**).[51]

Acute interstitial pneumonia

AIP, frequently referred to as acute bovine pulmonary edema and emphysema or, in the United Kingdom, fog fever,[5] occurs in pastured cattle moved to lush green

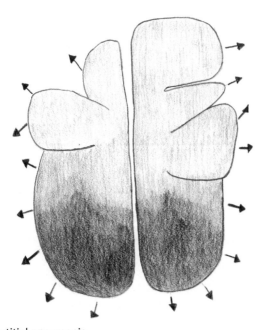

Fig. 9. Acute interstitial pneumonia.

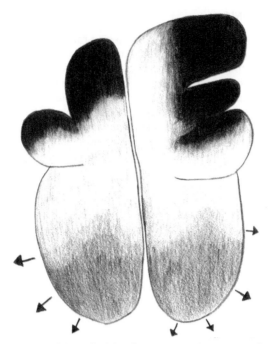

Fig. 10. Secondary interstitial (so-called feedlot interstitial pneumonia).

pastures or by exposure to chemicals, including plant toxins, such as *Perilla* mint ketone and 4-ipomeanol from moldy sweet potatoes.[53] Clinical signs usually develop within 2 to 3 weeks of pasture changes or as short as 1 to 2 days after exposure to plant toxins. Classically, movement of cattle to lush green pastures results in excess ingestion of L-tryptophan with conversion to 3MI by rumen flora.[51,52] Metabolism of

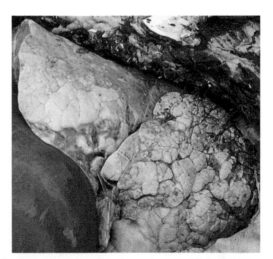

Fig. 11. AIP in a feedlot calf. Overinflated cranioventral lobules interspersed with darker pneumonic lobules (checkerboard). Caudal dorsal lung contains diffuse gray areas of pneumonia. (*Courtesy of* Dr Amelia Woolums, University of Georgia, Athens, GA.)

3MI in bronchiolar Clara cells and type I pneumocytes results in highly activated intermediates that cause pneumocyte necrosis and exfoliation setting in motion the pathologic processes resulting in interstitial pneumonia. This form of AIP is differentiable from AIP of feedlot cattle (discussed later) by epidemiology, known causative agents, and lesion characteristics.

At necropsy, cattle often have abundant subcutaneous emphysema over the dorsal subcutis, emphysema within the mediastinum, and frothy edema in the trachea. Lungs are diffusely wet, heavy, and fail to collapse. Lobules tend to be individualized (**Fig. 12**). Interlobular septa are distended with edema and gas bubbles. Palpable changes may be subtle to obvious and range from palpably normal to somewhat rubbery in a diffuse distribution. Palpation of single lobules provides critical assessment of lung texture. Parenchyma ranges from pink to tan. Clear, watery, edema fluid readily exudes from the cut surface.

Interstitial pneumonia in feedlot cattle

This form of interstitial pneumonia is a sporadic cause of death in North American feedlot cattle that usually occurs late within the feeding period.[6,51,52] Most surveys recognize the lesion in less than 10% of the total feedlot deaths with occasionally larger outbreaks reported.[6,41,42] Many causes have been investigated, and it is most likely that interstitial pneumonia in feedlot cattle results from one or combinations of several mechanisms. As in AIP of pastured cattle, a role for 3MI has been examined. In the feedlot disease, 3MI has been generally discounted because of the sporadic nature of the disease and lack of association with dietary change. In one feedlot study, however, blood levels of a 3MI metabolite were significantly higher in AIP than in control cattle suggesting a potential pathogenic role for 3MI.[54] Interstitial pneumonia also was described with some frequency in feedlot heifers fed melengestrol acetate to suppress estrus.[55] Several studies have investigated the association of BRSV and interstitial pneumonia with conflicting results; however, this may be because attempts to culture or demonstrate viral antigen is done using postmortem-collected specimens, and negative results may not accurately account for the virus' role in pathogenesis.[51,54,56,57] Lesions of small airway disease, such as bronchiolar necrosis and, more commonly, its healing stage, bronchiolitis obliterans, are frequently found histologically in feedlot cases of interstitial pneumonia.[4,6,57] It was suggested that feedlot interstitial pneumonia might result from the effects of increased proinflammatory cytokines within lungs due to chronic bronchiolar disease, and endotoxin from gram-negative

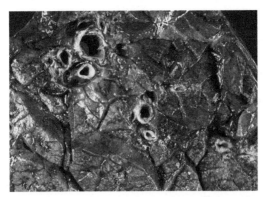

Fig. 12. AIP with lobules clearly separated by interlobular edema. Subtle differences are seen in various lobules. (*Courtesy of* Dr John King, Cornell University, Ithaca, NY.)

respiratory infections may contribute alveolar and bronchiolar damage leading to interstitial pneumonia.[52]

Gross patterns of interstitial pneumonia in feedlot cattle include that of acute diffuse distribution but more frequently interstitial pneumonia is in caudal lobes combined with bronchopneumonia cranially (see **Fig. 10**). In addition, interstitial pneumonia may occur in a patchy distribution, with pneumonic lobules separated by prominently pale, bulging, overinflated lobules or groups of lobules (so-called checkerboard pattern) (see **Fig. 11**).[51,56] Lesions of bronchopneumonia have been reported in 32% to 96% of fatal cases of feedlot AIP. Death due to AIP usually occurs from 21 to 73 days after onset of preceding respiratory illness, such as bronchopneumonia.[6,57,58]

Gross lesions of feedlot cases of interstitial pneumonia are typical. Bilaterally, lungs fail to collapse and are overinflated and heavy with variable amounts of interlobular edema and emphysema. The lesion may be diffuse, but it is usually more obvious in the caudal dorsal lobes. Cranioventral bronchopneumonia or fibrinous pneumonia is often visible. Palpation of caudal areas reveals a rubbery texture in a diffuse but more commonly a slightly lumpy pattern, wherein rubbery texture is confined to individual lobules separated by palpably normal lobules. Affected lobules range from pale red-gray, pink or tan, to clear fluid exudes or can be expressed from the cut surface unless concurrent suppurative bronchitis or bronchopneumonia is present. The so-called checkerboard pattern of rubbery, perhaps dark lobules interspersed with normal to pale, overinflated lobules may be seen; however, in many cases of interstitial pneumonia, the lesion is not visually obvious but palpably so.

Bronchointerstitial pneumonia

The bronchointerstitial form of interstitial pneumonia is used to describe uncomplicated viral infections of the lung due to BHV-1, PI-3, and BRSV infections.[4,5,31] Ellis and colleagues[8] also described pulmonary lesions associated with experimental BVDV type 2 infections as bronchointerstitial pneumonia. Although the lesions of bovine respiratory coronavirus infection are not well documented, and several investigators have failed to reproduce a lung disease with these viruses, experimental infection of calves with a winter dysentery bovine coronavirus resulted in small intestine villous atrophy and bronchointerstitial pneumonia.[59–61] Bronchointerstitial pneumonia is characterized by bronchiolar epithelial and pneumocytic damage resulting in bronchiolar necrosis, mild inflammatory cell influx, and type II pneumocyte hyperplasia. In the field, bronchointerstitial pneumonia is often complicated with secondary bacterial infection, which obscures and overshadows the primary viral lesion. Therefore, cases of true bronchointerstitial pneumonia are only occasionally recognized. For example, bronchointerstitial pneumonia was recognized in only 3 of 214 (1.4%) pneumonic lungs in a recent feedlot study.[42]

Gross lesions of bronchointerstitial pneumonia have been documented best in BRSV infections, are cranioventral distributed, and are often subtle ranging from reddened areas of atelectasis to rubbery gray lobules.[62] If exudate is expressible, it is usually mucoid to mucopurulent. Caudal lobes may be overinflated with emphysematous bullae.

SEVERE ANEMIA

As a differential for diffuse AIP, the gross appearance of lungs from severely anemic cattle must be considered. These lungs fail to collapse and are pale, overinflated, and markedly puffy (**Fig. 13**). A yellowish tint may occur in severe, acute hemolytic

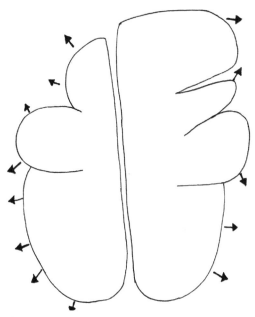

Fig. 13. Severe anemia.

crises and the lungs appear dry on cut surface. In subacute to chronic blood loss, pulmonary edema and pleural effusion may occur.

ASPIRATION PNEUMONIA

Inhalation of foreign material, in particular liquids, can result in aspiration pneumonia. The characteristics of the resulting pneumonic lesion are dependent on the nature and distribution of the material as well as the extent and type of bacterial contamination.[3–5] Aspiration due to faulty intubation, dysphagia, regurgitation, and infected large particles of necrotic mucosa from upper respiratory lesions can cause aspiration pneumonia. Pail- or bottle-fed calves, intubation and balling gun accidents, traumatic pharyngitis, rumenitis from ingesta of oilfield fluids, and prolonged recumbency have all been implicated in causing aspiration pneumonia. Aspiration of rumen contents is, by far, the most common cause of aspiration pneumonia of cattle. The resulting lesions are often unilateral, necrotizing to gangrenous, and predominantly cranioventral (**Figs. 14** and **15**). Another diagnostically useful feature of distribution exists when the pneumonic lesion is not only unilateral but also caudally situated without cranial lung involvement. Fibrinopurulent to suppurative pleuritis is commonly present and covers the necrotic foci; empyema may result from ruptured foci.[58] Pneumonic lesions are brown to green and may be hemorrhagic, often forming cystic cavities exuding malodorous brown fluid that may contain ingesta. Putrid odors are especially prevalent in the presence of aspirated rumen anaerobic bacteria. Foreign material may be readily visible within the airways, but terminal aspiration of rumen contents must not be mistaken for a lesion of aspiration pneumonia. If the inciting material is lipid-rich, lipid droplets are visible floating on bronchoalveolar fluids.

The least common form of aspiration pneumonia in cattle is lipid pneumonia, resulting from aspiration of lipid-rich material, such as mineral oil or other oil-based

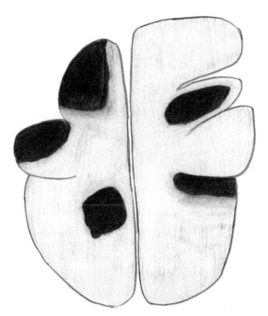

Fig. 14. Aspiration pneumonia.

compounds. Those compounds can stimulate an intense interstitial pneumonia with alveolar exudation of fibrin and leukocytes, type II pneumocyte hyperplasia, and interstitial fibrosis. Uncomplicated lesions may range from diffuse to cranioventral and are wet, rubbery, pale, yellowish, or mottled. Foci of necrosis or suppurative exudation can be present due to bacterial infection.

EMBOLIC PNEUMONIA

Embolic pneumonias consist of multiple, randomly distributed inflammatory foci throughout all lung lobes (**Fig. 16**).[3–5] In contrast, abscesses that develop in chronic suppurative bronchopneumonia and fibrinous pleuropneumonia maintain a cranioventral distribution. Embolic pneumonia is preceded by bacterial infection and suppuration at another location, which in cattle is most commonly liver, but other loci may

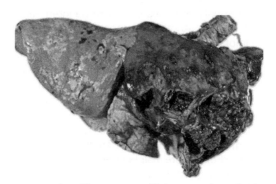

Fig. 15. Aspiration pneumonia with severe, multiple, necrotic cavitations.

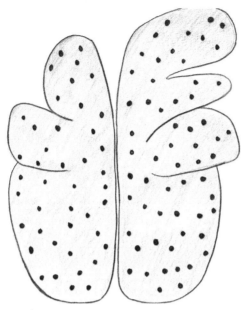

Fig. 16. Embolic pneumonia.

occur, such as traumatic reticulopericarditis, mastitis, endometritis, and jugular thrombophlebitis. Extension of infection into local veins causes thrombophlebitis, pulmonary thromboembolism, and disseminated foci of pulmonary inflammation. Right-side vegetative endocarditis may also be present. Hepatic abscesses, often caused by *Fusobacterium necrophorum*, may erode hepatic veins or caudal vena cava resulting in embolic showering of the lung. The earliest lesions are small foci of acute inflammation and necrosis that may progress to small- to moderate-sized abscesses of liquefactive to caseous necrosis. Lungs are usually edematous and perhaps emphysematous. Infected emboli may erode pulmonary artery branches causing pulmonary hemorrhage and leakage of free blood into major airways. With respiratory movements, redistribution of blood into small airways and alveoli occurs. Hemoptysis may also be present. In those cases, free blood is present in major airways, and on cut surface, aspirated blood is distributed in the lungs as feathery, lacy-appearing, red areas, which are particularly obvious within subpleural lobules **(Fig. 17)**. In contrast to aspirated free blood, intrapulmonary hemorrhage associated with trauma, septicemia, or endotoxemia appears as dark red petechia or ecchymoses that are discretely demarcated and might be more randomly distributed than are areas of aspirated blood.

VERMINOUS PNEUMONIA

Dictyocaulus viviparus is the cattle lungworm, and lesions are found in pastured cattle or in feedlots supplied primarily by cattle from Southern states.[3,5,63] Infection is acquired through ingestion of infective larvae from moist environments. Clinical signs of pneumonia may exist during various phases of infection (prepatent, patent, postpatent, and reinfection). Grossly visible lesions are seen primarily in the patent period.

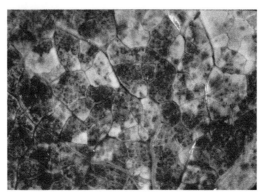

Fig. 17. Aspirated (inhaled) blood distributed as feathery, lacy-appearing dark areas throughout lobules.

During the prepatent period as larvae migrate and develop within the lung, small foci of interstitial pneumonia and eosinophilic bronchiolitis develop, which may appear grossly as small multifocal areas of lobular atelectasis and pulmonary edema. In the patent period, adult worms develop in bronchi and induce eosinophilic to mucopurulent bronchitis, resulting in atelectasis, emphysema and a verminous pneumonia.[3,4,64] Gross examination of patent infections reveals bilateral lesions first in the caudal lung lobes consisting of caudal-dorsal, wedge-shaped areas of moderate firmness (**Fig. 18**) and in severe infections throughout the lungs. Lesions vary from red and atelectatic to consolidated and gray or pale and overinflated. Emphysema due to forced expiration and bronchiolar lesions may be seen in severe cases. When severe, prominent

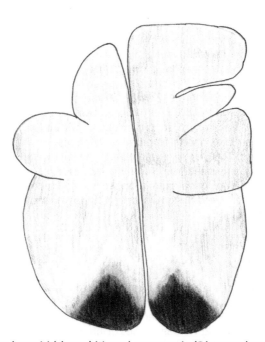

Fig. 18. Verminous (parasitic) bronchitis and pneumonia (*Dictyocaulus viviparus*).

emphysema may cause the prosector to miss the verminous lesions and incorrectly interpret the case as an AIP. Bronchi need to be carefully followed into the caudal-dorsal lobe, wherein distal bronchi contain cloudy to frothy mucus and slender adult white nematodes 4 to 8 cm long.

TUBERCULOUS PNEUMONIA

Bovine tuberculosis is a reportable disease, and current control programs in North America have limited the prevalence of disease. Endemic and sporadic tuberculosis in some wild and farm-reared cervids throughout the United States and occasional diagnoses in cattle, particularly in the northern Midwestern states and along the southern US border, are reminders that vigilance is still needed to accurately recognize and diagnose the disease.[65–70]

In cattle, M bovis causes caseous granulomas in the lungs and occasionally in other organs.[71] Regional lymph nodes, especially retropharyngeal and bronchial, particular targets of M bovis infection, are usually involved and help distinguish tuberculosis from other purulent to caseous pneumonias (**Fig. 19**). The classical lesion of tuberculosis is the tubercle. Tubercles are usually circumscribed, often encapsulated, 1- to 40-mm granulomatous foci containing white to pale yellow caseous necrosis with or without foci of mineralization.[4] Liquefaction may develop in some older lesions.[68] At necropsy, lesions may not be obvious even in an animal that reacted positively on a tuberculin skin test. Careful examination of lymph nodes, in particular retropharyngeal, bronchial, and mediastinal, may demonstrate granulomatous inflammation and tubercle formation. Lung lesions are present in approximately 10% to 20% of the cases. In rare generalized cases, small disseminated caseous to caseocalcareous tubercles are present throughout the lungs. More commonly, solitary or clusters of tubercles are present, particularly in the caudal lung lobe. Liquefaction may occur in large

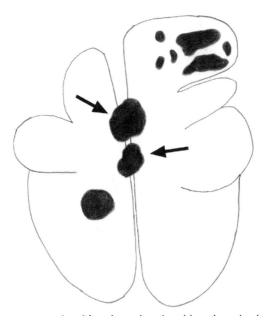

Fig. 19. Tuberculous pneumonia with enlarged regional lymph nodes (*arrows*).

lesions and could be misinterpreted as an abscess due to *A pyogenes*. Tuberculous lymphadenitis and pneumonia must be differentiated from mycotic lymphadenitis and granulomatous pneumonia, which is sometimes seen in slaughtered cattle.[72] Mycotic pneumonia is relatively rare in cattle but can occur due to *Coccidioides immitis*, *Aspergillus* spp, *H capsulatum*, and other opportunistic fungi.[73]

SUMMARY

Pneumonia is a major cause of death and economic losses to the cattle industry. Recognizing the patterns of pneumonic lesions and understanding the pathogenesis of the various types of pneumonia are important for correct diagnosis and interpretation of the lesions. Bacterial pneumonias consist of bronchopneumonia and fibrinous pneumonia and pleuropneumonia as well as caseonecrotic, aspiration, and tuberculous pneumonias. Two major patterns of interstitial pneumonia are recognized in cattle, and verminous pneumonia is associated with *Dictyocaulus viviparus* infection.

ACKNOWLEDGMENTS

The authors thank Heather Martin for providing drawings of the various patterns of pneumonia and Sarah Shields for assistance in manuscript preparation.

REFERENCES

1. Miles DG. Overview of the North American beef cattle industry and the incidence of bovine respiratory disease (BRD). Anim Health Res Rev 2009;10:101.
2. Patrick RL. A dairy producer's view of respiratory disease. Anim Health Res Rev 2009;10:111.
3. Andrews GA, Kennedy GA. Respiratory diagnostic pathology. Vet Clin North Am Food Anim Pract 1997;13:515.
4. Caswell JL, Williams KJ. Respiratory system. In: Maxie G, editor, Pathology of domestic animals, vol 2. Edinburgh (UK): Saunders; 2007. p. 523.
5. Lopez A. Respiratory system. In: McGavin MD, Zachari JF, editors. Pathologic basis of veterinary disease. St. Louis (MO): Mosby; 2007. p. 463.
6. Hjerpe CA. Clinical management of respiratory disease in feedlot cattle. Vet Clin North Am Large Anim Pract 1983;5:119.
7. Ellis JA. Update on viral pathogenesis in BRD. Anim Health Res Rev 2009;10:149.
8. Ellis JA, West KH, Cortese VS, et al. Lesions and distribution of viral antigen following an experimental infection of young seronegative calves with virulent bovine virus diarrhea virus-type II. Can J Vet Res 1998;62:161.
9. Lathrop SL, Wittum TE, Brock KV, et al. Association between infection of the respiratory tract attributable to bovine coronavirus and health and growth performance of cattle in feedlots. Am J Vet Res 2000;61:1062.
10. Confer AW. Update on bacterial pathogenesis in BRD. Anim Health Res Rev 2009;10:145.
11. Confer AW, Panciera RJ, Clinkenbeard KD, et al. Molecular aspects of virulence of *Pasteurella haemolytica*. Can J Vet Res 1990;54(Suppl):S48.
12. Corbeil LB. *Histophilus somni* host-parasite relationships. Anim Health Res Rev 2007;8:151.
13. Dabo SM, Taylor JD, Confer AW. *Pasteurella multocida* and bovine respiratory disease. Anim Health Res Rev 2007;8:129.

14. Rice JA, Carrasco-Medina L, Hodgins DC, et al. *Mannheimia haemolytica* and bovine respiratory disease. Anim Health Res Rev 2007;8:117.
15. Czuprynski CJ. Host response to bovine respiratory pathogens. Anim Health Res Rev 2009;10:141.
16. Rivera-Rivas JJ, Kisiela D, Czuprynski CJ. Bovine herpesvirus type 1 infection of bovine bronchial epithelial cells increases neutrophil adhesion and activation. Vet Immunol Immunopathol 2009;131:167.
17. Srikumaran S, Kelling CL, Ambagala A. Immune evasion by pathogens of bovine respiratory disease complex. Anim Health Res Rev 2007;8:215.
18. Thomson RG. Pathogenesis of pneumonia in feedlot cattle. In: Loan RW, editor. Bovine respiratory disease. A symposium. College Station (TX): Texas A&M University Press; 1984. p. 326.
19. Blackall PJ, Bojesen AM, Christensen H, et al. Reclassification of [*Pasteurella*] *trehalosi* as *Bibersteinia trehalosi* gen. nov., comb. nov. Int J Syst Evol Microbiol 2007;57:666.
20. Welsh RD, Dye LB, Payton ME, et al. Isolation and antimicrobial susceptibilities of bacterial pathogens from bovine pneumonia: 1994–2002. J Vet Diagn Invest 2004;16:426.
21. McNeil HJ, Shewen PE, Lo RY, et al. *Mannheimia haemolytica* serotype 1 and *Pasteurella trehalosi* serotype 10 culture supernatants contain fibrinogen-binding proteins. Vet Immunol Immunopathol 2002;90:107.
22. Confer AW, Clinkenbeard KD, Murphy GL. Pathogenesis and virulence of *Pasteurella haemolytica* in cattle: an analysis of current knowledge and future approaches. In: Donachie W, Lainson FA, Hodgson JC, editors. Haemophilus, Actinobacillus, and Pasteurella. London (UK): Plenum Press; 1995. p. 51.
23. Czuprynski CJ, Leite F, Sylte M, et al. Complexities of the pathogenesis of *Mannheimia haemolytica* and *Haemophilus somnus* infections: challenges and potential opportunities for prevention? Anim Health Res Rev 2004;5:277.
24. Czuprynski CJ, Welch RA. Biological effects of RTX toxins: the possible role of lipopolysaccharide. Trends Microbiol 1995;3:480.
25. Olson ME, Ceri H, Morck DW, et al. Biofilm bacteria: formation and comparative susceptibility to antibiotics. Can J Vet Res 2002;66:86.
26. Hoshinoo K, Sasaki K, Tanaka A, et al. Virulence attributes of *Histophilus somni* with a deletion mutation in the ibpA gene. Microb Pathog 2009;46:273.
27. Ruby KW, Griffith RW, Kaeberle ML. Histamine production by *Haemophilus somnus*. Comp Immunol Microbiol Infect Dis 2002;25:13.
28. Sandal I, Inzana TJ. A genomic window into the virulence of *Histophilus somni*. Trends Microbiol 2010;18:90.
29. Sandal I, Shao JQ, Annadata S, et al. *Histophilus somni* biofilm formation in cardiopulmonary tissue of the bovine host following respiratory challenge. Microbes Infect 2009;11:254.
30. Behrens A, Heller M, Rosenbusch R, et al. Immunoelectron microscopic localization of variable proteins on the surface of *Mycoplasma bovis*. Microbiology 1996; 142(Pt 7):1863.
31. Caswell JL, Archambault M. *Mycoplasma bovis* pneumonia in cattle. Anim Health Res Rev 2007;8:161.
32. Haines DM, Martin KM, Clark EG, et al. The immunohistochemical detection of *Mycoplasma bovis* and bovine viral diarrhea virus in tissues of feedlot cattle with chronic, unresponsive respiratory disease and/or arthritis. Can Vet J 2001; 42:857.

33. Pietrocola G, Valtulina V, Rindi S, et al. Functional and structural properties of CbpA, a collagen-binding protein from *Arcanobacterium pyogenes*. Microbiology 2007;153:3380.

34. Billington SJ, Jost BH, Cuevas WA, et al. The *Arcanobacterium* (*Actinomyces*) *pyogenes* hemolysin, pyolysin, is a novel member of the thiol-activated cytolysin family. J Bacteriol 1997;179:6100.

35. Rudnick ST, Jost BH, Billington SJ. Transcriptional regulation of pyolysin production in the animal pathogen, *Arcanobacterium pyogenes*. Vet Microbiol 2008;132:96.

36. Jost BH, Billington SJ. *Arcanobacterium pyogenes*: molecular pathogenesis of an animal opportunist. Antonie Van Leeuwenhoek 2005;88:87.

37. Ward AC, Weiser GC, DeLong WJ, et al. Characterization of *Pasteurella spp* isolated from healthy domestic pack goats and evaluation of the effects of a commercial Pasteurella vaccine. Am J Vet Res 2002;63:119.

38. McNeil HJ, Shewen PE, Lo RY, et al. Novel protease produced by a *Pasteurella trehalosi* serotype 10 isolate from a pneumonic bighorn sheep: characteristics and potential relevance to protection. Vet Microbiol 2003;93:145.

39. Davies RL, Lee I. Sequence diversity and molecular evolution of the heat-modifiable outer membrane protein gene (*ompA*) of *Mannheimia* (*Pasteurella*) *haemolytica*, *Mannheimia glucosida*, and *Pasteurella trehalosi*. J Bacteriol 2004;186:5741.

40. Tegtmeier C, Angen O, Ahrens P. Comparison of bacterial cultivation, PCR, in situ hybridization and immunohistochemistry as tools for diagnosis of *Haemophilus somnus* pneumonia in cattle. Vet Microbiol 2000;76:385.

41. Booker CW, Abutarbush SM, Morley PS, et al. Microbiological and histopathological findings in cases of fatal bovine respiratory disease of feedlot cattle in Western Canada. Can Vet J 2008;49:473.

42. Fulton RW, Blood KS, Panciera RJ, et al. Lung pathology and infectious agents in fatal feedlot pneumonias and relationship with mortality, disease onset, and treatments. J Vet Diagn Invest 2009;21:464.

43. Gagea MI, Bateman KG, van Dreumel T, et al. Diseases and pathogens associated with mortality in Ontario beef feedlots. J Vet Diagn Invest 2006;18:18.

44. Lopez A, Yong S, Shewen P. Effect of intratracheal inoculation of *Pasteurella haemolytica* cytotoxin on the integrity of rat lung. Can J Vet Res 1987;51:533.

45. Confer AW, McCraw RD, Durham JA, et al. Serum antibody responses of cattle to iron-regulated outer membrane proteins of *Pasteurella haemolytica* A1. Vet Immunol Immunopathol 1995;47:101.

46. Shahriar FM, Clark EG, Janzen E, et al. Coinfection with bovine viral diarrhea virus and *Mycoplasma bovis* in feedlot cattle with chronic pneumonia. Can Vet J 2002;43:863.

47. Gagea MI, Bateman KG, Shanahan RA, et al. Naturally occurring *Mycoplasma bovis*-associated pneumonia and polyarthritis in feedlot beef calves. J Vet Diagn Invest 2006;18:29.

48. Adegboye DS, Hallbur PG, Cavanaugh DL, et al. Immunohistochemical and pathological study of *Mycoplasma bovis*-associated lung abscesses in calves. J Vet Diagn Invest 1995;7:333.

49. Khodakaram-Tafti A, Lopez A. Immunohistopathological findings in the lungs of calves naturally infected with *Mycoplasma bovis*. J Vet Med A Physiol Pathol Clin Med 2004;51:10.

50. Rodriguez F, Bryson DG, Ball HJ, et al. Pathological and immunohistochemical studies of natural and experimental *Mycoplasma bovis* pneumonia in calves. J Comp Pathol 1996;115:151.
51. Woolums AR, Mason GL, Hawkins LL, et al. Microbiologic findings in feedlot cattle with acute interstitial pneumonia. Am J Vet Res 2004;65:1525.
52. Woolums ARL, Gould DH, McAllister TA. Etiology of acute interstitial pneumonia in feedlot cattle: noninfectious causes. Compend Cont Educ Pract Vet 2001;23:S86.
53. Kerr LA, Linnabary RD. A review of interstitial pneumonia in cattle. Vet Hum Toxicol 1989;31:247.
54. Loneragan GH, Gould DH, Mason GL, et al. Association of 3-methyleneindolenine, a toxic metabolite of 3-methylindole, with acute interstitial pneumonia in feedlot cattle. Am J Vet Res 2001;62:1525.
55. Stanford K, McAllister TA, Ayroud M, et al. Effect of dietary melengestrol acetate on the incidence of acute interstitial pneumonia in feedlot heifers. Can J Vet Res 2006;70:218.
56. Loneragan GH, Gould DH, Mason GL, et al. Involvement of microbial respiratory pathogens in acute interstitial pneumonia in feedlot cattle. Am J Vet Res 2001;62:1519.
57. Sorden SD, Kerr RW, Janzen ED. Interstitial pneumonia in feedlot cattle: concurrent lesions and lack of immunohistochemical evidence for bovine respiratory syncytial virus infection. J Vet Diagn Invest 2000;12:510.
58. King JM, Roth-Johnson L, Dodd DC, et al. The necropsy book. a guide for veterinary students, residents, clinicians, pathologists, and biological researchers. 4th edition. Gurnee (IL): Charles Louis Davis, D.V.M. Foundation; 2005.
59. Park SJ, Kim GY, Choy HE, et al. Dual enteric and respiratory tropisms of winter dysentery bovine coronavirus in calves. Arch Virol 2007;152:1885.
60. Reynolds DJ, Debney TG, Hall GA, et al. Studies on the relationship between coronaviruses from the intestinal and respiratory tracts of calves. Arch Virol 1985;85:71.
61. Saif LJ, Redman DR, Moorhead PD, et al. Experimentally induced coronavirus infections in calves: viral replication in the respiratory and intestinal tracts. Am J Vet Res 1986;47:1426.
62. Gershwin LJ. Bovine respiratory syncytial virus infection: immunopathogenic mechanisms. Anim Health Res Rev 2007;8:207.
63. Panuska C. Lungworms of ruminants. Vet Clin North Am Food Anim Pract 2006; 22:583.
64. Schnieder T, Kaup FJ, Drommer W. Morphological investigations on the pathology of *Dictyocaulus viviparus* infections in cattle. Parasitol Res 1991;77:260.
65. Cassidy JP. The pathogenesis and pathology of bovine tuberculosis with insights from studies of tuberculosis in humans and laboratory animal models. Vet Microbiol 2006;112:151.
66. Cassidy JP. The pathology of bovine tuberculosis: time for an audit. Vet J 2008; 176:263.
67. Humblet MF, Boschiroli ML, Saegerman C. Classification of worldwide bovine tuberculosis risk factors in cattle: a stratified approach. Vet Res 2009;40(5):50.
68. Palmer MV, Waters WR, Thacker TC. Lesion development and immunohistochemical changes in granulomas from cattle experimentally infected with *Mycobacterium bovis*. Vet Pathol 2007;44:863.
69. Prasad HK, Singhal A, Mishra A, et al. Bovine tuberculosis in India: potential basis for zoonosis. Tuberculosis 2005;85:421.

70. Wobeser G. Bovine tuberculosis in Canadian wildlife: an updated history. Can J Vet Res 2009;50:1169.
71. Rhyan JC, Saari DA. A comparative-study of the histopathologic features of bovine tuberculosis in cattle, Fallow Deer (Dama-Dama), Sika-Deer (Cervus-Nippon), and Red Deer and Elk (Cervus-Elaphus). Vet Pathol 1995;32:215.
72. Ortega J, Uzal FA, Walker R, et al. Zygomycotic lymphadenitis in slaughtered feedlot cattle. Vet Pathol 2010;47:108.
73. Maddy KT, Crecelius HG, Cornell RG. Distribution of *Coccidiodes immitis* determined by testing cattle. Public Health Rep 1960;75:955.

Innate Immunology of Bovine Respiratory Disease

Mark R. Ackermann, DVM, PhD[a],*, Rachel Derscheid, DVM[b],
James A. Roth, DVM, PhD[c]

KEYWORDS

- Bovine • Innate immunity • Lung • Pneumonia

Pneumonia is a leading cause of loss to the cattle industry in the United States and Europe. Of cattle diseases, it has the greatest economic impact. Respiratory pathogens can cause serious outbreaks of acute pneumonia in neonatal, weaned, and growing calves. Chronic infection leads to debilitation, decreased performance, and culling in older animals. The means to enhance effective and noninjurious immune responses are needed because of the high incidence of pneumonia in cattle, ubiquity of respiratory pathogens, the increasing frequency of antibiotic resistance, and the general expectation by consumers for producers to use antibiotics less frequently. The lung has a wide array of both innate and adaptive immune responses to airborne particulates, vapors, and microbial pathogens. Vaccines can effectively enhance resistance to some pathogens, but not all. More recently, additional attention has been given to innate immune responses and methods/regimens that increase innate immune activity. Despite advances in managerial practices, vaccines, and clinical therapies, pneumonia remains a widespread problem and methods to enhance host resistance to pathogen colonization and pneumonia are needed.

There are a variety of factors and conditions that predispose cattle to pneumonia. Cattle have anatomic and cellular differences from humans and other species and are managed in groups/herds, all of which can increase susceptibility to microbial pathogens. This article highlights the basic innate immune response of the respiratory tract and newer developments in the understanding of adaptive immune responses of the bovine respiratory tract, placing special emphasis on features unique to cattle.

Funding acknowledgment: MRA: NIH NIAID RO1 AI062787.

[a] Department of Veterinary Pathology, 2738, College of Veterinary Medicine, Iowa State University, 1600 South 16th Street, Ames, IA 50011-1250, USA
[b] Department of Veterinary Pathology, 2740, College of Veterinary Medicine, Iowa State University, 1600 South 16th Street, Ames, IA 50011-1250, USA
[c] Department of Veterinary Microbiology, 2156, College of Veterinary Medicine, Iowa State University, 1600 South 16th Street, Ames, IA 50011-1250, USA
* Corresponding author.
E-mail address: mackerma@iastate.edu

INNATE IMMUNE RESPONSES
Commensal Microflora

The upper respiratory tract is colonized by a variety of bacterial pathogens that are inhaled and/or replicate in the tonsillar crypts and nasal/sinus mucin. Colonization of these organisms within regions of the upper respiratory tract mucosa may occupy micronutrient and receptor sites resulting in reduced colonization by pathogens. In a study from 1964, bacterial isolates from trachea and lung were colonized by *Bacillus* sp, *Streptococcus* sp, *Streptomyces* sp, *Micrococcus* sp, and *Pseudomonas* sp.[1] A 1991 study demonstrated *Pasteurella (Mannheimia) haemolytica*, *Pasteurella multocida*, *Mycoplasma bovine*, and *M bovirhinis*, *Histophilus somni*, *Streptomycetes* sp, *Neisseria* spp, and *Bacillus* spp in nasopharyngeal swabs of healthy calves.[2] The deeper lung remains relatively sterile in healthy cattle; however, in a recent study of bronchoalveolar lavage fluid from cattle in Denmark,[3] 63% of healthy cattle harbored bovine bacterial pathogens (*Pasteurella multocida*, *Histophilus somni*, *Mannheimia haemolytica*, *Arcanobacterium pyogenes*, and *Mycoplasma* sp).

Pathogenic Microflora

Bovine respiratory disease complex (BRDC) is a complex infectious disease caused by the interaction of several microbial agents. These include viruses that have a tendency to infect immunocompromised lung: bovine herpesvirus-1 (BHV-1), bovine respiratory syncytial virus, bovine parainfluenza virus 3, bovine coronavirus, bovine adenovirus A-D, and bovine viral diarrhea virus 1 and 2. Many herds of cattle are colonized by *Mycoplasma* spp (*bovis, dispar, bovirhinis*), which inhibit function and activity of ciliated respiratory epithelial cells. Initial viral infections, toxins such as 3-methyl indole, or other immunosuppressive conditions allow increased replication of other bacterial pathogens: *Mannheimia haemolytica*, *Pasteurella multocida*, *Histophilus somni*, *Arcanobacterium pyogenes*, and Chlamydiaceae. *Mannheimia haemolytica*, *Pasteurella multocida*, and *Histophilus somni* can colonize the tonsil and mucous of the nasal meatus and sinuses. With stress, their replication increases and their area of colonization spreads.

Respiratory Airways

Cattle have a relatively long tracheobronchial tree, which increases the amount of dead space volume in comparison with dogs, pigs, and horses.[4] Increased dead space affects the amount of fresh oxygen that can be delivered to lung and increases the risk of alveolar hypoventilation with partial obstruction. The increased dead space in cattle may not affect respiratory tract immunity per se; however, it may allow increased surface area for particulate deposition and increased transit time of inhaled vapors, gases, and particulate matter.

Hairs

Hairs along the external nares provide a physical barrier to inhalation of large particulate matter. Squamous cells that line the anterior nares form a layer of stratified squamous epithelium that is more resistant to microbial adhesion compared with pseudostratified epithelium.

Mucociliary Apparatus

The air-surface liquid (ASL) lining the upper respiratory tract and pulmonary airways is generated largely from submucosal glands and goblet cells and provides a layer of protection against inhaled particulate matter, aerosols, vapors, and microbial pathogens (**Fig. 1**). The antimicrobial activity of the ASL is becoming increasingly

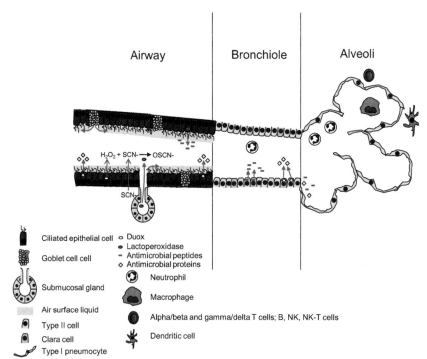

Fig. 1. Schematic illustration of the bovine respiratory immune system emphasizing the innate components. Depicted are immune systems within 3 main regions of the respiratory tract: the airways (upper respiratory tract to the bronchi), bronchiole, and alveoli. *Airway:* Conducting airways are lined by pseudostratified ciliated epithelium that transports the air-surface liquid (ASL) anteriorly toward the pharynx or nares. ASL is produced by secretion products from goblet cells and submucosal glands. Within the ASL are mucins (see text), as well as antimicrobial proteins (eg, lysozyme, lactoferrin, surfactant proteins A and D, SLPI, PLUNC, and others) and antimicrobial peptides (defensins and RNAase 7), which are produced by ciliated epithelial cells. The oxidative defense system (ODS) is composed of lactoperoxidase (LPO) produced by submucosal glands, dual function oxidases 1 and 2 (Duox1 and Duox2) produced by epithelia, and thiocyanate (SCN-) transport proteins produced by epithelia. Duox1 and 2 produce hydrogen peroxide (H_2O_2), which, in the presence of SCN-, is converted to OSCN-, which has potent antimicrobial activity. *Bronchioles:* Bronchioles are lined by Clara and Type II cells, both of which also produce antimicrobial proteins and peptides. Clara cells also produce CC10, an immunomodulatory protein, and express cytochrome P450 enzymes that biometabolize toxins. With injury, Type II and Clara cells proliferate and replace damaged cells. *Alveoli:* Type I pneumocytes line the alveolar lumen and are covered by surfactant phospholipids that are admixed with surfactant proteins, antimicrobial proteins, and antimicrobial peptides. With injury, Type I pneumocytes are replaced by Type II cells, which then differentiate into Type I cells. *Effector cells:* Neutrophils, alveolar and intravascular macrophages, alpha/beta T (CD4 and CD8) cells, and gamma/delta T cells along with B, NK, and dendritic cells are effector cells present along the respiratory tree for induction of adaptive immune responses. With inflammation, neutrophils and macrophages are present in the alveolar lumen, bronchioles, and airways. Other immune responses such as pattern recognition receptors as well as cytokine, interferon, and chemokine responses are not included in this figure.

understood. The ASL has 2 layers, a periciliary sol layer close to the apical cell surface and a gel/mucus layer that is toward the airway lumen. Ciliary beat occurs principally within the sol layer, which is less viscous than the gel layer. Dehydration can enhance the viscosity of the ASL as can aggregates of DNA and filamentous actin that accumulate from degraded neutrophils, leukocytes, and necrotic epithelial cells along with bacterial biofilms. Sneezing and coughing help to expel particulates and ASL/mucin aggregates and also induce some dilation of the airway lumens.

Air Surface Liquid

Once considered simply a lubricant for airway function, the ASL has a very active role in innate defense. Water accumulates within the periciliary sol layer after secretion of chloride ions by epithelial cells, submucosal glands, and serous cells and water is resorbed as sodium is removed from the layer by epithelial Na+ channels (ENaC). In addition to providing a microenvironment for ciliary activity, the periciliary sol layer maintains a proper pH (slightly more acidic than blood). The gel layer of the ASL is composed of mucin glycoproteins and proteoglycans secreted by goblet cells and submucosal glands. The amount of this layer can increase with chronic inflammatory conditions, allergic conditions, and cholinergic stimulation. The mucin glycoproteins are either tethered to the apical membrane of the subjacent epithelial cell or secreted. The protein backbone of the mucin glycoproteins encoded by *MUC* genes contain repeating serine and threonine amino acids that form O-linkages with oligosaccharides. In humans, MUC1 and MUC4 (and also MUC 11, 13, 15, and 20) proteins are associated with the apical surface, whereas MUC5AC is secreted from goblet cells and MUC5B is secreted from mucous cells of submucosal glands.[5] Variations of *MUC* gene expression change with inflammation and lung injury. MUC proteins serve as receptors and signaling molecules and can bind bacteria. For example, MUC1 is a receptor for *Pseudomonas aeruginosa* flagellin protein, activates Src tyrosine kinases, and activates phospholipase C and protein kinase C. MUC7 is a non–gel-forming secreted mucin.

The ASL contains numerous molecules that mediate antimicrobial as well as pro- and anti-inflammatory activity, immunomodulation, and wound healing.[6] The osmotic gradient is maintained by sodium and chloride levels regulated by sodium and chloride transport pumps and channels, which allows proper protein, enzyme, and peptide activity. The presence and activity of some of these, such as lactoferrin and lysozyme have been known for many years. Lactoferrin binds and sequesters iron from microbial agents, whereas lysozyme can disrupt membranes of bacteria. Additional components of the ASL have been indentified in cattle and other species and increasingly appreciated for the immune and immunomodulatory role. These include antimicrobial peptides such as defensins, cathelicidins, and larger proteins.[7] There are 3 major subclassifications of defensins and 2, the alpha and beta defensins, are present in cattle.

Three beta-defensins of cattle include tracheal antimicrobial peptide (TAP), lingual antimicrobial peptide (LAP), and enteric antimicrobial peptide. TAP and LAP are produced by respiratory epithelia and TAP has the highest level of expression. In fact, TAP was the first mammalian defensin identified, being isolated and cloned by Gill Diamond and colleagues in 1991.[8] Both TAP, LAP, and other defensins can form pores in the membranes of bacteria, enveloped viruses, and other microbial agents resulting in rapid lysis. Beta defensins have numerous other activities that range from exacerbating the acute inflammatory reaction by triggering histamine release from mast cells, to triggering the adaptive immune response through their chemotactic properties to dendritic cells, to inducing wound healing via their mitogenic function in epithelial cells. Cercropin is an antimicrobial peptide from insects that, when delivered by vector to bovine mucosa, reduces colonization by *Mannheimia haemoyltica*.[9] Bovine neutrophils have numerous alpha defensins as well; however, these are produced in neutrophils and are present in the ASL only after neutrophil recruitment and degranulation. Cathelicidin antimicrobial peptides are also produced in neutrophils and can be released by lung epithelia; however, epithelial expression is apparently low and limited. Airway epithelial cells also produce RNAase 7, an RNA helicase with antimicrobial properties; however, the expression levels of RNAase in cattle are not known. Bovine neutrophils express 13 defensins that are released upon degranulation and contribute to microbial killing and the acute inflammatory reaction. Binding of defensins and other antimicrobial peptides to host membranes is limited, presumably because of the higher cholesterol content of mammalian cells and, thus, autotoxicity by these peptides is not a feature of the their activity.

In alveoli of deep lung, alveolar macrophages engulf particulate matter and pathogens that manage to be inhaled into the deep lung. Once activated, the macrophages release cytokines, chemokines, and other soluble mediators that stimulate an inflammatory and/or immune response. Cells lining alveoli (type I pneumocytes) are covered by a layer of surfactant, composed of phosphatidylcholine and other phospholipids, which prevents alveolar collapse by its effect on apical membrane surface tension. Surfactant is secreted by airway type II cells and Clara cells along with surfactant proteins. Intracellularly, surfactant proteins B and C are associated with surfactant and maintain surfactant folding/structure until release. Surfactant proteins A and D are also associated with surfactant and released by pseudostratified ciliated, type II, and Clara cells into the airway and/or alveolar lumen and have very potent antimicrobial and immunomodulatory roles. Surfactant protein A (SP-A) and D (SP-D) can bind and inactivate microbial agents. Both of these proteins have a carbohydrate recognition domain (CRD) that binds to mannose residues of microbial pathogens. Once bound, the pathogen and surfactant protein complex can aggregate and be taken up by alveolar macrophages. This is well documented for respiratory syncytial virus (RSV) in humans,[6] and individual altered surfactant proteins A and/or D attributable to nucleotide polymorphisms have increased numbers of RSV infection and increased severity. Once released, SP-A can activate macrophages and enhance macrophage uptake and killing of microbial pathogens. In addition, SP-A present within the alveolar lumen liquid can be taken up by the pulmonary lymphatic drainage system and enter the blood. Increased levels of SP-A in blood is associated with pneumonia and could be a useful biomarker of pneumonia severity.

Airway and Lung Alveolar Epithelia

As indicated previously, the ASL is produced by subjacent airway and lung epithelial layer that is specialized along the respiratory tract. The inner nares is lined by stratified squamous epithelium that transitions into pseudostratified ciliated epithelium that lines the nasal meatus and conchae (turbinates). Intervening within the pseudostratified ciliated epithelium are goblet cells that release mucin products discussed earlier and also submucosal glands. In the ethmoid region, additional nerve sensory fibers enter the respiratory epithelia and mediate olfactory sensations. Pseudostratified ciliated epithelia, along with submucosal glands, line the frontal and ethmoid sinuses, trachea, and bronchi. Lung bronchiole mucosa has a thinner epithelial layer (1 cell-layer thick) lined by both type II and Clara cells (see **Fig. 1**). Both cell types produce surfactant and surfactant proteins and can serve as progenitor cells; type II cells are progenitors for other type II cells and type I cells that line lung alveoli. Clara cells produce daughter cells that can be Clara cells or type II cells. Clara cells also express mixed function oxidases (cytochrome p450 isoenzymes such as CYP1A1 and CYP1A2) that detoxify inhaled toxins and/or toxins that are spread hematogenously. This is a beneficial feature for some toxins; however, for others, such as 3-methyl indole (3 MI), a toxic metabolite, 3-methylindololamine is formed that causes Clara and airway epithelial cell injury and necrosis. With loss of these cells, there is concomitant loss of the epithelial barrier and the overlying air-surface liquid containing antimicrobial factors. The 3 MI is present in certain feedstuffs such as foggage, rape, and kale. Clara cells also produce Clara cell secretory protein 10 (CC10). CC10 is an important, yet subtle, immunomodulator of lung physiology, influencing synthesis, secretion, and function of molecules such as phospholipase A2, interferon gamma, and locally produced IgA. Generally, it is an immunosuppressive and anti-inflammatory protein that is important in limiting the collateral damage caused by inflammatory cells such as neutrophils.

Microbial Pattern Recognition Molecules

Epithelial cells are central to respiratory systems sensing of the external environment. Most particulate matter and microbial agents are removed from the inhaled air in the nares, nasal conchae, and trachea leaving the deeper lung sterile and relatively free from particulate material. These substances, along with mists, vapors, and gases once through the ASL can bind the lung epithelia and trigger activation, cell injury, metaplasia, or cell death. Microbial agents produce a number of conserved molecular patterns, termed pathogen-associated molecular patterns (PAMPs) that include substances such as teichoic acid from gram-positive bacteria, lipopolysaccharide (LPS) from gram-negative bacteria, cytokine-phosphate-guanine (CpG) DNA, single- and double-stranded RNA (dsRNA), flagellin, fungal zymosan, and lipopeptides from mycobacteria. Major pathogens of cattle, *Histophilus somni, Mannheimia haemolytica, Pasteurella multocida, Mycoplasma bovis*, bovine herpesvirus-1 (BHV-1; infectious bovine rhinotracheitis), parainfluenza virus, bovine respiratory syncytial virus, and bovine viral diarrhea virus (BVD), all produce some type of PAMP that are recognized by epithelia, alveolar macrophages, and intravascular macrophages. Intravascular macrophages are macrophages within the small capillaries of alveolar walls, attached to the underlying endothelial cells that are very active in metabolic generation of inflammatory mediators such as prostaglandins and leukotrienes. With acute inflammation, neutrophils also recognize PAMPs, and with adaptive immune responses, the various lung dendritic cells (DCs), including plasmcytoid DCs, natural killer (NK) cells, NK T cells, alpha/beta and gamma/delta T cells, and B cells, all interact with microbial PAMPs.

The lung, like other organs, expresses a wide variety of extracellular, cell surface, endosomal, and cytoplasmic receptors that recognize microbial PAMPs, termed pattern recognition receptors (PRRs). Extracellular PRRs include LPS binding protein, mannan-binding lectins such as ficolin and collectins, and also C-reactive protein and serum amyloid protein. In swine, single nucleotide polymorphisms (SNP) in these mannan-binding lectin C are associated with increased respiratory disease.[10]

Cell surface PRR on respiratory epithelia include Toll-like receptors (TLRs), which are transmembrane receptors that have outer leucine-rich repeats (LRR) and cytoplasmic TII/interleukin-1 (IL-1) receptor homology domains that transmit signals to the nucleus once the outer LRR are activated by PAMPs. The TLR activate nuclear factor (NF)-kappa B or the interferon regulatory factors (IRF)-3 and -7. Cattle have 10 TLRs that have specific and sometimes overlapping PAMP affinities. In short, TLR 1 has affinity for triacyl lipopeptide of mycobacteria; TLR 2 has affinity for peptidoglycans of gram-positive organisms and lipoarbinomannan of mycobacteria and zymosan of fungi; TLR 3 has affinity for dsRNA; TLR 4 has affinity for LPS; TLR 5 has affinity for flagellin; TLR 6 has affinity for diacyl lipopeptides of mycoplasma; TLR 7 and 8 have affinity for single-stranded RNA (ssRNA); TLR 9 has affinity for CpG; and TLR 10 is not yet fully assessed. As indicated, several TLRs[1,2,5–9] signal through MyD88, which leads to NF-kappa B activity and inflammatory reactions, whereas other TLRs[3] are MyD88 independent (signaling through TRIF/TRAF) and induce IRF-3 and -7 and type I interferon genes. TLR 4 can signal through MyD88 or TRIF/TRAF, depending on the stimulus. LPS, a bacterial component of *Histophilus somni, Mannheimia haemolytica,* and *Pasteurella multocida*, first binds LPS binding protein, soluble CD14, and the TLR 4 cofactor MD2 before fully activated TLR 4. TLR 4 is also bound by the F protein of RSV.

Bovine respiratory viruses, BHV-1, PI-3, RSV, and BVD, can infect lung epithelial cells. Viruses can induce formation of noncapped, 5' triphosphated RNA, long dsRNA, ssRNA, and viral DNA, along with their capsids, matrix proteins, and nonstructural proteins. These signal through TLR 3, 7, 8, and 9 as indicated previously but recent work has also characterized cytosolic viral pathogen recognition receptors, retinoic acid–induced gene-I (RIG-I), and melanoma differentiation associated gene-5 (MDA-5). These proteins have an RNA helicase and caspase recruitment (CARD) structural domains and recognize noncapped 5' triphosphated RNAs (RIG-I) and dsRNA (MDA-5). RIG-I and MDA-5 activate NF-kappa B and IRF-3 and -7 via mitochondrial antiviral signaling adaptor (MAVS), interferon-beta promoter stimulator (IPS-1), virus-inducing signaling adaptor, and Cardif.

Other cytosol receptors include the nucleotide-binding domain, leucine-rich repeat (NOD)-like receptors that can detect viral, bacterial, and other pathogens that enter the cytoplasm. Over 20 NOD-like receptors have been identified. NOD 1 and 2 bind peptidoglycan, linterleukin 1β-converting enzyme and protease activating factor (IPAF) recognizes flagellin, and NACHT, LRR, and PYD contain protein3 (NALP3) recognizes a very broad range of exogenous and endogenous molecules including viruses, low intracellular potassium, toxins, ultraviolet light, asbestos, silica aluminum, and urate crystals. NOD-like receptors have leucine-rich repeat domains that recognize pathogens. The NOD-like receptors stimulate cell activation. In macrophages, NALP3, IPAF, and NALP1 are components of the inflammasome. The inflammasomes induce activity by triggering caspase 1 activation that results in cleavage of pro-interleukin 1 beta (IL-1 beta) to active IL-1 beta and active IL-18. IL-1 beta and IL-18 bind their respective receptors on leukocytes and other cells, which triggers proinflammatory responses.

Although NF-kappa β and IRF-3 or -7 can be activated by TLR, RIG-I, MDA-5, and NOD-like proteins, endogenous molecules such as heat shock proteins 60 and 70, urates, adenosine, and other molecules can also activate epithelial cells, macrophages, and other inflammatory cell types in the lung. These are termed danger-associated molecular patterns (DAMPs) or alarmins. Although DAMPs activate these inflammation transcription factors, their activation signal is modulated by simultaneous binding to CD24, which interacts with Siglec, which reduces the intensity of NF-kappa B activation.

Oxidative Killing by Respiratory Epithelia

More recently, an oxidative defense system (ODS) has been identified in the human and ovine respiratory tracts. Because it is active in sheep, it is likely also present in cattle. The ODS requires activity of epithelial enzymes dual oxidases1 and 2 (Duox1 and Duox2), which are members of the nicotinamide adenine dinucleotide phosphate (NADPH) oxidase family and generate hydrogen peroxide production onto the ASL. In the presence of thiocyante (SCN-), the hydrogen peroxide that is weakly microbicidal is then converted to a more toxic compound, hypothiocyanite (OSCN-), which is short-lived but highly microbicidal.

Cytokines, Chemokines, Interferons

Acute inflammatory cytokines such as IL-1, tumor necrosis factor (TNF), and IL-6 invoke activation of nearby cells including endothelial cells, epithelial cells, alveolar macrophages, and lung dendritic cells. With activation there is release of chemokines that attract migration of neutrophils and monocytes into the affected area and with time also attract DCs and NK, T, and B cells. Inflammatory chemokines include IL-8 (CXCL8), GCP-2 (CXCL6), ENA-78 (CXCL5), Gro (CXCL1-3), IP-10 (CXCL10), I-Tac (CXCL11), RANTES (CCL5), MIP-alpha (CCL3) and -beta (CCL4), MCP 1-5 (CCL7, 8, 12, 13), and eotaxins 1-3 (CCL24, 26) depending on the stimulus with receptors that include CXCR1, 2, and 3 and CCR1, 2, 3, and 5. Lymphocytes that home to the lung use a different set of chemokines (eg, naïve cells express CCR1-10, CSCR1-3 and memory cells express CCR8-10, CSCR1, 2, 4, and 5). Chemerin is a chemotactic factor for DCs and macrophages through binding of chemokine-like receptor 1 (CMKLR1).

Some viral infections activate viral receptors that invoke IRF-3 and -7, which stimulate production of type I interferons (IFN alpha and beta) that are released by numerous cells types. These interferons bind Jak/Stat receptors of adjacent cells to induce expression of antiviral substances that include the ISGlyation pathway, which complexes with IRF-3 and prevents degradation; MxA protein, which binds and traps viruses; 2′,5′-oligoadenylate synthetase 1 (OAS1) activates RNaseL, which cleaves viral RNA; and protein kinase R (PKR), which dimerizes in the presence of viral RNA and inhibits eukaryotic translation initiation factor 2 alpha (EIF2 alpha) to reduce viral replication.

Effector Cells

In addition to respiratory epithelia, major innate immune effector cells include the vascular endothelium, neutrophils, alveolar and intravascular macrophages, dendritic cells, NK cells, NK T cells, eosinophils, and mast cells. With acute inflammatory responses, endothelial cells become activated by inflammatory mediators, open gaps, and allow passage of serum factors into the lung, especially alveolar lumens. This fluid contains dilute microbial agents and toxins physically, and contains numerous molecules with protective immune function such as complement, hydrolytic enzymes, IgG, IgM, IgA, IgE, collectins, acute phase proteins, and others. Endothelial cells also release inflammatory mediators and express adhesion molecules that mediate passage of leukocytes into sites of infection/injury. Neutrophils internalize microbial agents, foreign substances, and other particulates, release their granule contents, and upon death release neutrophil extracellular traps (NETs) composed of DNA, histones, and antimicrobial peptides (alpha defensins) that entrap microbes. NK cells do not require previous antigenic exposure to kill virus-infected cells. They express CD161 and CD56 and are activated by interferon and macrophage cytokines to produce interferon gamma and release perforin to kill virus-infected cells. In many species, activation of macrophages occurs in a classical, proinflammatory cell–mediated Th1-type response induced by interferon gamma and TNF; an alternative Th2-type response induced by IL-4, and an anti-inflammatory, regulatory response induced by IL-10. In cattle, however, the Th1/Th2 paradiagm is not as clearly distinct, functionally, as in other species. Despite this, alveolar and intravascular macrophages of the bovine do function in generation of cell-mediated, humoral, and regulatory (inhibitory) responses. In allergic (Th2-type) conditions, eosinophilic and mast cell infiltration occurs with release of granule content. Once established, inhaled antigen can cross-link IgE receptors on mast cells and basophils resulting in cellular activation.

Factors That Can Alter Respiratory Immunity

The bovine lung has anatomic features that predispose cattle to respiratory infections. This is reviewed elsewhere.[4] Briefly, cattle have a relatively increased area of dead space, as indicated, and they also have a right tracheal bronchus. The bovine lung has interlobular septae with limited interdependence, increased resistance, and decreased compliance, and collateral ventilation is reduced because of a lack of (1) bronchoalveolar communication (channels of Lambert), (2) alveolar pores (pores of Kohn), and (3) interbronchiolar connections (channels of Martin). Because of the lack of collateral ventilation, atelectasis occurs readily and these areas of lung remain consolidated and lack functional gaseous exchange. Regions of atelectasis are also under hypoxic vasoconstriction whereby arterioles shunt blood flow away from these areas to better perfused regions with adequate gaseous exchange. Thus, these anatomic and physiologic conditions increase the demands for protective immune responses.

There are several environmental factors and managerial issues that also can lower respiratory tract immunity. These include transportation, weaning, overcrowding, changes in social structure, precipitation, fluctuations in temperature, humidity, air exchange, lighting, sounds, changes in feedstuffs, feedlot floor conditions, and other microbial agents. These can affect even basic aspects of the immune system. For example, although corticosteroids (dexamethasone), catecholamines, acetylcholine, and substance P do not affect basal level of TAP and LAP expression by respiratory epithelial cells, dexamethasone exposure reduces TAP and LAP expression on exposure to LPS.[11] In addition, infection with type 2 bovine viral diarrhea virus (BVDV) also reduces LPS-induced expression of TAP (and lactoferrin) but a type 1 noncytopathic BVD strain had no effect.[12]

Other conditions that impair immune responses may include single nucleotide polymorphisms within genes encoding innate and adaptive immune responses of the lung as studied in swine; however, no large-scale studies have been completed in cattle, to date.

Diagnostic Biomarkers

Some innate immune molecules have use or potential use in assessing respiratory tract function/activity or stage/severity of clinical disease. Surfactant protein A (SP-A) production by lung epithelia increases markedly in fetal lung near term and thus roughly delineates the level of lung maturation at birth. SP-A production can also be increased with viral pneumonia and enters the pulmonary lymphatic vessels where it is carried by the thoracic duct to the systemic blood circulation. Thus, serum SP-A measurement has potential to be a marker of respiratory tract maturation and also pneumonia severity.

Recent work has shown that acute-phase proteins are clinical markers of pneumonia severity. Serum-associated amyloid (SAA), haptoglobin, alpha 1-acid glycoprotein produced by liver in response to IL-1, and TNF alpha are produced during pneumonia. SAA and haptoglobin can differentiate acute and chronic pneumonia and alterations in haptoglobin and apolipoprotein A1 are associated with viral infections.[13] Metabolic and elemental compounds are biomarkers of viral infection (glucose, low density lipoprotein [LDL], valine, phosphorus, and iron) and disease outcome (lactate, glucose, iron).[13]

RECENT DEVELOPMENTS IN ADAPTIVE IMMUNE RESPONSES

Several excellent reviews of respiratory adaptive immune responses to bovine pathogens have detailed advanced concepts in cellular and molecular immunology in this text series[14] and other journals.[15,16] These pathogens can evade respiratory immune responses by modulating (1) the host immune response, and/or (2) the microbial phenotype or location.[15] In addition, it is commonplace for investigators to study neutrophils, alveolar macrophages, and other airway cells retrieved by bronchoalveolar lavage. In contrast, few investigative studies have examined the precise role of adaptive immune cells (dendritic, gamma/delta T, alpha/beta T, B, NK, and NK-T cells) in the respiratory mucosa, bronchus-associated lymphoid tissue (BALT), and tracheobronchial lymph nodes in response to bovine pulmonary pathogens. Such studies could be completed with laser capture microdissection coupled with flow cytometric analysis and microarray. Moreover, the dynamic interaction among these cells and their migration to and from the tracheobronchial lymph node have not been fully assessed. Clearly, there is antigen exposure in the lung airways that triggers differentiation, maturation, and responses by these cells that have a kinetic progression with time. The progression and cellular/molecular responses are likely very different in neonatal lung upon initial encounter to a newly inhaled antigen and repeated exposure of an antigen in an older animal. This dynamic is further complicated by vaccination.

Passive Transfer (Colostrum)

Adaptive responses of the bovine neonate including failure of passive transfer (FPT) have been reviewed.[17,18] With FPT there are inadequate levels of maternal IgG, particularly IgG1, which comprises 80% of IgG, and other immunoglobulins that increase risk of respiratory infection. More recently, additional components of colostrum appear to influence the development and activity of the neonatal calf immune system. Maternal colostral leukocytes reduce CD11a+ lymphocytes in neonatal calf blood and these calves have higher CD25-, CD26-, and MHC I–expressing lymphocytes. Thus, maternal colostral leukocytes accelerate fetal lymphocyte development.[19]

Proinflammatory cytokines are also present in colostrum. IL-beta, IL-6, TNF alpha, and IFN gamma are significantly increased in colostrum but reduced to zero or nearly zero by day 5 of lactation. The high colostral levels of these cytokines correspond to increased levels in the serum of neonatal calves.[20] Serum cytokine levels of IL-1 beta, IL-1 alpha, TNF alpha, IL-6, and IFN gamma peak at 12–24 hours after birth and progressively decrease to zero or near zero by day 21. One study has shown high levels of IL-18 in colostrum and increased serum levels of IL-18 in neonates by 6 hours post colostral ingestion.[21] The increased colostral cytokines appear to trigger neutrophil function, as colostral whey enhances neutrophil functional assays (cytochrome C reduction and iodination).[22] This finding suggests that the colostral cytokines are important for neutrophil "readiness" in newborn animals. This likely has a systemic protective effect because neutrophil function is vital for the protection of respiratory airways, intestine, and other mucosal surfaces against microbial pathogens.

Gamma/Delta T Cells

The generation of humoral and cellular responses of the adaptive immune system by the bovine are described by Srikumara and colleagues[15] and Kindt and collegues.[23] These occur simultaneously with innate immune responses. The adaptive responses are contingent upon antigen recognition, antigen processing and presentation by dendritic cells, and involvement of gamma/delta T cells and alpha/beta (CD 4 and CD8) cells. Of these, gamma/delta T cells of cattle are of special interest for at least two reasons. First, newborn calves have an unusually high number of circulating gamma/delta T cells and second, gamma/delta T cells of ruminants express WC-1 antigen. Gamma/delta T cells account for 60% of the peripheral blood mononuclear cells in young calves. WC1+ gamma/delta T cells are considered an inflammatory population, whereas CD1- gamma/delta T cells are regulatory with myeloid cell features. Within the WC1+ phenotype are WC1.1+ and WC1.2+ subsets that differ in their IFN gamma production and proliferative responses to stimuli.[24,25] The role of WC protein is not fully understood but it may be a homolog of CD4 and CD8 antigens on alpha/beta T cells by regulating gamma/delta T-cell responses or transmission of signals from the outside into the cell.[26] It is possible that WC protein binds microbial PAMPs similar to other proteins with similarities to WC.

CLINICAL IMPLICATIONS

A 2009 study of bovine respiratory disease (BRD) in an Oklahoma feedlot underscores the complexity of this disease and its clinical impact.[27] BRD morbidity was 14.7% in that herd with 0.7% mortality. The mean fatal disease onset was 32.6 days and mean treatment interval was 29 days, mean number of antibiotic treatments were 2.6 days, and mean day of death was 61.8 days. All of the agents listed at the beginning of this article were isolated from the cattle. These agents were correlated with mortality, treatment, lesion, and association with other agents. Also correlated were the type of lesions with mortality, treatment, and infectious agent. Interestingly, along with BVDV-1a and 2b, BVDV-1b was identified in fatal cases and this was considered note-worthy because most current BVDV vaccines contain BVDV-1a and 2b but not BVDV1b. The work also identified BVDV-2b for the first time. This study confirms the continued presence of and damage caused by these microbial agents in 2009. Thus, despite advancements in managerial practices, vaccine development, antimi-crobial agents, medicine, and molecular diagnostics, each of these agents remains a significant concern.

The innate immune response can be viewed as the basal, most basic immune response to pathogen but it is a response that is difficult to enhance therapeutically. As with adaptive immune responses, there is redundancy and overlap in the function of innate immune products that protect the respiratory tract. However, loss of some innate factors is clearly associated with increased incidence and/or severity of respi-ratory disease. Factors that influence this include dehydration, genetic changes result-ing in altered expression of innate immune factors, stress, and primary infection.

Dehydration

It is well known that dehydration causes increased viscosity of respiratory secretions. The sol layer of the respiratory air-surface liquid is reduced resulting in increased mucinous material that can allow increased colonization of bacterial pathogens and accumulation of inhaled particulate matter because of reduced mucociliary function.

Genetic Changes Resulting in Altered Expression of Innate Immune Factors

Single nucleotide polymorphisms (SNPs) are single nucleotide changes in a particular animal that can result in production of a different amino acid in a protein. Although this is a very slight change, a single amino acid change may greatly change the function of an innate immune factor. As indicated, studies in pigs have demonstrated that SNPs in mannan-binding lectin C are associated with increased susceptibility to respiratory disease. Humans with SNPs in surfactant protein A and D have increased incidence and severity of respiratory syncytial virus pneumonia. Identifying an association between SNPs and increased respiratory disease often requires large-scale genetic studies matched to clinical disease scores and thus are often expensive. However, SNPs within a cattle herd that has minimal genetic variation could have profound effects.

Stress

Causes of stress are varied but include overcrowding, lack of shade in the hot summer, rapid and extreme fluctuations in temperature, wind, shipping, persistent startling (eg, dogs, coyotes, traffic noise), and other situations that change the physical and/or mental homeostasis of cattle. Stress affects cortisol levels, among other endogenous stress responses, and corticosteroids (dexamethasone) can reduce innate immune expression of defensin genes in response to LPS, as indicated. Thus, there appears to be a direct effect of stress on certain innate immune factors.

Primary Infection

As indicated, all animals have commensal microflora in the upper respiratory tract and nasopharynx. Changes in these secondary to stress, dehydration, or SNPs can allow increased proliferation of pathogens. For example, stressed cattle can have increased proliferation of *Mannheimia haemolytica* in the nasopharynx and tonsil. In addition, with reduced innate immune responses, organisms such as *Mycoplasma bovis* and viruses (PI-3, RSV, BVDv) have enhanced opportunities to colonize, proliferate, and damage the respiratory epithelia setting the stage for secondary bacterial pathogens with increased virulence.

Reducing the effects and duration of these factors are a first step in enhancing innate immune activity. With time, therapies aimed toward enhancing activity of some innate immune responses may become a viable option and adjunct to management, vaccination, and antimicrobial agents.

SUMMARY

The bovine respiratory tract immune response is sophisticated and shaped by anatomic and cellular features unique to cattle/ruminants, management practices, and interactions with specific microbial pathogens. Because extensive inflammatory reactions impair gaseous exchange and lung function, innate immune responses are vital for sensing and handling pulmonary exposures to particulates, vapors, microbial agents, and other inhaled substances without invoking a marked inflammatory reaction. Cattle have anatomic features such as reduced collateral ventilation that reduce the effectiveness of the innate immune response and current managerial practices sometimes weaken the innate immune response. With persistence or repeated exposure to antigens or insults, adaptive immune responses are generated. Neonatal calves require colostrum for fully functional adaptive responses and have high levels gamma/delta cells that contribute significantly to adaptive responses in concert with dendritic cells, NK cells, macrophages, alpha/beta T cells, and B cells.

REFERENCES

1. Collier JR, Rossow CF. Microflora of apparently healthy lung tissue of cattle. Am J Vet Res 1964;25:391–3.
2. Allen JW, Viel L, Bateman KG, et al. The microbial flora of the respiratory tract in feedlot calves: associations between nasopharyngeal and bronchoalveolar lavage cultures. Can J Vet Res 1991;55:341.

3. Angen O, Thomse J, Larsen LE, et al. Respiratory disease in calves: microbiological investigations on trans-tracheally aspirated bronchoalveolar lavage fluid and acute phase protein response. Vet Microbiol 2009;137(1–2):165–71.
4. Kirschvink N. Respiratory function in cattle: impact of breed, heritability, and external factors. Dtsch Tierartzl Wochenschr 2008;115:265–70.
5. Linden SK, Sutton P, Karlsson NG, et al. Mucins in the mucosal barrier to infection. Mucosal Immunol 2008;1(3):183–97.
6. Grubor B, Meyerholz DK, Ackermann MR. Collectins and cationic antimicrobial peptides of the respiratory epithelia. Vet Pathol 2006;43:595–612.
7. Bartlett JA, Fischer AJ, McCray PB Jr. Innate immune functions of the airway epithelium. Contrib Microbiol 2008;15:147–63.
8. Diamond G, Zasloff M, Eck H, et al. Tracheal antimicrobial peptide, a cysteine-rich peptide from mammalian tracheal mucosa: peptide isolation and cloning of cDNA. Proc Natl Acad Sci U S A 1991;88:3952–6.
9. Boudreux CM, Corstvet RE, Cooper RK, et al. Effects of cercropin B transgene expression on *Mannheimia haemolytica* serotype 1 colonization of the nasal mucosa of calves. Am J Vet Res 2005;66(100):1922–30.
10. Lillie BN, Keirstead ND, Squires EJ, et al. Gene polymorphisms associated with reduced hepatic expression of porcine mannan-binding lectin C. Dev Comp Immunol 2007;31:830–46.
11. Mitchell GB, Al-Haddawi MH, Clark ME, et al. Effect of corticosteroids and neuropeptides on expression of defensins by tracheal epithelial cells. Infect Immun 2007;75(3):1325–34.
12. Al-Haddawi M, Mitchell GB, Clark ME, et al. Impairment of innate immune response of airway epithelium by infection with bovine viral diarrhea virus. Vet Immunol Immunopathol 2007;116:153–62.
13. Aich P, Babiuk LA, Potter AA, et al. Biomarkers for prediction of bovine respiratory disease outcome. OMICS 2009;113:199–210.
14. Ellis JA. The immunology of the bovine respiratory disease complex. Vet Clin North Am Food Anim Pract 2001;17(3):535–50.
15. Srikumaran S, Kelling CL, Ambagala A. Immune evasion by pathogens of bovine respiratory disease complex. Anim Health Res Rev 2008;8(2):215–29.
16. Makoschey B, Lekeux P, Lacroux C, et al. Concepts in the prevention of bovine respiratory disease. Berl Munch Tierarztl Wochenschr 2008;121(11/12):446–9.
17. Barrington GM, Parish SM. Bovine neonatal immunology. Vet Clin North Am Food Anim Pract 2001;17(3):463–76.
18. Cortese VS. Neonatal immunology. Vet Clin North Am Food Anim Pract 2009;25:221–7.
19. Reber AJ, Donovan DC, Gabbard J, et al. Transfer of maternal colostral leukocytes promotes development of the neonatal immune system. Part II. Effects on neonatal lymphocytes. Vet Immunol Immunopathol 2008;123:305–13.
20. Yamanaka J, Hagiwara K, Kirisawa R, et al. Transient detection of proinflammatory cytokines in sera of colostrum-fed newborn calves. J Vet Med Sci 2003;65(7):813–6.
21. Muneta J, Yoshihara K, Minagawa Y, et al. Bovine IL-18 ELISA: detection of IL-18 in sera of pregnant cow and newborn calf, and in colostrums. J Immunoassay Immunochem 2005;26:203–13.
22. Roth JA, Frank DE, Weighner P, et al. Enhancement of neutrophil function by ultrafiltered bovine whey. J Dairy Sci 2001;84:824–9.
23. Kindt TJ, Goldsby RA, Osborne BA. Kuby immunology. 5th edition. New York: W.H. Freeman and Company; 2007.

24. Rogers AN, Vanburen DC, Hedblom E, et al. Function of ruminant gammadelta T cells is defined by WC1.1 or WC1.2 isofomr expression. Vet Immunol Immunopathol 2005;108:211–7.
25. Rogers AN, Vanburen DB, Hedblom EE, et al. Gammadelta T cell function varies with the expressed WE1 coreceptor. J Immunol 2005;174:3386–93.
26. Chen C, Herzig CTA, Telfer JC, et al. Antigenic basis of diversity in the gamma/delta cell co-receptor WC-1 family. Mol Immunol 2009;46:2565–75.
27. Fulton RW, Blood KS, Panciera RJ, et al. Lung pathology and infectious agents in the fatal feedlot pneumonias and relationships with mortality, disease onset, and treatments. J Vet Diagn Invest 2009;21:464–77.

Prevention of Respiratory Disease in Cow/Calf Operations

Gerald L. Stokka, DVM, MS

KEYWORDS

• Respiratory disease • Cow • Calf • Risk factors

Respiratory disease of calves from birth until weaning in cow/calf operations is common, yet sporadic in occurrence and usually with low prevalence. Dewell and colleagues[1] reported a 12% overall morbidity in a group of 1556 calves, of which 39% (4.7% case specific) was due to respiratory disease. In a survey of 520 cow/calf producers in Canada the incidence of preweaning mortality (5.4%–5.6%) attributed to pneumonia ranges from 12.8% to 17.5%, with greater losses occurring on larger operations.[2] The diagnosis of pneumonia in calves between the age of 1 month and weaning is generally termed nursing calf pneumonia, or in the case of spring calving herds, summer pneumonia. Although the common risk factors associated with bovine respiratory disease (BRD) in postweaned calves, such as commingling, transportation stress, and dietary changes, can be identified in cases of nursing calf pneumonia, they may not be of primary importance.

RISK FACTORS

Identification of risk factors associated with calf pneumonia in beef herds is an important step in attempts to manage this disease. An acceptable way to consider and quantify the causative factors with clinical disease is in the form of a logistic regression equation. This type of equation represents the relationship between the probability of disease and the presence or absence of one or more risk factors.[3–6] Risk factors associated with a clinical disease (ie, nursing calf pneumonia) should include

1. Failure or partial failure of passive transfer
2. Any type of commingling of different groups, even those belonging to the same operation, such as in extended calving intervals or 2 different calving seasons
3. Environmental risk, extreme cold or heat along with precipitation
4. Nutritional risk, such as a change in diet, energy, and protein deficiency

Pfizer Animal Health, 11551 2nd Street SE, Cooperstown, ND 58425, USA
E-mail address: gerald.stokka@pfizer.com

Vet Clin Food Anim 26 (2010) 229–241
doi:10.1016/j.cvfa.2010.04.002   vetfood.theclinics.com

5. Exposure to pathogens such as bovine herpesvirus 1 (BHV-1), bovine virus diarrhea virus (BVDV), bovine respiratory syncytial virus (BRSV), bovine respiratory corona-virus (BRCV), and *Mycoplasma bovis*
6. Trace mineral deficiency
7. Handling stress
8. Other operation-specific risk factors.

Each one of these risk factors or a combination of several can result in enough stress to allow clinical disease to manifest itself. A regression equation $Y = b0 + b1X1 + b2X2 + ... + bkXk$, for respiratory disease may resemble this model: $Y = 0.2 + 0.2(X1) + 0.1(X2) + 0.1(X3) + 0.15(X4) + ...$, where Y is the probability of respiratory disease, X1 is the degree of failure of passive transfer, X2 is the nutritional status of the cow and newborn calf, X3 is environmental influences such as rain or snow and cold temperatures, and X4 is exposure to pathogens. Although this approach helps to provide an understanding of the risk factors and explain the cause of the disease, the diagnostic ability to identify or even influence some of these factors is not always apparent. Producers can become frustrated with control programs that focus on only 1 or 2 factors. In herd investigations each risk factor must be considered.

EFFECT OF MATERNAL IMMUNITY

The role of maternal immunity and its relationship to health in calves is clear. Its role as a risk factor with respiratory disease in nursing calves is not so clearly defined. Wittum and Perino[7] showed that calves with failure of passive transfer were 3.2 to 9.5 times more likely to become sick and 5.4 times more likely to die before weaning than calves with normal passive transfer. Faber and colleagues[8] reported on the role of passive transfer in reducing risk of illness and mortality and on lifetime effects in dairy cattle. Dewell and colleagues[1] reported that calves with serum IgG concentrations of at least 2700 mg/dL weighed an estimated 3.34 kg (7.38 pounds) more at 205 days of age than calves with lower serum IgG concentration. The effect on performance was also noted in lambs, in which there was a significant association with IgG concentration at 24 hours of age and mean daily gain.[9] The research makes it clear that a partial or complete failure of passive transfer is one of the most important risk factors leading to the development of clinical disease and a negative effect on performance. How does maternal immunity play a role in preventing clinical disease in neonatal and young calves? In the bovine, with syndesmochorial placentation, transfer of immunity does not take place during gestation. Although the fetus is able to mount an active immune response during gestation, the newborn is essentially lacking protection against common organisms that in the adult cause no clinical disease.[10] Other immune factors also seem to play a role in disease protection and production performance in the young bovine.

Antibodies, Cytokines, and Maternal Cell Transfer

Disease protection for the newborn is conferred by the transfer of antibody, primarily through the absorption of IgG1. All classes of immunoglobulins IgG, IgM, and IgA are absorbed, with IgA and IgG1 being resecreted to provide mucosal protection. In addition to immunoglobulins, other immune-protective components are part of passive transfer.

Hirako and colleagues[11] showed that proinflammatory immune cytokines interleukin 1β (IL1β), IL1 receptor antagonist, and tumor necrosis factor α (TNF-α) were lower in postcolostrum-fed calves that became clinically ill in the first 4 months of life. Proinflammatory cytokines are necessary to activate innate and active immunity.

Lymphocytes from the dam are passed to the neonate via the colostrum. These lymphocytes may survive for a period of time in the intestinal lumen but may also penetrate the mucosa and find residence in the mesenteric lymph nodes. This transfer may allow for cell-mediated immunity to be passed to the newborn from the dam. Archambault and colleagues[12] reported that cell-mediated immune transfer to neonates could be enhanced by maternal vaccination. Although Donovan and colleagues[13] showed that transfer of live maternal cells from colostrum to neonatal calves enhanced responses to antigens against which the dams had previously responded (BVDV), but not to antigens to which the dams were naive, our complete understanding of the role of lymphocyte transfer is still not clear. What is clear is there is no true substitute for the passage of maternal immunity from dam to the neonate. Colostral supplements, substitutes, and frozen colostrum, although valuable as an addition to fresh colostrum, cannot match the quality of the dam's fresh colostrum.[14]

Quality, Concentration, and Volume

Measurement of maternal immunity is centered on the measurement of the amount of immunoglobulins in the bloodstream. Measurement of total proteins with the refractometer can give a qualitative measurement of passive transfer.[15] Total proteins in the serum that are equal to or greater than 5.5 provide a yes or no answer to whether passive transfer has occurred. Dewell and colleagues[1] showed that quantitative differences in passive transfer may result in differences in outcomes of disease and performance. Calves with serum IgG1 levels up to 2500 mg/dL were 1.5 times more likely to get sick before weaning and 2.4 times more likely to die before weaning than calves with higher IgG1 levels. Calves need to acquire as much protection as possible from the dam's colostrum. Anything less than maximum absorption seems to increase health and performance risk.

Absorption

The volume intake of colostrum is positively correlated with passive transfer, but how does adequate transfer occur in beef cattle with at times a very low volume of colostrum? In a Canadian study, colostrum production in beef cows ranged from 0.9 to 5 L. In the same study the production of colostral immunoglobulins ranged from 103 to 525 g.[16] If the requirement of the calf to achieve adequate transfer is 300 g, then with a concentration of 150 g/L, the neonate would need to consume 2 L at an efficiency of absorption at 100%. Estimates of absorption range from 6% to 88%, although most estimates fall in the range of 20% to 35%.[17,18] If one assumes an efficiency of absorption of 35% and a colostral concentration value of 100 g/L, then to achieve a serum concentration of 20 g/L, with a total serum volume of 4 L (serum volume 59.6% of body weight), the calf would have to consume approximately 2.3 L.

Consumption in grams of Ig's $(100 \times 2.3 \text{ L}) \times$ %AEA/plasma volume

(Body weight $\times$ 9.6%) $(0.35/4\text{L})$ = expected Ig concentration 20.125 g/L

With this knowledge it becomes imperative that any investigation of respiratory disease in suckling calves must begin with an analysis of factors that influence the passage of immunity from dam to calf.

GENETIC RISK

Calving ease is an important genetic trait that affects passive transfer via stress level at birth. Besser and colleagues[19] reported that calves experiencing dystocia had lower absorption of IgG1 from colostrum associated with respiratory acidosis. Calves born after experiencing calving difficulty have a physiologic acidosis. In addition, increased calving difficulty is associated with extended time to nursing.[20] Because time to first nursing is associated with efficiency of absorption, this too is a factor related to efficiency of passive transfer. It is important to recognize the role of calving ease in the equation of long-term health of calves. A second genetic trait associated with passive transfer is that of udder and teat conformation. The mechanics of transfer are critical to passive transfer, that is, teat size and length, and udder attachment. Goonewardene and colleagues[21] reported that pendulous udders coupled with large teat size can complicate the suckling process. This situation reduces the probability of good immune transfer, which increases the risk of clinical disease and decrease growth rates. A third genetic trait is the selection for increased growth rates in calves. Muggli and colleagues[22] reported that calves from Hereford lines selected for performance had lower IgG1 concentration than calves from the randomly selected control line. Field observations seem to support this research observation. Herds with selection pressure exclusively on performance tend to experience a higher level of clinical disease, often in the form of respiratory disease. The reason for this may not be evident; however, it may seem logical that selection for performance also leads to an increase in birth weight, calving difficulty, longer period of time to standing and nursing, or perhaps greater milk production leading to a higher incidence of mastitis or udder and teat problems, thus leading to decreased absorption of immunity.

HANDLING RISK

Maternal stress is another risk factor that must be considered. Tuchscherer and colleagues[23] reported the effect of maternal stress in sows and its subsequent negative effect on passive transfer with the sequelae of higher morbidity and mortality in suckling pigs. Lay and colleagues[24] reported on stress in pregnant cows exposed to repeated transportation and the negative effect on the progeny to respond to stress. It is evident from these studies that repeated stress in the pregnant female can have a detrimental effect on the health of offspring. The application of this directly relates to adopting low-stress handling methods of pregnant females.

COMMINGLING RISK

Commingling risk in postweaned calves has been well documented to be a major risk factor in the development of BRD.[25–27] On the other hand, commingling stress is not usually a prime risk factor in respiratory disease of young calves. When calves are moved to new pastures during the grazing season or combined with different groups, or sorted during estrous synchronization procedures, this stressor can be involved. Thus, any investigation of respiratory disease in young calves must include this potential risk factor.

ENVIRONMENTAL RISK

Environmental risk is a third risk factor.[28] The stress of heat and humidity as described by the temperature humidity index has been associated with an increase in early embryonic loss in dairy cattle.[29] Environmental risk can affect transfer of maternal immunity. Calves born in extremely harsh environmental conditions such as cold or heat have delayed time to nursing, and the stress associated with controlling homeostasis. Carstens[30] states calf mortality increases with decreases in ambient temperature or when precipitation occurs on the day of birth.

NUTRITIONAL RISK

Nutritional restriction of energy and protein in the beef cow can have profound effects on the developing fetus. Long and colleagues[31] showed that restriction of the cow resulted in a decrease in placentation area. Larson and colleagues[32] reported an increase in calf weaning weight from cows on winter range receiving adequate protein supplementation in late gestation versus cows on restricted protein diets. Late gestation protein supplementation of cows also improved carcass quality in steers born to protein-supplemented cows. These effects are analogous to the detrimental effects of nutritional restriction in gestating sows on fetal myogenesis, birth weight, and postnatal growth.[33] Odde[20] reported that body condition score (BCS) influenced time to standing for a newborn calf. Calves born to cows with BCS 4 took approximately 60 minutes to stand in contrast to calves born to cows with BCS 5, which took 43 minutes to stand. Time to standing has a direct influence on intake and absorption of colostral immune factors.

PATHOGEN RISK

The most common approach when dealing with respiratory outbreaks in suckling calves is to identify the most likely viral and/or bacterial pathogens as the cause. Although this is an important part of prevention and treatment strategies, the cause may be more symptomatic rather than a major risk factor, particularly as it applies to secondary bacterial pathogens. Most cow/calf herds are maintained in multiple pasture units on a single operation. Exposure within these units to potential pathogens is common. In many herds, pathogens such as BRSV have likely become endemic and are not likely to cause significant clinical disease in well-vaccinated herds. In herd situations with exposure to BVDV persistent infection (PI) animals in the absence of other risk factors may result in clinical disease.[34] Exposure to cattle from other operations may present a pathogen risk because naive cattle exposed to the common viral pathogens such as infectious bovine rhinotracheitis (IBR), BRSV, BVDV, and BRCV as well as the bacterial pathogen such as *Mycoplasma bovis*[35,36] may cause clinical disease in the absence of other apparent risk factors. The risk posed by these viral pathogens is readily reduced by herd vaccination programs. The use of modified live virus (MLV) vaccines greatly decreases shedding of these viruses and reduces the risk of clinical disease. The pathogen previously characterized as *Pasteurella trehalosi* and recently renamed *Bibersteinia trehalosi* has long been recognized as a cause of ovine respiratory disease in small ruminants.[37,38] Its role in acute cases of respiratory disease in young dairy and stocker calves seems to be increasing and may be influenced by the use of prophylactic antibiotics given to control other pathogens.[39] Vaccination to control bacterial pathogens gives mixed results in the field. This finding could be due to timing of vaccination, not given before pathogen exposure, lack of booster doses, and lack of attention to the primary causative risk factors.

COST OF ILLNESS

The cost of respiratory disease in nursing calves is not easily measurable, therefore some assumptions must be made. Weaning weights are generally assumed to be less with any clinical disease such as calf scours. With respiratory disease the assumption is that weaning weights are reduced by as much as 15.87 kg (35 pounds) on average.[7] This loss does not include treatment costs or time and labor associated with treatment or death loss. If the value of gain at the calf level until weaning is approximately $1.10/kg ($0.50/pound), then a loss of weaning weight of 15.87 kg (35 pounds) would be worth $17.50. If treatment costs including labor are $20/calf, and assuming no death loss, then the cost of one calf needing treatment would be $37.50. If the percentage of calves becoming ill during the suckling phase is 10%, then the cost of illness for each calf in the herd would be $3.75. When death loss occurs and is included in this calculation the cost of illness increases dramatically. If the value of each calf lost is equal to the cost of keeping a cow on an annual basis (eg, $500), then each 1% death loss increases the cost of respiratory disease for each surviving calf by $5.00/calf. Thus, if the percentage of calves needing treatment is 10% and death loss is 1%, then the total cost of respiratory disease would be $8.75 for each surviving calf. With proper herd health management, attention to common risk factors, and the use of specific vaccines most herd outbreaks of respiratory disease in suckling calves can be reduced or prevented.

MANAGEMENT OF RESPIRATORY DISEASE IN SUCKLING CALVES

Management of respiratory disease in suckling calves requires knowledge of all the risk factors contributing to the signs and symptoms of clinical disease. Signs and symptoms of respiratory disease in calves include increased respiratory rates, increased rectal temperature, a single or both ears drooped, and depression. It is difficult to distinguish the causative agents based on clinical signs. It is also likely that most cases of respiratory disease are the result of infections by multiple pathogens. For the veterinarian to manage and prevent these cases, it is necessary to logically create a list of risk factors most likely involved in the outbreak.

VACCINATION

Vaccination of young calves (30–60 days) to prevent respiratory disease has become a common management practice. Beef calves are commonly vaccinated against clostridial diseases at a young age. Although reports suggest that vaccination produces a limited antibody response in young calves,[40] this practice seems to be an effective management strategy as the prevalence of clostridial diseases such as blackleg, malignant edema, and gas gangrene become rare in vaccinated populations. The addition of viral vaccines and bacterins to prevent respiratory disease is also now commonly included. Their efficacy has come under some scrutiny as even in well-vaccinated herds cases of respiratory disease may still occur. Vaccines are given to prevent clinical disease and pathogen transmission caused by specific pathogens. IBR vaccine is given to prevent IBR. It is not possible to vaccinate against every pathogen known to cause respiratory disease. Nor do all vaccines provide equal levels of protection or efficacy. It becomes critical to prioritize vaccines given to young calves. To do this the veterinarian must have a guiding principle regarding vaccination. It is helpful to ask 3 questions:

1. Is there a substantial risk of disease caused by a specific pathogen?
2. Is there a commercial vaccine that has shown efficacy against the specific pathogen?
3. Does management of the herd allow for the proper use of the vaccine within the constraints of handling times?

If the answer is no to any of these questions, then it begs the questions, why recommend their use at all and will other risk management strategies prove to be as effective?

VACCINE INTERFERENCE

A common practice among cattle producers is to use combination vaccines, which combine several different antigens into a single injection. The advantage of this approach is to reduce the number of injections given to animals yet achieve the same level of immunity as if each antigen had been given independently. Biologics manufacturers must prove to the United States Department of Agriculture that there is no interference among individual antigens when given together in a single dose. What is not well understood is the potential for interference when different vaccines are given concurrently. As was stated earlier, it is a common practice to give MLV vaccines along with bacterins. Studies have shown that vaccine interactions may occur when giving an MLV vaccine along with bacterins.[41] Immune interaction, defined by a diminished immune response to one or more of the antigens given concurrently, was recently reported in 2 separate trials.[42] This interaction seems to be confined to animals that are naive to the antigens given.

MATERNAL IMMUNITY AND VACCINATION

What is the role of maternal immunity on vaccination of the young calf? Does the presence of maternal antibody interfere with an active immune response? Woolums and Smith[43] reviewed and described reasons for lack of protection following vaccination in young calves: age of calf at vaccination, amount of maternal antibody, type of vaccine, virulence of the pathogen challenge, and the outcome that was used to describe the success or failure of the vaccination. With BHV-1, the antibody response in the presence of antibody is negligible; however, on receiving a second dose even months later the response was greater than calves receiving their initial dose at this same time.[44] In BVDV, the literature is less clearly defined.[45–47] What is clear is that calves without maternal immunity to BVDV can respond to MLV vaccine, whereas at higher levels of maternal antibody, antibody production is blocked and cell-mediated immune (CMI) responses are primed.[48] Vaccination of young calves with BRSV has shown a CMI response in the presence of maternal antibody.[49] In a recent study intranasal vaccination with BRSV showed protection against BRSV challenge as measured by virus shedding.[50] The data indicate that young beef calves can respond to vaccination, and response as measured by antibody production is affected in the presence of maternal immunity. A population of memory cells can be generated and when either vaccination or exposure occurs, immunization has provided a degree of protection not seen in nonvaccinated animals.

POPULATION DYNAMICS

Methods to control disease in beef cattle populations have traditionally been focused on immunization to prevent clinical disease. Whereas prevention of clinical disease is a direct effect of immunization, the indirect effect of disease prevention by decreasing transmission is of primary importance with pathogens that are transmitted from animal to animal.[51]

In human medical literature, the concept of population/herd immunity has successfully been used to implement vaccination programs designed to protect populations against specific pathogens. Specifically, they include diphtheria, tetanus, and pertussis, and also measles, mumps and rubella, as well as poliomyelitis.[52] Although we are concerned about each individual being protected against disease, the greater purpose is to immunize as many as possible within the population such that susceptible individuals within a population are also protected. A greater level of population protection can be achieved by

1. Reducing the number of animals shedding disease pathogens
2. Decreasing the amount of pathogens shed by infected animals

3. Decreasing the duration of shedding
4. Increasing the infectious dose necessary to cause infection.

The percentage of immune individuals in a population to achieve herd protection varies by pathogen, but ranges from 83% to 94%.[53] This concept is the basic premise of herd vaccination programs.

In the veterinary medicine community there is some debate about the practice of annual booster vaccinations in companion animals because some boosters may no longer be necessary for clinical disease prevention because of low risk.[54] For veterinarians in food animal practice there are questions as to efficacy, duration of immunity, and number of doses needed to achieve significant population and individual animal protection.[55,56] Veterinarians are called on to make recommendations concerning vaccination protocols for multiple diverse livestock businesses. To do so they require in-depth herd knowledge regarding some assessment of risk for specific diseases, management, genetics, nutrition status, and handling facilities. For example, in beef cattle breeding herds, purchased females or bulls may be introduced into new herds without benefit of a quarantine period, biosecurity testing, or knowledge of purchased animals' herd disease status. Even when vaccination programs are specifically outlined, it is rare for buyers to seek veterinary advice as to the quality of the program.

In IBR-vaccinated animals, protective immunity is assumed regardless of type of vaccine, with MLV vaccines providing better protection.[57] Although the issue of duration of immunity and protection may be debated, the real issue is one of risk analysis and risk management. What is the risk of the herd being exposed to a field challenge with either IBR or BVDV? In most commercial operations this risk exists, but is difficult to quantify. In most purchases this approach does not have negative consequences; however, in a quality control system with responsibility for disease control, the veterinarian will likely seek to lower the risk of exposure and increase specific immunity to the pathogens considered to be of greatest risk.

In most livestock businesses the risk of exposure to common pathogens is not known. However, there is information as to the number of immune animals necessary to prevent spread of disease. By using this information the veterinarian can make informed recommendations regarding the type of vaccine, the timing of boosters, and the frequency of vaccination. The spread of disease depends on the basic reproductive rate (R_0). The basic reproduction number R_0 is the number of secondary infections resulting from one primary case in a totally susceptible population. The basic reproduction number is a feature of the infectious agent and the host population without a control measure being active.

If R_0 in a vaccinated population is larger than 1, then the vaccine cannot totally prevent the spread of infection and additional biosecurity principles must be used.[58] It has been estimated that for BHV-1 infections R_0 is approximately 7.0. After using 2 different vaccines it was estimated that R_0 was 2.4 and 1.1.[59] This finding means that within a susceptible population, 2.4 or 1.1 new cases will arise from 1 case. In this immunized population transmission cannot effectively be prevented. Within real populations these numbers must be considered within the context that as animals become infected and are contagious, the number of susceptible animals declines and the number of recovered and immune animals increases. It has been estimated that the critical proportion of immune animals is expressed by the equation critical proportion = $1 - 1/R_0$. The higher the R_0 the greater the number of animals that must be immune to prevent spread of the infectious agent. If $R_0 = 7.0$ for a specific pathogen, then the proportion of immune animals within that population must be $1 - (1/7)$. This calculation means that approximately 86% of the population must be immune to prevent transmission. Estimates for limiting the spread of BVDV within a population have been made based on mathematical models. In herds without PI animals, 57% of the animals must be immune to stop transmission. For herds with animals that are persistently infected with BVDV, 97% must be immune.[60] This issue of herd immunity to BVDV is further complicated by the amount of cross-protection afforded by commercial vaccines, as strain differences can exist between vaccine virus and wild virus.[61] A sound recommendation for vaccines can be made based only on actual challenge model and field trials using sound science and proper design.

The challenge of making sound vaccination recommendations as part of an overall herd health program is the responsibility of food animal veterinarians. Making those recommendations requires an in-depth knowledge of the risk of disease, management ability, facilities, nutritional requirements, and in breeding herds the current genetic base. In addition, veterinarians must have a working knowledge of the relative efficacy, duration of immunity, and the effect on transmission of the available commercial vaccines. With this as a working tool, the veterinarian can use the concept of population dynamics and herd immunity when making specific herd recommendations regarding the timing and frequency of vaccination administration.[62]

SUMMARY

When investigating outbreaks of respiratory disease in young calves, it is important to review all of the risk factors that could potentially contribute to the clinical disease. A list of risk factors should include

1. Failure or partial failure of passive transfer. This may be due to
   Cows in low body condition score
   Udder and teat conformation
   Genetic type, selection for moderate growth versus high performance (select for type based on resources available to the operation)
2. Genetic risk
   Dystocia
   Mothering ability
   Udder and teat conformation
2. Any type of commingling of different groups, even those belonging to the same operation
   Moving long distances to new pastures
   Combining different pasture groups together before weaning
3. Environmental risk
   Heat risk
   Cold risk
   Snow and freezing rain
4. Nutritional risk, such as a change in diet
   Creep feeding
   Lush pastures
   Drought-stressed pastures
5. Exposure to pathogens such as IBR, BVDV, BRSV, BRCV, and *Mycoplasma bovis*
   Within-herd exposure or exposure to other populations
6. Trace mineral deficiency or toxicity
   Cu, Se, Zn
   Sulfur
7. Other risk factors
   Lack of adequate quality and quantity of labor

Practitioners ultimately give advice and make recommendations based on 3 principles

1. Research
2. Experience
3. Observations by veterinary peers.

Although this approach can be less than ideal, it is evident even from the literature that not all answers to questions regarding nursing calf pneumonia can be found. Nor can all questions be answered through research. For this reason, in investigation of outbreaks of clinical disease in beef herds, the use of a well-constructed list of risk factors is essential. The list of risk factors to be ruled out should become evident and recommendations for intervention and ultimately prevention can be implemented.

REFERENCES

1. Dewell RD, Hungerford LL, Keen JE, et al. Association of neonatal serum immunoglobulin G1 concentration with health and performance in beef calves. J Am Vet Med Assoc 2006;228:914–21.
2. Dutil L, Fecteau G, Bouchard É, et al. A questionnaire on the health, management, and performance of cow-calf herds in Québec. Can Vet J 1999;40:649–56.
3. Gay E, Barnouin J. A nation-wide epidemiological study of acute bovine respiratory disease in France. Prev Vet Med 2009;89:265–71.
4. Svensson C, Hultgren J, Oltenacu PA. Morbidity in 3–7-month-old dairy calves in south-western Sweden, and risk factors for diarrhoea and respiratory disease. Prev Vet Med 2006;74:162–79.
5. Virtala AM, Gröhn YT, Mechor GD, et al. The effect of maternally derived immunoglobulin G on the risk of respiratory disease in heifers during the first 3 months of life. Prev Vet Med 1999;39:25–37.
6. Perez E, Noordhuizen JP, van Wuijkhuise LA, et al. Management factors related to calf morbidity and mortality rates. Livest Prod Sci 1990;25:79–93.
7. Wittum TE, Perrino LJ. Passive immune status at postpartum hour 24 and long-term health and performance of calves. Am J Vet Res 1995;56:1149–54.
8. Faber SN, Faber NE, McCauley TC, et al. Case study: effects of colostrum ingestion on lactational performance. The Professional Scientist 2005;21:420–5.
9. Massimini G, Britti D, Peli A, et al. Effect of passive transfer status on preweaning growth performance in dairy lambs. J Am Vet Med Assoc 2006;229:111–5.
10. Tizard IR. Veterinary immunology: an introduction. In: Tizard IR, editor. Veterinary immunology an introduction. 6th edition. Philadelphia: WB Saunders; 2000. p. 210–21.
11. Hirako T, Hisaeda K, Uumi K, et al. Serum cytokine levels evaluated in neonatal calves in relation to disease incidence up to 4 months after colostrum ingestion. Journal of Rakuno Gakuen University Natural Science 2005;29:171–5.
12. Archambault D, Morin G, Elazhary Y, et al. Immune response of pregnant heifers and cows to bovine rotavirus inoculation and passive protection to rotavirus infection in newborn calves fed colostral antibodies or colostral lymphocytes. Am J Vet Res 1988;49:1084–91.
13. Donovan DC, Reber AJ, Gabbard JD, et al. Effect of maternal cells transferred with colostrum on cellular responses to pathogen antigens in neonatal calves. Am J Vet Res 2007;68:778–82.

14. Berge AC, Besser TE, Moore DA, et al. Evaluation of the effects of oral colostrum supplementation during the first fourteen days on the health and performance of preweaned calves. J Dairy Sci 2009;92:286–95.
15. Calloway C, Tyler J, Tessman R, et al. Comparison of refractometers and test endpoints in the measurement of serum protein concentration to assess passive transfer status in calves. J Am Vet Med Assoc 2002;221:1605–8.
16. Petrie L, Acres SD, McCartney DH. The yield of colostrum and colostral gamma-globulins in beef cows and the absorption of colostral gammaglobulins by beef calves. Can Vet J 1984;25:273–9.
17. Francisco SF, Quigley JD. Serum immunoglobulin concentrations after feeding maternal colostrum or maternal colostrum plus colostral supplement to dairy calves. Am J Vet Res 1993;54:1051–4.
18. Quigley JD III, Kost CJ, Wolfe TM. Absorption of protein and IgG in calves fed a colostrum supplement or replacer. J Dairy Sci 2002;85:1243–8.
19. Besser TE, Szenci O, Gay CC. Decreased colostral immunoglobulin absorption in calves with postnatal respiratory acidosis. J Am Vet Med Assoc 1990;196: 1239–43.
20. Odde KG. Reducing neonatal calf losses through selection, nutrition and management. Large Animal Practice 1996;17:12–5.
21. Goonewardene LA, Wang Z, Price MA, et al. Effect of udder type and calving assistance on weaning traits of beef and dairy X beef calves. Livest Prod Sci 2003;81:47–56.
22. Muggli NE, Hohenboken WD, Cundiff LV, et al. Inheritance of maternal immuno-globulin G1 concentration by the bovine neonate. J Anim Sci 1984;59:39–48.
23. Tuchscherer M, Kanitz E, Otten W, et al. Effects of prenatal stress on cellular and humoral immune responses in neonatal pigs. Vet Immunol Immunopathol 2002; 86:195–203.
24. Lay JDC, Randel RD, Friend TH, et al. Effects of prenatal stress on suckling calves. J Anim Sci 1997;75:3143–51.
25. Gupta S, Earley B, Ting ST, et al. Effect of repeated regrouping and relocation on the physiological, immunological, and hematological variables and performance of steers. J Anim Sci 2005;83:1948–58.
26. Mitchell G, Clark M, Siwicky M, et al. Stress alters the cellular and proteomic compartments of bovine bronchoalveolar lavage fluid. Vet Immunol Immunopa-thol 2008;125:111–25.
27. Step DL, Krehbiel CR, DePra HA, et al. Effects of commingling beef calves from different sources and weaning protocols during a forty-two-day receiving period on performance and bovine respiratory disease. J Anim Sci 2008;86:3146–58.
28. Nienaber JA, Hahn GL. Livestock production system management responses to thermal challenges. Int J Biometeorol 2007;52:149–57.
29. Santolaria P, Lopez G, Garcia I, et al. Effects of cumulative stressful and acute variation episodes of farm climate conditions on late embryo/early fetal loss in high producing dairy cows. Int J Biometeorol 2010;54:93–8.
30. Carstens GE. Cold thermoregulation in the newborn calf. Vet Clin North Am Food Anim Pract 1994;10:69–106.
31. Long NM, Vonnahme KA, Hess BW, et al. Effects of early gestational undernutri-tion on fetal growth, organ development, and placentomal composition in the bovine. J Anim Sci 2009;87:1950–9.
32. Larson DM, Martin JL, Adams DC, et al. Winter grazing system and supplemen-tation during late gestation influence performance of beef cows and steer progeny. J Anim Sci 2009;87:1147–55.

33. Foxcroft GR, Dixon WT, Novak S, et al. The biological basis for prenatal programming of postnatal performance in pigs. J Anim Sci 2006;84:E105–12.
34. Stevens ET, Thomson DU, Loneragan GH, et al. Effects of short-term exposure of feeder cattle to calves persistently infected with bovine viral diarrhea virus. Bov Pract 2007;41:151–5.
35. Gulliksen SM, Jor E, Lie KI, et al. Respiratory infections in Norwegian dairy calves. J Dairy Sci 2009;92:5139–46.
36. Tschopp R, Bonnemain P, Nicolet J, et al. [Epidemiological study of risk factors associated with Mycoplasma bovis infections in fattening calves]. Schweiz Arch Tierheilkd 2001;143:461–7 [in German].
37. González SJM, Arcaute RMRd. Prevention of the ovine respiratory syndrome by means of vaccination. Portal Veterinaria Albeitar 2009;123:42–3.
38. Villard L, Gauthier D, Maurin F, et al. Serotypes A1 and A2 of Mannheimia haemolytica are susceptible to genotypic, capsular and phenotypic variations in contrast to T3 and T4 serotypes of *Bibersteinia (Pasteurella) trehalosi*. FEMS Microbiol Lett 2008;280:42–9.
39. Weiser GC, Miller DS, Drew ML, et al. Variation in *Pasteurella* (*Bibersteinia*) and *Mannheimia* spp following transport and antibiotic treatment in free-ranging and captive Rocky Mountain bighorn sheep *Ovis canadensis canadensis*. Journal of Zoo and Wildlife Medicine 2009;40:117–25.
40. Harcourt SJ, Buddle BM, Hamel K, et al. Influence of maternal and sire effects on antibody response following clostridial vaccination of Friesian-Jersey crossbred calves. Proc N Z Soc Anim Prod 2004;64:110–4.
41. Harland RJ, Potter AA, van Drunen-Littel-van den Hurk S, et al. The effect of subunit or modified live bovine herpesvirus-1 vaccines on the efficacy of a recombinant *Pasteurella haemolytica* vaccine for the prevention of respiratory disease in feedlot calves. Can Vet J 1992;33:734–41.
42. Seeger JT, Stokka G, Cortese V, et al. Interactions between concurrent modified-live viral and Mannheimia haemolytica vaccination. AJVR 2010, submitted for publication.
43. Woolums AR, Smith RA. Vaccinating calves: new information on the effects of maternal immunity. Stillwater (OK): American Association of Bovine Practitioners; 2007. p. 10–7.
44. Menanteau-Horta AM, Ames TR, Johnson DW, et al. Effect of maternal antibody upon vaccination with infectious bovine rhinotracheitis and bovine virus diarrhea vaccines. Can J Comp Med 1985;49:10–4.
45. Cortese VS, West KH, Hassard LE, et al. Clinical and immunologic responses of vaccinated and unvaccinated calves to infection with a virulent type-II isolate of bovine viral diarrhea virus. J Am Vet Med Assoc 1998;213:1312–9.
46. Ellis J, West K, Cortese VS, et al. Effect of maternal antibodies on induction and persistence of vaccine-induced immune responses against bovine viral diarrhea virus type II in young calves. J Am Vet Med Assoc 2001;219:351–6.
47. Ridpath JE, Neill JD, Endsley J, et al. Effect of passive immunity on the development of a protective immune response against bovine viral diarrhea virus in calves. Am J Vet Res 2003;64:65–9.
48. Platt R, Widel P, Kesl L, et al. Comparison of humoral and cellular immune responses to a pentavalent modified live virus vaccine in three age groups of calves with maternal antibodies, before and after BVDV type 2 challenge. Vaccine 2009;27:4508–19.

49. van der Sluijs MT, Kuhn E, Makoschey B. A single vaccination with an inactivated bovine respiratory syncytial virus vaccine primes the cellular immune response in calves with maternal antibody. BMC Vet Res 2002;6:2.
50. Kimman TG. The immune response to and pathogenesis of BRSV (bovine respiratory syncytial virus) infections. Vet Med 1993;88:1196–204.
51. Halloran ME, Haber M, Longini IM Jr, et al. Direct and indirect effects in vaccine efficacy and effectiveness. Am J Epidemiol 1991;133:323–31.
52. Anderson RM. The concept of herd immunity and the design of community-based immunization programmes. Vaccine 1992;10:928–35.
53. May T, Silverman R. 'Clustering of exemptions' as a collective action threat to herd immunity. Vaccine 2003;21:1048–51.
54. Horzinek M. Vaccine use and disease prevalence in dogs and cats. Vet Microbiol 2006;117:2–8.
55. Ellis J, Waldner C, Rhodes C, et al. Longevity of protective immunity to experimental bovine herpesvirus-1 infection following inoculation with a combination modified-live virus vaccine in beef calves. J Am Vet Med Assoc 2005;227:123–8.
56. Fulton R, Johnson B, Briggs R, et al. Challenge with Bovine viral diarrhea virus by exposure to persistently infected calves: protection by vaccination and negative results of antigen testing in nonvaccinated acutely infected calves. Revue canadienne de recherche vétérinaire. Can J Vet Res 2006;70:121–7.
57. Bosch JC, Kaashoek MJ, Kroese AH, et al. An attenuated bovine herpesvirus 1 marker vaccine induces a better protection than two inactivated marker vaccines. Vet Microbiol 1996;52:223–34.
58. Graat EAM, Frankena K, Noordhuizen JPTM, et al. Introduction to theoretical epidemiology. Application of quantitative methods in veterinary epidemiology. Wageningen (The Netherlands): Wageningen Pers; 1997. p. 249–69.
59. Bosch JC. Bovine herpesvirus 1 marker vaccines: tools for eradication?. Utrecht (The Netherlands): University of Utrecht; 1997.
60. Cherry BR, Reeves MJ, Smith G. Evaluation of bovine viral diarrhea virus control using a mathematical model of infection dynamics. Prev Vet Med 1998;33:91–108.
61. Thurmond MC, Goyal SM, Ridpath JT. Viral transmission. Bovine viral diarrhea virus: diagnosis management and control. Oxford (UK): Blackwell Publishing; 2005. p. 91–4.
62. Stokka GL. Population dynamics and herd immunity. 39th Annual Convention Proceedings American Association of Bovine Practitioners 2006;39:88–9.

Control, Management, and Prevention of Bovine Respiratory Disease in Dairy Calves and Cows

Patrick J. Gorden, DVM[a],*, Paul Plummer, DVM, PhD[b]

KEYWORDS

- Bovine respiratory disease • Control • Management
- Dairy calves • Dairy cows

Despite advances in veterinary medicine, animal husbandry, and animal welfare, respiratory disease among dairy calves and cows continues to be a major problem for dairy producers. Although much of the effort is concentrated on controlling bovine respiratory disease (BRD) in young calves, also known as enzootic calf pneumonia (ECP), outbreaks of respiratory disease in adult animals can have negative effects on bovine welfare and production, resulting in devastating economic outcomes for dairy owners.

The United States Department of Agriculture National Animal Health Monitoring Service (NAHMS) has examined the incidence of respiratory disease in calves for more than 20 years (**Table 1**).[1] When evaluating respiratory disease statistics among dairy cattle, it becomes apparent that incidence of respiratory disease has not changed much since the early 1990s. Pre-weaned calf mortality has essentially been unchanged, ranging from a low of 7.8% in 2006 to 10.8% in 1996. The percentage of deaths attributed to respiratory disease in pre-weaned calves has also remained essentially unchanged during the same time period. A similar trend for mortality rate (range of 1.8%–2.2%) has been seen in weaned calves. There has been a substantial increase in the percentage of deaths credited to respiratory disease in weaned calves (34.8% to 46.5%).[1] In a separate study, Sivula and colleagues[2] reported a 7.6% morbidity rate and a 2.3% mortality rate from respiratory disease among calves between birth and 16 weeks of age. The attack rate of respiratory

[a] Food Supply Veterinary Medicine, Veterinary Diagnostic and Production Animal Medicine Department, Iowa State University College of Veterinary Medicine, 2432 Lloyd Veterinary Medical Center, 1600 South, 16th Street, Ames, IA 50011, USA
[b] Food Supply Veterinary Medicine, Veterinary Diagnostic and Production Animal Medicine Department, Iowa State University College of Veterinary Medicine, 2426 Lloyd Veterinary Medical Center, 1600 South, 16th Street, Ames, IA 50011, USA
* Corresponding author.
E-mail address: pgorden@iastate.edu

Vet Clin Food Anim 26 (2010) 243–259
doi:10.1016/j.cvfa.2010.03.004
0749-0720/10/$ – see front matter © 2010 Elsevier Inc. All rights reserved.

Table 1 Changes in respiratory disease incidence 1991 to 2007				
	1991	1996	2002	2007
Pre-weaned calf mortality	8.4	10.8	10.5	7.8
Percentage of deaths caused by respiratory disease pre-weaned calves	21.3	24.5	21.3	22.5
Weaned calf mortality	2.2	2.4	2.8	1.8
Percentage of deaths caused by respiratory disease–weaned calves	34.8	44.8	50%	46.5

Data from USDA. Dairy 2007, Part V: Changes in dairy cattle health and management practices in the United States, 1996–2007. Fort Collins (CO): USDA: APHIS:VS, CEAH; 2009 #519.0709.

disease development in Minnesota dairy calves was 0.1 cases per 100 calf days during the same age range.

The costs associated with respiratory disease include prevention, treatment, and lost productivity. Several researchers have attempted to use available NAHMS data from their state to calculate a local cost of respiratory disease and respiratory disease prevention for specific management groups. For unweaned calves, estimates range from $9.84 to $16.35 per calf whereas weaned calf estimates range from $2.05 to $2.22 per calf.[3,4] Respiratory disease in the early stages of the calf's life can have significant effects on subsequent productivity and survivability, thus adding to these costs. A diagnosis of pneumonia during the first 6 months of life resulted in slower growth rates later in life[5] and decreased productivity.[2,6] Heifers followed through first calving that were diagnosed with respiratory disease as young calves were 2 or more times more likely to die before calving[7,8] and calve at an older age when compared with heifers that did not develop respiratory disease before 90 days of age.[8]

Diagnosis of pneumonia in adult dairy cattle is not as common as diseases such as mastitis, lameness, metabolic disease, and reproductive disorders. Annually, 3.3% of dairy cows develop owner-reported pneumonia and those pneumonia cases account for 11.3% of cow deaths.[9] Losses and prevention costs were estimated at $4.31 per cow in Michigan herds to $9.08 per cow in Ohio herds.[3,10] The Ohio study reported an estimated annual prevalence per 100 cow-years for pneumonia of 19% among adult dairy cattle.[10]

The lack of progress in controlling respiratory disease demonstrates that there continues to be significant room for improvement in controlling this multifactorial syndrome, and that dairy producers need assistance in applying evolving husbandry practices to improve dairy cattle health.

This article focuses on biosecurity programs to prevent respiratory disease in dairy calves and cows. Effective disease identification and treatment strategies are addressed.

PREVENTION OF RESPIRATORY DISEASE IN DAIRY CALVES

Prevention practices associated with respiratory disease control in calves include the development and maintenance of a robust immune system through delivery of adequate good-quality colostrum, sound nutrition, proper vaccination, biosecurity, and provision of adequate ventilation.

Minimizing Failure of Passive Transfer

The newborn calf is born with a naïve but functional immune system. Immune protection is dependent on consumption of preformed antibody. Failure of passive transfer (FPT) is a major factor in the development and severity of respiratory disease in calves.[5,11–17] Despite the significant effort placed on colostrum delivery to newborn calves, NAHMS Dairy 2007 determined that nearly 1 in 5 (19.2%) newborn heifer calves had FPT.[18] As part of complete program for respiratory disease control, practitioners must continually focus on colostrum management and monitor the incidence of FPT.

Associated with FPT are the environments that the calves are placed into, as these can have significant impacts on pneumonia as well. Assuring maternity pens are kept clean and dry and that calves are moved from maternity pens immediately after birth are important aspects of newborn care. Delivery of calves into a heavily contaminated maternity pen and leaving newborn calves in the maternity pen increases the risk that calves are orally exposed to bacterial pathogens.[19] Incidental consumption of environmental bacteria by the newborn calf is a risk factor for the development of enteric disease, and limits colostrum immunoglobulin absorption across the gut wall.[20,21]

Colostrum Collection and Storage

Colostrum must be collected, processed, and stored in a manner that limits bacterial contamination and minimizes bacterial incubation. Bacteria counts in colostrum can be assessed by performing a total plate count (TPC) and coliform counts. The goal is to have the TPC less than 1 million colony-forming units (CFU)/mL and the coliform count less than 10,000 CFU/mL.[22] Several methods have been used to reduce bacteria counts in colostrum while still maintaining adequate passive transfer, including pasteurization and acidification of colostrum using formic acid.[23–25] It should be noted that use of pasteurization and formic acid to control *Mycobacterium avium* subsp *paratuberculosis* (MAP) remains controversial and may not be appropriate for herds attempting to control Johnes disease.[23–28] Until further research is completed to more thoroughly characterize the importance of low numbers of MAP in treated colostrum samples, producers who are actively attempting to control or eradicate Johnes disease may wish to consider the use a colostrum replacement. For a more thorough discussion of colostrum replacers, readers are referred to an earlier issue of *Veterinary Clinics of North America*.[23]

Colostrum Delivery

An adequate volume of high-quality colostrum must be fed in a timely manner. Colostrum should contain at least 50 g IgG/L.[21] For typical Holstein calves (~85–90 lbs [38.5–40 kg]), 4 quarts (3.78 L) of colostrum should be fed as soon as possible after birth, preferably within 1 to 2 hours of birth.[29] Smaller calves such as Jerseys should be limited to 3 quarts (2.83 L) delivered in the same time frame. Colostrum delivered by a nurse bottle or esophageal feeder will result in adequate passive transfer[30–32] and provides assurance that the calf has consumed an adequate volume.

Navel Dipping

Navel dipping can play an important role in controlling diseases in newborn calves. Proper disinfection of navels has been shown to reduce calf mortality by half and reduce the percentage of calves treated for respiratory disease from nearly 19% in the nondisinfected group to 5% in the disinfected group (Donald Sockett, DVM, presentation notes, Land O Lakes, Webster City, IA, January 2010). To properly perform naval disinfection, spraying of navels should be avoided, as this procedure does not provide adequate disinfection of the interior portion of the umbilical cord (Donald Sockett, DVM, presentation notes, Land O Lakes, Webster City, IA, January 2010). Dipping of the navel into a clean vessel containing fresh disinfectant provides better coverage of both the internal and external surface of the umbilicus.

Nutrition and Immune System Function

Adequate nutrition is essential for rapid growth and development of the young calf. Unfortunately, the definition of adequate has been somewhat blurred in the past in order to minimize the cost of milk-feeding programs. The immune system's nutrient consumption increases dramatically when responding to microbial challenges. Rates of gluconeogenesis increase 150% to 200% during moderate infections, and the basal metabolic rate has been shown to increase 25% to 55% during periods of sepsis in the human. Sepsis in laboratory rodents has resulted in a loss of approximately 40% of total body protein and reduction in rates of protein synthesis.[33] If nutrient intake is not optimal, calf growth and immune system functionality will be negatively affected.

Recent research has shown the potential growth ability of young calves and has demonstrated the importance of adequate nutrient intake on the function of the immune system. Godden and colleagues[34] compared the feeding of waste milk and milk replacer (MR), and demonstrated a reduction in respiratory disease mortality by feeding an equal volume of pasteurized waste milk compared with 0.45 kg of a 20% protein, 20% fat (20:20) MR per day. This finding should not be taken as endorsement of whole milk or pasteurized waste milk as the only liquid sources of increased energy and protein. There are several MR formulations on the market that will provide increased energy and protein compared with a 20:20 MR.

The effect of cold stress (4.7°C and 68.2% humidity) during the milk-feeding period has also been shown to increase respiratory disease scores and antibiotic treatments compared with calves not experiencing cold stress (15.5°C and 59% humidity).[35] Although further research is needed to fully understand the relationship between nutrient consumption and immune function, nutrition programs should be designed to maximize lean muscle gain and skeletal growth in order to fully support immune function and minimize respiratory disease.

Feeding Waste Milk

Feeding of waste milk increases growth rates of calves compared with the same volume of 20:20 MR.[34] However, feeding raw waste milk is a risk factor for *Mycobacterium bovis* colonization of the pharynx.[36] Pasteurization of waste milk has been shown to effectively reduce pathogenic bacteria associated with respiratory disease[37,38] but like colostrum, pasteurization remains controversial for the control of MAP.[27,34] Producers who are trying to control Johnes disease should avoid feeding waste milk until research is available that more completely characterizes the importance of low numbers of MAP in heat-treated milk.

Farms that use pasteurization of waste milk should monitor the effectiveness of the pasteurization process by using time- and temperature-monitoring equipment to assure a thorough process. In addition, TPC and coliform counts can be performed on pre- and post-pasteurization samples to assure adequate reduction in bacterial numbers. If pasteurized waste milk is not going to be fed immediately, particular attention needs to be paid to rapid and complete cooling followed by proper storage, because bacterial numbers can rapidly increase in warm milk.

Housing and Ventilation

Risk factors associated with housing calves and an increased incidence of respiratory disease include contact with or shared air space with older animals, relative humidity levels greater than 75%, poor air quality, increased stocking density, bedding type, bedding density, and power washing of calf facilities while calves are still present in the immediate area.[39,40] Housing management should be designed or modified to minimize risk factors associated with respiratory disease development.

The individual calf hutch placed in an outdoor environment often provides the best environment for the prevention of respiratory and other diseases of calves.[36,39,41] Calf hutches should be situated to minimize weather effects and should not be placed in proximity to other objects that can contaminate the calf's environment, such as building exhaust fan vents or runoff from neighboring animal lots. Hutches should be placed at least 4 feet (1.22 m) apart and thoroughly sanitized between uses. Ideally, hutches should be moved between groups to minimize bacterial contamination of the surface beneath the hutch.[36] Feeding and management practices should be organized to assure that animal contact moves sequentially from younger to older calves. Personnel who have been working with older animals should thoroughly disinfect clothing and hands before proceeding back into areas that house younger animals.

Ventilation of Unweaned Calf Barns

In an effort to improve worker comfort and reduce cold stress on animals, there has been an increase in the use of barns to house calves, especially on operations in the northern United States. Unfortunately, many of these barns have been designed to maximize calf numbers, resulting in space available per calf well below current recommendations of 2.2 to 3 m^2.[42] Ventilation systems are often designed with minimal regard for or understanding of the microenvironments created by individual housing of calves.[40] Investigations of risk factors for development of respiratory disease have demonstrated that there is often an association between increased bacteria counts in the air in the calf's microenvironment and increased incidence of respiratory disease.[40,43-46] Traditional tools used for evaluation of air quality, such as air meters to sense ammonia levels or manometers, have been found to be of little value in assessing risk for the development of respiratory disease.[40] Association between high bacteria counts in the air and the development of respiratory disease do not prove a causal relationship. In studies that have identified bacteria found in air it was determined that the majority of airborne bacteria are nonpathogenic, but even dead airborne bacteria can provide a burden on respiratory tract defenses that would make lung tissues more susceptible to infections.[47] Human work environments with high levels of nonpathogenic bacteria have been associated with a higher risk of the development of respiratory disease.[48]

Risk factors for increased bacteria counts in the air include high ambient temperatures, the use of solid-pen dividers and solid ends on calf pens, the use of bedding materials that provide a higher nesting score allowing calves to nest down into the bedding material to conserve heat (ie, straw), and smaller pen sizes per calf (<3 m^2). Humidity and ammonia levels were not found to have an effect on bacteria concentration in the air. Factors that were shown to decrease the prevalence of respiratory disease in calves include:

- Decreasing age of the individual calf
- Lower airborne bacteria counts
- Presence of solid dividers between calves
- Increased nesting score.[40]

The previous sentence is contradictory to an earlier sentence concerning risk factors of increased bacteria counts. Despite the fact that solid dividers and increased nesting score increased airborne bacteria counts, these factors are still protective as they reduce nose-to-nose contact and help the calf conserve energy.

Barns that are designed to house unweaned calves in individual hutches should be planned to provide the calf with at least 2.2 to 3 m^2 of total area per calf,[36,40,42] have solid dividers between calves, but maintain an open front and rear of the area where possible. Hutches should be bedded with material that allows the calf to adequately nest during periods of cold stress.[40,49] Addition of a positive pressure ventilation system that provides approximately 15 cubic feet per minute (CFM; 1 CFM = 0.028 m^3/min) of additional air per calf may help improve air quality enough to provide disease control similar to calf hutches and provide a comfortable work environment for workers.[49]

Ventilation of Group-Housed Calves

Although not commonplace in the United States, group housing of unweaned calves is becoming more prevalent, especially with the increased awareness of animal welfare and with computer milk-feeding stations being more readily available. Previous work has associated the use of computer milk feeders with an increased incidence of respiratory disease, although the role of stocking density was not evaluated in those trials.[50] More recent work has suggested that housing computer-fed calves in groups of 10 or less results in improved growth and less morbidity associated with respiratory disease.[51] These findings agree with others that have suggested limiting group size in both unweaned and weaned calves to groups of less than 7 results in the best overall welfare for the calves.[52] Further research is needed to determine whether this apparent group size effect is related to better social welfare of the calves in smaller groups or an effect of stocking density as a factor of barn volume. Stocking rate in a given volume of area is an important variable in total airborne pathogen load,[53,54] with a lower stocking rate reducing respiratory morbidity[6] (Thomas Earlywine, PhD, presentation notes, Land O Lakes, Webster City, IA, January 2010). Ventilation requirements do not have a linear relationship with stocking density. A twofold increase in stocking density requires nearly a tenfold increase in ventilation capacity to maintain pathogenic bacteria levels at similar concentrations.[54] This layout proves to be especially problematic in calf barns that are designed to be naturally ventilated or ventilated by negative pressure. These types of barns may not provide adequate ventilation at the level of the calf's environment. Positive pressure ventilation systems similar to those described in the previous section may be necessary to adequately ventilate buildings housing groups of unweaned and weaned calves.[49] Calves housed in buildings should have 2.3 to 2.8 m^2 or more of space available per calf.[42]

As calves age, positive pressure ventilation systems may become unnecessary as long as the ventilation system can provide even airflow throughout the building, and provide 4 air turns per hour in the winter and a minimum of 30 air turns per hour in the summer.[36,55]

Minimizing Weaning Stress

The process of weaning calves from milk and moving them into group housing is a very stressful period and often results in outbreaks of respiratory disease.[36,52,56,57] Weaning age is variable between calf raisers. Average weaning age in the United States is 8.2 weeks, with the majority of calves being weaned between 6 and 8 weeks of age.[18] There are various recommendations for determining when a calf is ready to be weaned, with most sources suggesting the calf is ready when consuming 1.5 to 2.5

lbs (680–1134 g) of calf starter per day for at least 2 to 3 consecutive days.[18,56] Using this benchmark will require that feed intake is monitored in calves approaching the intended weaning age.

There has been little work published on the best method to wean calves to minimize stress and associated respiratory disease. Some sources recommended not to move calves into group pens at the same time they are weaned but to give them 1 to 2 weeks in the individual pen after weaning to adjust fully to starter consumption.[57] A Minnesota trial saw no difference in growth rate between grouping calves immediately versus leaving calves in individual pens.[58] In contrast, an Italian trial reported that weaning calves at 49 days and immediately moving the calves to group housing resulted in higher growth rates and reduced respiratory treatments by one-half compared with weaning the calves and leaving them in individual hutches for 1 week.[56] In a separate trial, calves that were grouped at 49 days and fed MR 1 time per day for 1 week had a reduced incidence of respiratory disease compared with calves that were weaned at 49 days and then left in individual housing for 1 week (respective respiratory incidence = 20% vs 34%).[56] When calves are moved into group pens, it is important to allow them adequate space per calf, plenty of fresh air, and ready access to feed and water.[57]

An additional consideration when weaning calves should be to screen calves for signs of sickness. Calves that are clinically sick will be shedding large numbers of pathogenic organisms into the environment and are likely an important reservoir for introduction of disease to other calves.[36] Application of a screening method to consistently evaluate calves for sickness prior to weaning will reduce the number of calves that are inadvertently weaned with active respiratory disease.[59]

Metaphylaxis at Weaning

In beef feedlot production, the use of metaphylaxis at the time of movement to the feedlot has been successfully used to reduce the incidence of BRD.[11] Little work has been done regarding metaphylaxis in dairy calves until recently. Calves treated at weaning with a full dose of tulathromycin (Draxxin) were 50% less likely to develop BRD than calves administered approximately two-thirds the label dose of sustained-release oxytetracycline (Biomycin 200).[60] Veterinarians and producers should carefully evaluate the effectiveness of this practice, as it may lead to increased antimicrobial resistance. There were no negative controls in the study. For more information about metaphylaxis in cattle, see the article by Nickell and White elsewhere in this issue for further exploration of this topic.

Vaccine Programs in Young Calves

Effective vaccine programs for young dairy calves are difficult to develop because of the complex nature of the immature immune system of calves and the complexities of management systems in which the calves live. When developing vaccine programs, a risk assessment should be completed to determine the need for certain vaccines based on pathogen risks and breaks in immunity, such as FPT. The newborn calf has a functional immune system that is able to respond to antigens, provided maternal antibody is not present. Many of the native defense mechanisms have decreased activity in the first weeks to months of life.[61] If calves are at high risk for the development of disease due to high incidence of FPT in the herd, vaccination in the first month of life to develop antibody protection may be warranted.

One method for overcoming maternal antibody is to use vaccines administered at the mucosal surface, that is, intranasal (IN) vaccines. IN vaccines will result in the development of immune proteins (primarily IgA) on the mucosal surface where potential pathogens will be invading. This antibody will neutralize infectious agents at the mucosal surface; thus preventing infection rather than just reducing severity of disease as is expected with parenteral vaccine administration. IN vaccine will also induce interferon release at the mucosal surface, which will provide a nonspecific antiviral environment and may stimulate maturation of the immune system.[61]

There is some consensus amongst calf consultants that the use of modified live vaccines in the first months of life will benefit the calf through the development of cell-mediated immunity; however, there is very little evidence to support this practice.[61] In these programs, calves are vaccinated several times during the first months of life, sometimes at intervals as close as 1 week. Extrapolating from research from other species, overvaccinating calves may lead to negative outcomes such as immunologic tolerance or autoimmunity.[61] A small body of evidence exists to support this immunologic response, but much more research is needed in this area to explore this practice.[62]

Vaccination programs should be designed to address the continuous-flow nature of most dairy operations as compared with seasonal vaccination patterns used in beef operations. It may be important to incorporate vaccines into breeding-age heifers prior to pregnancy if vaccines are not approved for pregnant animals. In addition, modified live infectious bovine rhinotracheitis (IBR) vaccines can cause necrosis of the corpus luteum, so IBR vaccines should not be administered close to breeding season in IBR-naïve animals.[63]

Immunology and vaccinology are rapidly developing fields of veterinary medicine, which should help answer some of the essential questions veterinarians have regarding development of effective vaccination programs for dairy calves. Readers are referred to the article by Ackermann and colleagues elsewhere in this issue for further exploration of this topic.

Quarantine Procedures for New Arrivals and Sick Animals

Off-site heifer raising and purchasing herd replacements represents a significant risk for the introduction of disease to the resident herd. At present, 9.3% of all dairy herds, representing 11.5% of heifers raised in the United States, are raised off-site. When heifers are raised off-site, approximately 63% of those heifers are comingled with cattle from other farms.[9] Approximately 39% of dairy operations brought some outside animals onto their farm during the previous year, including heifers raised off-site. On those operations, just over 20% of the farms quarantined animals from the resident population on arrival.[9] Incorporating quarantine facilities into dairy farm design plans is often overlooked even though it could provide insurance against disease proliferation. A written quarantine plan should be established that addresses caretaker and animal movement plans; and protocols for feeding, vaccination, disease testing, and facility disinfection to minimize the spread of disease between newly-arriving groups and the resident herd. If the dairy is purchasing lactating dairy cows, plans for milking cows in an isolated facility will also need to be made. Ideally, animals should be quarantined for a minimum of 14 to 21 days.[36]

Introduction of bovine viral diarrhea (BVD) into a dairy herd is often through a new heifer entering the herd, either home-raised or purchased.[41] Control of BVD outbreaks has been fairly well achieved through vaccination and other control programs. Persistently infected (PI) animals are an important reservoir of disease transmission.[36,64,65] As part of a complete biosecurity program for the prevention of respiratory disease, all new and returning herd arrivals should be tested by an appropriate screening test for the presence of virus in the submitted tissue as part of the quarantine process. In addition, in herds purchasing pregnant animals and herds trying to achieve BVD-negative status, calves should be tested at birth. For more information about BVD control programs, readers should consult the article by Julia Ridpath elsewhere in this issue for further exploration of this topic.[66]

Housing of sick animals in a location away from healthy animals is an essential method for the control of disease spread on dairy farms. Animals that are clinically sick will be shedding large numbers of pathogenic organisms into the environment and are likely an important reservoir for introduction of disease to other animals,[36] especially immunocompromised animals such as young calves and peri-parturient cows. When selecting a site for the hospital facility, care must be taken to minimize contact with healthy animals and assure that the predominant airflow does not move toward clinically normal animals.

CONTROL AND MANAGEMENT OF RESPIRATORY DISEASE OUTBREAKS IN DAIRY CALVES

Veterinarians are not usually asked to evaluate individual sick calves unless there has been a history of respiratory disease in the past or there currently is an outbreak in which several calves are affected. To completely evaluate the disease process, a complete examination including collection of a thorough history should be completed, even if examining only one calf. Collection of history should facilitate the development of a list of all calf-rearing practices that could potentially have a negative impact on calf health. All responses should be validated with physical examinations, record analysis, and facilities evaluation, if possible. Record analysis can be used to determine previous morbidity and mortality rates and to assess whether there are patterns associated with certain seasons of the year or stocking rates. To complete the workup, the nutritional program, vaccination schedules, and treatment protocols should be examined. The calf caretakers' abilities to detect cases of respiratory disease should also be assessed.

Physical examinations should be performed on as many clinically-affected animals as are available to determine the range of clinical signs and to validate the true presence of respiratory disease. Many dairy producers do not recognize early signs of respiratory disease. Dairymens' diagnoses of pneumonia have been reported to have a sensitivity of 56% and a specificity of 100%.[2] Use of a screening system, such as the Calf Respiratory Scoring Chart, developed by veterinarians at the University of Wisconsin (UW) School of Veterinary Medicine (http://www.vetmed.wisc.edu/dms/fapm/fapmtools/calves.htm), can provide a more objective evaluation of clinical signs and provide a guideline for disease treatment. This screening system evaluates rectal temperature, nasal discharge, cough and ocular discharge, and ear position to assign an individual respiratory severity score for each calf. Validation of the screening system has been completed based on bronchoalveolar lavage (BAL) fluid cytology and culture. Calves that have a composite score of more than 4 are considered to have respiratory disease and should be treated accordingly.[59] Application of the UW screening system across all ages of available animals allows for the determination of age of onset of the respiratory problems, encouraging the calf caretaker to initiate therapy earlier in the course of the disease. The screening system can also be used to determine which calves need therapy, monitor treatment efficacy, and evaluate calf caretakers' ability to diagnose and treat calves. If used correctly, greater than 85% of calves that need to be treated should be correctly identified by calf caretakers.[59]

Selection of Therapeutic Agents

Selection of a therapeutic agent should be based on isolated or suspected etiologic agents based on previous experience with the herd. The most common bacterial agents associated with ECP include *Pasteurella multocida, Mannheimia haemolytica, Histophilus somni,* and various *Mycoplasma* species.[2,17,36,39,65,67] Bovine respiratory syncytial virus (BRSV) and bovine coronavirus have been incriminated as primary agents in outbreaks of ECP.[17,39,65,67] Respiratory viruses (IBR, BVD, PI3, and BRSV) invade the upper respiratory tract tissues, resulting in the development of rhinitis, tracheitis, and/or bronchitis; this sometimes leads to the development of secondary bacterial invasion of the lower respiratory tract and the subsequent development of pneumonia.[41] However, there are many cases of ECP in which no virus pathogens are isolated from affected animals,[2,65] suggesting that viruses are not always involved in the development of ECP or that sampling occurs after optimal ability to detect virus.[2]

Diagnostic Methods to Assist Treatment Decisions

Necropsy can be an important diagnostic tool, but too often the wrong calves are selected to provide accurate diagnostic and therapeutic information. Performing necropsies on animals that are chronic poor doers or animals that would be classified as treatment failures should be avoided. Necropsies on such animals may result in the isolation of resistant strains of bacteria that may not truly represent the bacterial ecology of the initial pathogens. A more appropriate approach to using necropsy examinations would be to sacrifice acutely-affected animals. However, this should not be construed as a suggestion that necropsy examinations should not be completed if acutely-affected animals are not available for necropsy. Results of these examinations can provide critical information to determine deficiencies in management, such as nutritional insufficiency, and can be an important tool in client education. Necropsy examinations are essential for the diagnosis of aspiration pneumonia, which may be common in herds that are incorrectly using esophageal feeders to deliver colostrum, milk, or oral electrolytes.

Alternative methods to isolate the agents responsible for acute cases of ECP would be to use deep pharyngeal swabs, transtracheal wash (TTW), or BAL. Six acutely-affected animals should be selected for sampling based on physical examinations or the use of another screening method, such as the UW Calf Respiratory Scoring Chart.

Deep pharyngeal swabs can be done rapidly and are less invasive than TTW or BAL. Two or three individual swabs should be collected from each calf as described by McGuirk.[59] The number of swabs that should be collected per calf depends on type of diagnostic tests that will be performed; bacterial culture and sensitivity, mycoplasma culture, or viral detection. Presence of bacterial pathogens in high numbers, significant viral agents, or 2 or more swabs from the group of 6 testing positive for *Mycoplasma* spp is considered significant and can be used to direct treatment and management decisions. Comparative analysis between nasopharyngeal swabs and postmortem lung lavage has been used to validate the use of nasopharyngeal swabs in this manner. Positive predictive value for *M haemolytica* and *M bovis* was determined to be 100%. The negative predictive values were determined to be 67% and 33% for *M hemolytica* and *M bovis*, respectively. Genotypic analysis of matched isolates from nasopharyngeal swabs and lung lavage shows high degrees of similarity, demonstrating that the presence of bacteria on nasopharyngeal swabs is highly representative of lung etiology.[68] These results were obtained on clinical animals selected as described, and similar results would likely not be seen without appropriate case selection.

BAL or TTW can also be used to collect samples for culture, sensitivity, and viral detection, and can provide samples for cytologic evaluation of respiratory secretions.

Bacterial isolation of a homogeneous bacterial growth in excess of 10^6 CFU/mL or a positive *M bovis* culture is considered significant. Determination of leukocyte population by cytologic evaluation showing a decreased proportion of macrophages (<61%) or increased proportion of neutrophils (>39%) is considered indicative of an inflammatory response in the lung, even with a negative culture result.[59]

RESPIRATORY DISEASE IN ADULT DAIRY CATTLE

Despite the vast amount of literature concerning BRD in the dairy calf, there is nearly a complete paucity of information concerning adult dairy cattle. Incidence of pneumonia in the adult dairy animal is relatively low (3.3%)[9] but the proportional contribution to overall mortality on the dairy farm is 11.3%, indicating that response to therapy is relatively low. This lack of response may be caused by failure to recognize clinical disease early, or that these cases represent recrudescence of latent cases of ECP.

The concepts of control and prevention are very similar to the calf, but there are notable aspects that differ. Similarities include the maintenance of a functional immune system through delivery of sound nutrition, proper vaccination and minimal stress; biosecurity; and provision of adequate ventilation. The most notable difference between the 2 groups is the increased metabolic demand placed on the dairy cow through lactation.

Immune stress associated with parturition and lactation plays an important role in disease development.[69] Lymphocyte and neutrophil function decrease around the time of parturition[70,71] even though neutrophil numbers in the systemic circulation are increased.[69] The proportion of T lymphocytes is also altered, resulting in higher expression of T-suppressor cells around the time of calving and slower clearance of altered cells.[72,73] Stress introduced by negative energy balance and diseases such as ketosis[74–77] and hypocalcemia[72,78] make cows more susceptible to new and more severe infections during early lactation, including respiratory disease. Conditions that negatively affect dry matter intake and nutrient absorption, such as heat stress, subacute respiratory acidosis (SARA), and the inadvertent inclusion of mycotoxins in the diet may result in altered immune function and increased susceptibility to respiratory disease.[79–82] SARA can also have a direct effect on respiratory disease via caudal vena caval syndrome.[81]

Etiologic Agents and Diagnostic Procedures

The etiologic agents in the adult animal are similar to those mentioned for calves except that *M haemolytica* plays a more significant role in adult animals.[36,39] Herd workup procedures and diagnostic testing methods are also similar to those for the calf. Clinicians should pay particular attention to attempting to collect samples from acutely-affected animals in order to return results that are clinically relevant.[39,83] Clinicians should also assess overall herd health by doing a complete farm assessment to assure that conditions such as excessive negative energy and protein balance, ketosis, hypocalcemia, or SARA are not contributing to an increased incidence of respiratory disease.

Preventative Practices for Adult Dairy Cattle

Prevention practices associated with respiratory disease control in adult dairy cattle include immune system maintenance through sound nutrition, proper vaccination, and minimizing stress; biosecurity; and provision of adequate ventilation. Biosecurity practices for adult animals are similar to those in dairy calves. Readers should refer to the section on biosecurity earlier in this article for more discussion on the topic.

Maintenance of the Immune System

As discussed earlier, immune suppression is a major complication for disease prevention in adult dairy cattle. In addition to nutrition and management practices to minimize the effects of negative energy and protein balance as well as mineral insufficiency, husbandry practices must be maintained to maximize cow comfort and minimize stress. Such practices include prevention of overcrowding, minimizing pen moves, and averting social stress by incorporating management practices such as housing first-lactation cows separately from older cows. Discussion of nutritional and management practices that support a strong immune system and reduce stress are beyond the scope of this article. Readers should consult the article by Ackermann and colleagues elsewhere in this issue for further exploartion of this topic.

When designing vaccine programs for adult animals, a risk assessment of each individual dairy operation should be completed to determine the need for certain vaccines. These decisions should be based on pathogen risks and potential breaks in immunity, such as immune suppression associated with the periparturient period. To avoid immune suppression in the post-parturient period, it would be prudent to avoid administration of vaccines for at least 3 to 4 weeks after calving.[63] Consideration must be given to the need for transfer of colostral antibodies against disease threats of importance for the dairy. Vaccines should be administered at least 2 to 4 weeks before the expected calving date to avoid immune suppression,[70,71,77] thus providing sufficient time for immunoglobulin transfer to the colostrum to provide for adequate passive transfer.[23]

Ventilation

Ventilation systems need to be designed to limit the buildup of microbial agents, dust particles, noxious gases, heat, and humidity. Adult dairy cattle are minimally affected by cold stress caused by typical winter temperatures seen in the northern United States.[36] Barns may be underventilated during winter months to prevent freezing of water and manure systems, resulting in an increased incidence of respiratory disease. Ventilation systems should provide 36 CFM per 1000 lbs (454 kg) of body weight in cold weather and 335 CFM per 1000 lbs of body weight during hot weather.[84] An alternative method to assess ventilation function would be to determine the number of air exchanges per hour. During cold weather, 4 air exchanges must occur per hour whereas a minimum of 30 air exchanges per hour are needed during summer months.[36,55] Supplemental cooling will be necessary to minimize the effects of heat stress when the temperature heat index exceeds 72.[80,85]

SUMMARY

Incidence rates for BRD in dairy cattle have remained essentially unchanged over the last 20 years. Dairy calves are more commonly affected than adult animals, with BRD being the principal cause of death in weaned dairy calves. The lack of progress in controlling respiratory disease demonstrates that there continues to be significant room for improvement in controlling this multifactorial syndrome, and that dairy producers need assistance in applying evolving husbandry practices to improve the health of dairy cattle. Calf management programs that focus on the development of a robust immune system through adequate passive transfer, adequate energy and protein supply, sound biosecurity practices, and vaccination programs have helped alleviate problems on some herds. There is minimal information regarding control of respiratory problems in adult dairy cattle. Therefore, it seems prudent to focus the management strategies on preventing disease through sound management of the transition period, along with sound vaccination and biosecurity programs.

ACKNOWLEDGMENTS

The authors would like to thank Drs Reneé Dewell and Leo Timms for their technical assistance in preparing the manuscript.

REFERENCES

1. USDA. Dairy 2007, Part V: changes in dairy cattle health and management practices in the United States, 1996–2007. Fort Collins (CO): USDA: APHIS:VS, CEAH; 2009 # 519.0709.
2. Sivula NJ, Ames TR, Marsh WE, et al. Descriptive epidemiology of morbidity and mortality in Minnesota dairy heifer calves. Prev Vet Med 1996;27:155–71.
3. Kaneene JB, Hurd S. The national animal health monitoring system in Michigan. III. Cost estimates of selected dairy cattle diseases. Prev Vet Med 1990;8:127–40.
4. Sischo WM, Hird DW, Gardner LA, et al. Economics of disease occurrence and prevention on California dairy farms: a report and evaluation of data collected for the National Animal Health Monitoring System, 1986–1987. Prev Vet Med 1990;8:141–56.
5. Donovan GA, Dohoo IR, Montgomery DM, et al. Calf and disease factors affecting growth in female Holstein calves in Florida, USA. Prev Vet Med 1998; 33:1–10.
6. Bach A, Ahedo J, Kertz A. Using growth monitoring in heifer management and research [abstract]. J Dairy Sci 2008;91(E-Suppl 1):602.
7. Waltner-Toews D, Martin SW, Meek AH. The effect to early calfhood disease on survivorship and age at first calving. Can J Vet Res 1986;50:314–7.
8. Correa MT, Curtis CR, Erb HN, et al. Effect of calfhood morbidity on age at first calving in New York Holstein herd. Prev Vet Med 1988;6:253–62.
9. USDA. Dairy 2007, Part I: reference of dairy cattle health and management practices in the United States, 2007 Fort Collins (CO): USDA-APHIS-VS, CEAH; 2007 #N480.1007.
10. Miller GY, Dorn CR. Costs of dairy cattle diseases to producers in Ohio. Prev Vet Med 1990;8:171–82.
11. Van Donkersgoed J, Ribble C, Boyer LG, et al. Epidemiological study of enzootic pneumonia in dairy calves in Saskatchewan. Can J Vet Res 1993;57:247–54.
12. Blom JY. The relationship between serum immunoglobulin values and incidence of respiratory disease and enteritis in calves. Nord Vet Med 1982;34:276–84.
13. Thomas LH, Swann RG. Influence of colostrum on the incidence of calf pneumonia. Vet Rec 1973;92:454–5.
14. Williams MR, Spooner RL, Thomas LH. Quantitative studies on bovine immunoglobulins. Vet Rec 1975;96:81–4.
15. Davidson JN, Yancey SP, Campbell SG, et al. Relationship between serum immunoglobulin values and incidence of respiratory disease in calves. J Am Vet Med Assoc 1981;179:708–10.
16. Corbeil LB, Watt B, Corbeil RR, et al. Immunoglobulin concentrations in serum and nasal secretions of calves at the onset of pneumonia. Am J Vet Res 1984; 45:773–8.
17. Virtala AM, Grohn YT, Mechor GD, et al. The effect of maternally derived immunoglobulin G on the risk of respiratory disease in heifers during the first 3 months of life. Prev Vet Med 1999;39:25–37.

18. USDA. Dairy 2007, Heifer calf health and management practices on U.S. dairy operations, 2007. Fort Collins (CO): USDA: APHIS:VS, CEAH; 2010 #550.0110.

19. Villarroel A, Dargatz DA, Lane VM, et al. Suggested outline of potential critical control points for biosecurity and biocontainment on large dairy farms. J Am Vet Med Assoc 2007;230:808–19.

20. Poulsen KP, Hartmann FA, McGuirk SM. Bacteria in colostrum: impact on calf health. In: Proceedings of the 2002 American College of Veterinary Internal Medicine Forum, Dallas (TX). Ontario (CA): Content Management Corp 2002. p. 773.

21. Stewart S, Godden S, Bey R, et al. Preventing bacterial contamination and proliferation during the harvest, storage, and feeding of fresh bovine colostrum. J Dairy Sci 2005;88:2571–8.

22. McGuirk SM, Collins M. Managing the production, storage, and delivery of colostrum. Vet Clin North Am Food Anim Pract 2004;20:593–603.

23. Godden S. Colostrum management for dairy calves. Vet Clin North Am Food Anim Pract 2008;24:19–39.

24. Quirk Z, West J, Gorden PJ. Efficacy of formic acid as a means of controlling *Mycoplasma bovis* and *Mycobacterium avium* subspecies paratuberculosis in dairy cattle. In: Proceedings of the 41st Annual Meeting of the American Association of Bovine Practitioners, Charlotte (NC). Stillwater (OK): Frontier Printers Inc 2008. p. 279.

25. Anderson N. Experiences with free-access acidified-milk feeding in Ontario. In: Proceedings of the 41st Annual Meeting of the American Association of Bovine Practitioners, Charlotte (NC). Stillwater (OK): Frontier Printers Inc, 2008. p. 12–24.

26. Godden S, McMartin S, Feirtag J, et al. Heat-treatment of bovine colostrum. II: effects of heating duration on pathogen viability and immunoglobulin G. J Dairy Sci 2006;89:3476–83.

27. Peterson J, Godden S, Bey R. Relationship between bacteria levels in colostrum and efficiency of absorption of immunoglobulin G in newborn dairy calves. In: Proceedings of the 41st Annual Meeting of the American Association of Bovine Practitioners, Charlotte (NC). Stillwater (OK): Frontier Printers Inc 2008. p. 248.

28. Donahue M, Godden S, Bey R, et al. Preliminary results on the effect of feeding heat-treated colostrum on health and growth in pre-weaned dairy calves. In: Proceedings of the 42nd Annual Meeting of the American Association of Bovine Practitioners, Omaha (NE). Stillwater (OK): VM Publishing Co 2009. p. 187.

29. Bovine Alliance on Management and Nutrition. A guide to colostrum and colostrum management for dairy calves. revision. Available at: http://www.aphis.usda.gov/vs/ceah/ncahs/nahms/dairy/bamn/BAMNColostrum.pdf. 2001. Accessed January, 2010.

30. Molla A. Immunoglobulin levels in calves fed colostrum by stomach tube. Vet Rec 1978;103:377–80.

31. Adams GD, Bush LJ, Horner JL, et al. Two methods for administering colostrum to newborn calves. J Dairy Sci 1985;68:773–5.

32. Besser TE, Gay CC, Pritchett L. Comparison of three methods of feeding colostrum to dairy calves. J Am Vet Med Assoc 1991;198:419–22.

33. Lochmiller RH, Deerenberg C. Trade-offs in evolutionary immunology: just what is the cost of immunity? Oikos 2000;88(1):87–98.

34. Godden SM, Fetrow JP, Feirtag JM, et al. Economic analysis of feeding pasteurized nonsaleable milk versus conventional milk replacer to dairy calves. J Am Vet Med Assoc 2005;226(9):1547–54.

35. Nonnencke BJ, Foote MR, Miller BL, et al. Effects of chronic environmental cold on growth, health, and select metabolic and immunologic responses of pre-ruminant calves. J Dairy Sci 2009;92:6134–43.

36. Callan RJ, Garry FB. Biosecurity and bovine respiratory disease. Vet Clin North Am Food Anim Pract 2002;18:57–77.

37. Butler JA, Sickles SA, Johanns CJ, et al. Pasteurization of discard Mycoplasma mastitic milk used to feed calves: thermal effects on various *Mycoplasma*. J Dairy Sci 2000;83:2285–8.

38. Stabel JR, Hurd S, Calvente L, et al. Destruction of *Mycobacterium paratuberculosis*, *Salmonella* spp and *Mycoplasma* spp in raw milk by a commercial on-farm high-temperature, short-time pasteurization. J Dairy Sci 2004;87(7): 2177–83.

39. Woolums AR, Ames TR, Baker JC. The bronchopneumonias (respiratory disease complex of cattle, sheep, and goats). In: Smith BP, editor. Large animal internal medicine. 4th edition. St. Louis (MO): Mosby Elsevier; 2007. p. 602–52.

40. Lago A, McGuirk SM, Bennett TB, et al. Calf respiratory disease and pen micro-environments in naturally ventilated calf barns in winter. J Dairy Sci 2006;89: 4014–25.

41. Maunsell F, Donovan GA. Biosecurity and risk management for dairy replacements. Vet Clin North Am Food Anim Pract 2008;24:155–90.

42. Federation of Animal Science Societies. Dairy cattle. In: Guide for the care and use of agricultural animals in teaching and research. 3rd edition. Champagne (IL): Federation of Animal Science Societies 2010. p. 74–88.

43. Webster J. Environmental needs. In: Calf husbandry, health and welfare. Boulder (CO): Westview; 1984. p. 71–97.

44. Pritchard DG, Carpenter GA, Morzaria SP, et al. Effect of air filtration on respiratory disease in intensively housed veal calves. Vet Rec 1981;109:5–9.

45. Hillman P, Gebremedhin K, Warner R. Ventilation system to minimize airborne bacteria, dust, humidity, and ammonia in calf nurseries. J Dairy Sci 1992;75: 1305–12.

46. Blom JY, Madsen EB, Krogh HV, et al. Numbers of airborne bacteria and fungi in calf houses. Nord Vet Med 1984;36:215–20.

47. Wathes CM, Howard K, Jones CDR, et al. The balance of airborne bacteria in calf houses. J Agric Eng Res 1984;30:81–90.

48. Eduard W, Heederik D. Methods for quantitative assessment of airborne levels of noninfectious microorganisms in highly contaminated work environments. Am Ind Hyg Assoc J 1998;59:113–27.

49. Nordlund K. Practical considerations for ventilating calf barns in winter. In: Proceedings of 40th Annual Meeting of the American Association of Bovine Practitioners—Preconference Seminar 7B, Vancouver. Stillwater (OK): Frontier Printers Inc, 2007. p. 85–93.

50. Maatje K, Verhoeff J, Kremer WDJ, et al. Automated feeding of milk replacer and health control of group-housed veal calves. Vet Rec 1993;133:266–70.

51. Svensson C, Liberg P. The effect of group size on health and growth rate of Swedish dairy calves housed in pens with automatic milk-feeders. Prev Vet Med 2006;73:43–53.

52. Willard C, Losinger MS, Heinrichs AJ. Management variables associated with high mortality rates attributable to respiratory-tract problems in female calves prior to weaning. J Am Vet Med Assoc 1996;209:1756–9.

53. Nardell EA, Keegan J, Cheney SA, et al. Airborne infection: Theoretical limits of protection achievable by building ventilation. Am Rev Respir Dis 1991;144:302–6.

54. Wathes CM, Jones CD, Webster AJ. Ventilation, air hygiene and animal health. Vet Rec 1983;113:554–9.
55. Bates DW, Anderson JF. Calculation of ventilation needs for confined cattle. J Am Vet Med Assoc 1979;174(6):581–9.
56. Bach A, Ahedo J, Ferrer A. Optimizing weaning strategies of dairy replacement calves. J Dairy Sci 2010;93(1):413–9.
57. Quigley J. Calf Note #16—Stress at weaning. Available at: http://www.calfnotes.com. 2001. Accessed February, 2010.
58. Ziegler D, Ziegler B, Raeth-Knight M, et al. Performance of post weaned Holstein heifer calves transitioned to group housing using different management strategies while fed a common diet [abstract TH191]. J Dairy Sci 2008; 91(E-Suppl 1). F.
59. McGuirk SM. Disease management of dairy calves and heifers. Vet Clin North Am Food Anim Pract 2008;24:139–53.
60. Stanton AL, Kelton DF, LeBlanc SJ, et al. The effect of treatment with long-acting antibiotic at postweaning movement on respiratory disease and on growth in commercial dairy calves. J Dairy Sci 2010;93(1):574–81.
61. Chase CL, Hurley DJ, Reber AJ. Neonatal immune development in the calf and its impact on vaccine response. Vet Clin North Am Food Anim Pract 2008;24: 87–104.
62. Platt R, Widel PW, Kesl LD, et al. Comparison of humoral and cellular immune responses to a pentavalent modified live virus vaccine in three age groups of calves with maternal antibodies, before and after BVDV type 2 challenge. Vaccine 2009;27:4508–19.
63. Cortese V. Bovine vaccines and herd vaccination programs. In: Smith BP, editor. Large animal internal medicine. 4th edition. St. Louis (MO): Mosby Elsevier; 2007. p. 1591–603.
64. Shelton T, Hoffman B. Determining the prevalence of bovine viral diarrhea virus persistently infected calves originating from a number of modern western well-vaccinated dairy herds In: Proceedings of the 42nd Annual Meeting of the American Association of Bovine Practitioners, Omaha (NE). Stillwater (OK): VM Publishing Co 2009. p. 182.
65. Angen O, Thomsen J, Larsen LE, et al. Respiratory disease in calves: microbiological investigations on trans-tracheally aspirated bronchoalveolar fluid and acute phase protein response. Vet Microbiol 2009;137:165–71.
66. Smith S. BVD control for the dairy practitioner: Strategies and implementation. In: Proceedings of the 42nd Annual Meeting of the American Association of Bovine Practitioners, Omaha (NE). Stillwater (OK): VM Publishing Co 2009. p. 98–102.
67. Baker JC, Werdin RE, Ames TR, et al. Study on the etiologic role of bovine respiratory syncytial virus in pneumonia of dairy calves. J Am Vet Med Assoc 1986; 189:66–70.
68. Godinho KS, Sarasola P, Renoult E, et al. Use of deep nasopharyngeal swabs as a predictive diagnostic method for natural respiratory infections in calves. Vet Rec 2007;160:22–5.
69. Kimura K, Goff JP, Kehrli ME Jr. Effects of the presence of the mammary gland on expression of neutrophil adhesion molecules and myeloperoxidase activity in periparturient dairy cows. J Dairy Sci 1999;82:2385–92.
70. Kehrli ME Jr, Nonnecke BJ, Roth JA. Alterations in bovine neutrophil function during the periparturient period. Am J Vet Res 1989;50(2):207–14.
71. Kehrli ME Jr, Nonnecke BJ, Roth JA. Alterations in bovine lymphocyte function during the periparturient period. Am J Vet Res 1989;50(2):215–20.

72. Kimura K, Goff JP, Kehrli ME Jr, et al. Effects of mastectomy on composition of peripheral blood mononuclear cell populations in periparturient dairy cows. J Dairy Sci 2002;85:1437–44.
73. Shafer-Weaver KA, Sordillo LM. Bovine CD8$^+$ suppressor lymphocytes alter immune responsiveness during the postpartum period. Vet Immunol Immunopathol 1997;56:53–64.
74. Goff JP, Horst RL. Physiological changes at parturition and their relationship to metabolic disorders. J Dairy Sci 1997;80(1):176–86.
75. Perkins KH, VandeHaar JM, Burton JL, et al. Clinical responses to intramammary endotoxin infusion in dairy cows subjected to feed restriction. J Dairy Sci 2002; 85:1724–31.
76. Moyes KM, Drackley JK, Salak-Johnson JL, et al. Dietary-induced negative energy balance has minimal effects on innate immunity during a *Streptococcus uberis* mastitis challenge in dairy cows during mid-lactation. J Dairy Sci 2009; 92:4301–16.
77. Kremer WD, Noordhuizen-Stassen EN, Grommers FJ, et al. Severity of experimental *Escherichia coli* mastitis in ketonemic and nonketonemic dairy cows. J Dairy Sci 1993;76:3428–36.
78. Kimura K, Reinhardt TA, Goff JP. Parturition and hypocalcemia blunts calcium signals in immune cells of dairy cattle. J Dairy Sci 2006;89:2588–95.
79. National Research Council. Dry matter intake. In: Nutrient requirements of dairy cattle. 7th edition. Washington, DC: National Academy Press 2001. p. 3–12.
80. Collier RJ, Dahl GE, VanBaale MJ. Major advances associated with environmental effects on dairy cattle. J Dairy Sci 2006;89:1244–53.
81. Kleen JL, Hooijer GA, Rehage J, et al. Subacute rumen acidosis (SARA): a review. J Vet Med A Physiol Pathol Clin Med 2003;50:406–14.
82. Whitlow L. Mold and mycotoxin issues in dairy cattle: effects, prevention, and treatment. Available at: http://www.extension.org/pages/Mold_and_Mycotoxin Issues_in Dairy_Cattle:_Effects,_Prevention_and_Treatment. 2009. Accessed January, 2010.
83. Divers TJ. Respiratory disease. In: Divers TJ, Peek SF, editors. Rebhun's diseases of dairy cattle. 2nd edition. St. Louis (MO): Saunders Elsevier; 2008. p. 78–129.
84. Midwest Plan Service. Mechanical ventilating systems for livestock housing. 1st edition. Ames (IA): Midwest Plan Services-32. Iowa State University; 1990. 50011.
85. Brouk MJ, Smith JF, Harner III JP. Managing the cow environment for improved animal health and milk quality. In: NMC 43rd Annual Meeting Proceedings, Charlotte (NC). Madison (WI): Omnipress 2004. p. 271–81.

Control Methods for Bovine Respiratory Disease in Stocker Cattle

Shaun H. Sweiger, DVM, MS[a,b,c,*], Michael D. Nichols, DVM[d]

KEYWORDS
• Respiratory • Stocker • Control • Bovine • Disease

There is a segment of today's beef industry that procures calves to grow for a period of time until they enter a feedyard. These calves are generally light in weight and are often immunologically naive to respiratory pathogens. These calves are called stockers. The intent of this step in the process of beef production is to develop the immune repertoire and increase the size of calves before entry into the intensive feeding period.

Cattle health can affect every aspect of a stocker operation. Cattle procurement and marketing decisions, the ability to completely optimize the use of available pens and pastures, the efficient management of labor and facilities, the performance of the cattle, and ultimately the profitability of the enterprise are determined by an operation's ability to effectively manage cattle health. In addition, data exist that demonstrate that subclinical disease, and the performance effects resulting from this disease, can have a similar economic impact as the easily recognizable and profound effect of clinical disease.[1] This substantial impact has been referred to by many analysts as the "hidden cost" of disease.

Because bovine respiratory disease (BRD) is characterized by a complex interaction of many different factors, no one practice for reducing the effect of this disease exists. There are, however, strategies or approaches that contain basic foundations for intervention that can minimize the effect of this economically significant disease.

Effective stocker health management should focus on these foundational practices and avoid the constant distractions inherent in managing the health of calves at high

[a] Veterinary Diagnostic and Production Animal Medicine Department, Iowa State University's College of Veterinary Medicine, 2235 Lloyd Vet Med Center, Ames, IA 50011-1250, USA
[b] Sweiger Enterprises, LLC, 9421 North Robinson, Oklahoma City, OK 73114, USA
[c] CATTLE STATS, LLC, 9421 North Robinson, Oklahoma City, OK 73114, USA
[d] US Beef Veterinary Operations, Pfizer Animal Health, PO Box 542, Vega, TX 79092, USA
* Corresponding author. Veterinary Diagnostic and Production Animal Medicine Department, Iowa State University's College of Veterinary Medicine, 2235 Lloyd Vet Med Center, Ames, IA 50011-1250.
E-mail address: ssweiger@iastate.edu

Vet Clin Food Anim 26 (2010) 261–271
doi:10.1016/j.cvfa.2010.04.008
0749-0720/10/$ – see front matter © 2010 Published by Elsevier Inc.

risk of developing BRD. Implementing a systems approach specific for the operation and focusing on the details of that system will maximize the effect of any health management protocol. Although BRD control is focused in this article, establishing health protocols with the perspective of providing proper management before treatment is fundamental to implementing a successful health protocol. In addition, simplicity in protocol design is consistently superior to complex health programs, which provide too many opportunities for error. Finally, consistency is paramount in implementing, effectively monitoring, and efficiently making adjustments to stocker health programs.

PURCHASING FACTORS

The management history and overall health status of purchased calves is often unknown. If the calves have a documented preventative health history, control of BRD typically involves fewer challenges. It is the calf of unknown origin with little to no health history that is focused for the remainder of this discussion. Although information on the specifics of origin such as the time elapsed from removal from the cow to arrival at the farm of destination, the degree of commingling, and the time spent in transit is desired, it is rarely available. Nonetheless, it must be acknowledged that this unknown history is not only a complicating and determining factor in cattle health but also an opportunity for the next owner of these calves to procure them at a discounted price relative to the market. These discounted prices are a major driver in profitability for producers in this segment of the industry.

ARRIVAL PRIORITIES

Immediately after arrival, calves should have access to fresh water and have a dry place to lie down and rest. Although feed is important, perhaps the most critical need in the first 24 hours is ensuring adequate rest and water consumption. Just because water is present, it does not ensure that it is consumed. For many calves, it will be their first exposure to water in tanks or automatic waterers, and they will have to learn how to drink from these devices. Most high-risk calves do not know how to eat a mixed feed from a feed bunk or drink from a water trough. Easy access to high-quality grass hay and water placed next to the fence aids calves in eating and drinking soon after arrival. Allowing the water to overflow the automatic waterer, trough or tank creates sights and sounds that attract calves and is hoped to stimulate water intake. A properly balanced ration should be fed at consistent times beginning from day 1. It is preferred that calves are fed in bunks, and they should be managed to prevent overconsumption and facilitate a steady increase in feed intake.

NUTRITIONAL MANAGEMENT

Proper nutrition is a major management component in preventing and minimizing disease. Balancing performance and health in calves is critical. Rations should be formulated that best align with the management of the operation. For example, high-starch diets should not be fed to grazing cattle. High-fiber, low-starch, coproduct commodity feeds are better suited for grazing cattle. Also, starting calves on feed too aggressively can contribute to health problems. Delivering a ration inadequate in energy and protein can negatively affect health and performance as well. Varied feeding times and poor bunk management are 2 components of nutrition that frequently contribute to health challenges during the receiving period. Calves are creatures of habit; therefore, the goal should be to deliver the feed at or near the same time each day. The bunks should be clean (free of debris, old feed, wet feed, and others) before delivery of new feed. Providing fresh, high-quality feed is key in getting calves off to a good start.

Meeting the nutritional requirements of freshly weaned calves or newly arrived stockers is critical. If calves are to remain healthy, they must be fed a ration that meets their requirements for protein, energy, vitamins, and minerals. Rations for starting calves should be formulated for intake level of these nutrients rather than for percentage of feed composition. The diets for newly received cattle should be formulated to adjust nutrient concentrations for low-feed intake and to provide optimal performance during the receiving period.[2] It is important to recognize that there can be differences between the rations that are formulated, mixed, delivered, and actually consumed. Mixing and delivery can present opportunities for feeding errors. A common finding when responding to health challenges during the arrival period is improper nutrition. These challenges may present as inadequate nutrition as well as pushing the cattle too aggressively. Deficiencies of nutrients can significantly suppress the immune system, resulting in a poor response to vaccines administered to build immunity and prevent disease, as well as calves that cannot mount an immune response to an infection. The result is calves that continue to experience morbidity as a group well past the goal of experiencing only isolated cases of morbidity after 4 to 6 weeks post-arrival. These groups of calves with continuing morbidity are described by producers as "wont straighten out" and "not responding well to treatment with anti-infectives." Conversely, pushing calves too aggressively in the early receiving period develops digestive challenges that impair a steady increase in feed intake, reduces the intake of nutrients needed to make an immune response, and in some instances, causes digestive upsets that are difficult to clinically differentiate from the ones in the early stages of BRD. The management challenge during the receiving period is balancing optimum health and top performance. A ration during the early receiving period that does not promote good health and a steady, consistent increase in feed intake can result in poor health and performance for the entire stocker period.

It is important to understand that high-risk calves on arrival can have a poorly functioning rumen that wont respond to feed like a normally functioning rumen. In addition to mounting an immune response, a recently weaned, stressed calf has the highest need for protein than it will have in its lifetime to meet its maintenance and growth requirements. To stimulate a return to normal rumen function it requires high-quality protein and trace minerals. These are best provided in a total mixed ration that includes a vitamin and mineral supplement. In addition, the primary negative effect of parasites is to reduce appetite.[3] Therefore, even if an adequate ration or high-quality pasture is available to calves that have not been relieved of the parasite burden they carry when purchased, they do not optimally use the nutrition that is available to them.

Feed management can be important in the timely identification of disease.[2] Good early intakes are necessary not only for nutritional reasons but also because feeding behavior is a valuable indicator of health status. Animals in the early stages of BRD can often be accurately identified by their feeding behavior or lack thereof, as well as from the degree of "gut fill." This is also another important reason for not over-feeding. Feeding calves only what they will consume in a day keeps them slightly aggressive (hungry) and greatly enhances the ability to detect those individuals requiring treatment at feed delivery time.

Proper nutrition during the arrival period cannot prevent stress or infection, but it can decrease the effects of stress and enhance recovery from stressful periods. Nutritional failure when starting calves inhibits all other efforts at keeping cattle healthy during the arrival period. Providing a sound starter ration, managing the bunks well, and transitioning to a grower ration are necessary when the calves are consistently consuming feed at targeted intake levels.

CATTLE MOVEMENT MANAGEMENT

One of the biggest impacts on disease management in starting calves is the disease-challenge pressure brought on by the manner in which pens of cattle are purchased, assembled, and subsequently commingled in the process of building groups of calves to grow or graze. By controlling the movement of cattle into and within an operation during the receiving period, the movement and effects of disease causing pathogens in an operation can be managed.[4]

Exposure of calves to pathogens as they are gathered, sorted, weaned, hauled to market, and processed through the livestock market system can be substantial. There can also be additional negative effects when the calves pass through an order-buying facility and during the transportation process. What is frequently not recognized as having a similar effect is accumulation of cattle on 1 operation from multiple pastures, camps, or ranches. The questions that should be addressed in every operation are

- What pathogen challenges do calves face when they arrive at the operation?
- Where are newly arrived calves located or penned relative to other cattle of varying lengths of time postarrival?
- Where are the pathogens that are associated with BRD located in the operation?
- Where are the BRD pathogens located that should be most concerning with regard to exposing newly arrived calves?

Nearly every group of calves that arrive at any given operation contain potential BRD pathogens, and every group of commingled cattle may have multiple pathogens present in the group. Stocker operations have multiple opportunities to accumulate BRD pathogens, and when the number of pathogens exceeds a critical threshold, the challenge can and often will overwhelm the ability to protect cattle with any preventative or control program. Therefore, cattle movement in a stocker operation needs to be focused on operational efficiency and disease biocontainment. When managing large populations of high-risk cattle, pathogens that cause BRD are also managed. Commingling stocker calves, and consequently their pathogens, can have a profound negative effect on the attempt to control BRD in groups of calves. Timing is critical in deciding when to commingle groups of calves during the receiving period. Hospital pens can serve as an accumulation and dissemination point for pathogens in an operation. A study by Hessman and colleagues[5] demonstrated the effect of commingling on disease presence in a group of calves. This study examined the effects on health and performance as a result of exposure of cattle in a starter feedlot to calves that were persistently infected (PI) with bovine viral diarrhea (BVD) virus. The study involved 21,743 head and provided evidence that exposure of the general population of feedlot cattle to BVD-PI animals resulted in substantial costs attributable to negative effects on performance and increased fatalities. It is possible to complicate the health of calves during the receiving period exponentially when calves carrying different pathogens are commingled.

Epidemic disease curves demonstrate how many cattle are ill over a given time period. Stocker calves peak in the percentage of ill cattle in a herd at about day 14. When considering the effect that disease incidence or morbidity rate can have on the spread of diseases between groups at differing stages in the disease process, logical reasoning would explain why commingling of stocker calves frequently can have such a profound negative effect on the morbidity of groups of calves and why timing is critical when deciding to combine groups during the backgrounding period. Viral BRD pathogens are primarily transmitted from animal to animal, and the movement of pathogens between groups of cattle can be controlled to some degree by managing the movement of cattle within an operation and the timing of that movement. *When* BRD pathogens get introduced into a group of calves is more important and controllable than *if* they are introduced.

BRD pathogens are present in many groups of high-risk stocker calves. In addition, the pathogens can be selected for and multiplied in the process of moving cattle within an operation, and they can accumulate in certain locations within an operation. If these pathogens accumulate in areas of the operation where newly arrived calves are exposed, they can be effectively inoculated with BRD pathogens soon after arrival. It is must to gain an understanding that the critical period during which new groups of calves should not be exposed to accumulated pathogens is the first few weeks after arrival. Older groups of calves (2–6 weeks postarrival) may be shedding the most pathogens. Potentially, the most dangerous pathogens are in the calves that have failed to respond to treatment. Cattle movement within an operation should be planned with respect to the fact that both areas within an operation and cattle with potentially large numbers of pathogens need to be kept as far from newly arrived calves for as long as possible. The management of high-risk calves should include assembling small-to-moderate sized groups of new calves quickly, preferably within 1 to 2 days and not adding new cattle to a group during the backgrounding period, preferably 45 days. Cattle movement can be managed with a goal to keep calves less than 2 weeks post-arrival away from calves that have been at the operation for 2 to 6 weeks. Care should be taken when moving calves in and out of hospital pens, recovery pens, slow starter and buller pens, and other pens, because this movement provides an excellent avenue for pathogens to spread into groups. A common mistake that results in the regular exposure of newly received cattle to multiple pathogens is keeping chronically sick cattle penned near arrival areas and processing facilities.

Manage *what* happens and *when* it happens. A fence or an alley cannot stop disease, but they slow it down by minimizing the commingling of cattle and thus the pathogens they carry. Timing and challenge dose are critical with regard to exposure of recently arrived calves to BRD pathogens.

The inability to control or manage the movement of pathogens in an operation eventually results in increased time spent in the stocker operation. This inability can create a bottleneck that prevents buying as many new cattle as intended in a given period of time. The ability to identify, purchase, and handle the type and class of cattle that are available at an optimal price when other resources (ie, grass, feed, labor) are available is key to profitability in a stocker enterprise. Failure to manage cattle movement and thus pathogen movement affects this key aspect of operational efficiency and profitability.

PREVENTION TACTICS

Effective management methods for BRD in stocker calves must include an emphasis on prevention, and timing is critical. When weaning and preconditioning calves are at the ranch of origin, timing is the essential tool to use and maximize preventive efforts. Vaccines administered 2 to 4 weeks before weaning can consistently be an integral part of the approach to prevent BRD. The use of modified live viral vaccines and *Mannheimia* and *Clostridium* vaccines along with a parasiticide allows calves sufficient time to mount an initial immune response before the stress of weaning. A study by

Kirkpatrick and colleagues,[6] which was conducted by a collaboration between Oklahoma State University and The Noble Foundation, demonstrated equal results from vaccinating calves at approximately 2 months of age and again at weaning when compared with vaccinating them at approximately 3 weeks before weaning and again at weaning in terms of immunologic response and treatment costs. This is a good management procedure to save time and labor without sacrificing outcomes.

Calves begin to encounter risk factors for BRD even before they are separated from the cow at weaning. No prior immunization for recognized BRD pathogens as well as no prior exposure to cattle shedding BRD pathogens are risk factors when they are exposed postweaning. Postweaning risk factors include the stress of weaning, transportation to a livestock auction market, exposure to BRD-causing viruses and bacteria, changes in feed and water, dust, processing, the source and health status of other calves they are exposed to at a market, and the time and stress involved with transportation to the farm of destination. In addition, the frequent additional insult of first being transported to additional markets, or order-buyer gathering facilities, not to mention weather fluctuations, can also have a significant negative effect on health. Risk factors in the marketing process could last as little as 12 hours or as long as 2 weeks. The risk factors encountered by the calves on any given load of cattle can vary immensely. No 2 truckloads of cattle are alike, and seemingly minor changes (at the final destination for the calves) can have magnified effects as a result of the multiple risk factors and the time period over which those risk factors occur. It is important to realize that stocker calves are managed in groups and that no 2 groups are alike. The pathogen status of the individuals composing a group cannot be known. In addition, their vaccination or prior disease-exposure history are not typically known either. Cattle in which the history and source seem to be exactly the same will have widely different disease outcomes based on the presence or absence of pathogens and/or the resistance to those pathogens by individuals within the group.

When receiving sale barn–origin calves, timing is critical to effectively control BRD. Understanding when exposure occurs relative to when prevention and intervention can be implemented is fundamental to designing an effective BRD management protocol for stocker calves. Prevention should optimally begin at a minimum of 2 to 4 weeks before weaning. Vaccines administered to a calf for the first time in its life at 12 hours postarrival, as is the normal procedure with purchased stocker calves with an unknown history, puts true BRD prevention in question. Calves benefit from a 12- to 24-hour rest after arrival before processing to drink and rehydrate, as well as to eat and refill the rumen. A significant percentage of high-risk sale barn–origin calves may not be able to adequately respond to vaccines administered at arrival because of the multiple risk factors and stressors described earlier. A common approach to manage this suboptimal immune response is to revaccinate (not a vaccine label booster) at 7 to 14 days postarrival to attempt to stimulate an immune response in those calves that failed to respond to the initial vaccination. At 7 to 14 days postarrival, properly managed calves should respond in greater percentages to vaccines and make an immune response than is possible at 24 hours postarrival. Arrival vaccination remains valuable, even if a percentage of calves fail to mount an adequate immune response. An immune response with the associated individual, humoral and cell-mediated immunity protection, as well as the possible control of viremia and reduction in viral shedding from a percentage of calves in a group can play a critical role in controlling the spread of virus through the group. An immune response to vaccination by a percentage of calves in a group can have a positive impact on the pathogen dynamics within the group, even if many of the individual animal responses are incomplete or sometimes absent. An arrival vaccination followed by a revaccination 7 to 14 days postarrival is often implemented in an effort to enhance the level of herd immunity, while slowing the spread of virus through a group.

Parasite control should always be considered on arrival because internal parasites have been demonstrated to suppress vital components of the immune system, needed to respond to both viral and bacterial vaccines, as well as active infections.[7] This control includes using an efficacious parasiticide for internal parasites as well as a coccidiostat in either the feed or water. Internal parasites and coccidia can cause clinical disease as well as suppress the immune system.

Ideally, bull calves should be castrated before weaning.[8] In a report by Brazle[9] from the Kansas State University stocker research unit, data were produced to underscore the health benefit alone of early castration. However, a significant percentage of male calves purchased at an auction market are still intact and require castration once they arrive at the stocker operation. The purchased bull calves on arrival are castrated with a knife. Clean, surgical castration on arrival followed by placing the calves in properly maintained, clean pens is usually superior. Banding performed properly is a good alternative; however, banding must always include tetanus prophylaxis.

Vaccines are by no means a guarantee to prevent health problems in high-risk –origin calves due to the risk factors identified and quantified by multiple investigators. However, vaccines do give consistent enough results to be a valuable tool in controlling BRD and managing the health challenges associated with receiving stocker calves.

DISEASE CONTROL

Some groups of arriving calves have individual calves that are sick on arrival, or shortly after arrival, and frequently there can be significant morbidity in a group of high-risk stocker calves within the first 2 weeks postarrival. This morbidity pattern can be intensified and prolonged when the group has a BVD-PI calf. Testing calves at arrival processing and quickly removing BVD-PI calves is a disease control strategy that decreases morbidity and mortality, decreases treatment costs, and improves cattle performance.[10,11] Data collection and analysis to define the type and source of cattle to anticipate early morbidity with is a valuable tool in designing arrival health protocols. Purchased stocker calves should be assigned a risk category and treated and handled appropriately for their BRD risk. Some operations may not have the expertise and facilities to handle higher-risk cattle at all or in significant volume. Factors to be considered in risk categorization include source, commingling, sex, weight, shrink, time in transit, time of year, prior history, availability of resources, and current disease challenges observed in the operation. Groups at high risk for BRD losses should be considered for antiinfectives labeled for the control of BRD at the time of arrival processing.

Control antiinfectives are used to control respiratory disease in groups of cattle that can be classified on arrival as being at high risk of developing BRD. This type of control is also referred to as arrival metaphylaxis or arrival mass treatment. The primary reason to use control antibiotics is to reduce the morbidity or the number of cattle pulled due to illness and treated for BRD in the early receiving period.[12] Control antiinfectives also aid in reducing the number of chronics and mortalities in a group, thus having a significant positive effect on animal welfare. Identification of clinically ill animals in the immediate postarrival period is difficult because the early symptoms of BRD mimic those observed in animals that are simply stressed in the transition between market segments. Using an antiinfective at arrival processing can greatly assist management both by reducing the number of animals identified too late for therapy to be effective and by allowing a focus on other issues in the immediate post-arrival period.

A study by Wittum and colleagues[13] evaluated how ineffectively one is able to identify and treat cattle with BRD. This study, involving 469 steers, did not use a control antibiotic on arrival, and with a pull-and-treat protocol to address BRD in these calves, 35% had to be treated for BRD. Of the 35% treated, 78% had lung lesions at harvest indicating prior pneumonia. However, 68% of the steers that were never treated for BRD also had lung lesions at harvest. The presence of lung lesions versus no lung lesions in the cattle at harvest resulted in a 0.13 lb reduction in average daily gain throughout the entire feeding period. In high-risk calves, effectively and efficiently identifying and treating sick calves in a timely manner is a difficult endeavor. If significant morbidity is likely, administering an antiinfective labeled for control of BRD is a highly effective and economical tool for the control of BRD in stocker calves.

Another study that quantified the difficulty in properly identifying and caring for sick cattle was done at Oklahoma State University by Gardner and colleagues and was reported in the *Journal of Animal Science* in 1999.[14] This study placed 222 steer calves from a single herd into a commercial feedyard in Kansas. In Gardner's study, 50% of the steers were treated for BRD, of which 48% had lung lesions at harvest. Again, however, 37% of the steers that were never pulled and treated for sickness also had lung lesions at harvest. It was concluded that the calves that recovered from BRD never compensated for lost performance, and the high lung lesion incidence (37%) in steers never diagnosed as having BRD indicates that lung damage occurred during a respiratory infection not diagnosed by trained feedlot personnel. Also, the fact that 52% of the cattle treated for BRD had no lung lesions reflects imprecise clinical diagnoses. The imprecision of clinical diagnosis of BRD strengthens the argument for mass medications, particularly when significant morbidity in a group is anticipated.

TREATMENT PRINCIPLES

Treatment or therapy protocols for calves that develop clinical BRD should be developed and based on evidence obtained by randomized, controlled scientific studies available and then should be evaluated and altered based on data from treatment records collected at each operation.

Effective treatment must begin with a commitment to early identification and treatment of sick calves. All of the antiinfectives proved to be effective in treating BRD reach therapeutic levels within 2 hours of administration, and some of them much sooner. Therefore, early treatment is not primarily a function of the onset of therapeutic activity of a particular antiinfective but more accurately is an ability to consistently recognize sick calves early in the course of disease and administer a proven antiinfective. If finding a faster-acting antiinfective becomes a primary concern in treating calves with BRD, this foundational concept of identifying and treating calves early needs to be reviewed.

Treatment protocols for controlling BRD in clinically ill calves should be evidence based and consistent, with case definitions for calves that need to be treated for BRD, and implemented every time a calf is pulled for BRD. Treatment protocols should use proven, efficacious antiinfectives labeled for the treatment of BRD. If a calf is diagnosed as ill for the first time and needs treatment, it should be treated with the antiinfective designated in the protocol as the number 1 treatment. If an individual animal does not meet the case definition of a sick calf, it should not be treated. This approach is imperative to producing valid treatment records that can be analyzed to reliably evaluate existing treatment protocols and make effective changes based on those records.

Not all calves respond similarly to the same therapy. Typical of any biologic system, most calves requiring treatment respond well to an efficacious antiinfective that is administered in a timely manner and continued for an adequate period of time. With a biologic system there are always outliers, and calf response to treatment is no exception. Some calves seemingly respond to antiinfective therapy rapidly and completely because they would have recovered even without treatment. There is a percentage of calves in any population that do not respond well to treatment regardless of the antiinfective used because of poorly functioning immune system. Continuing to administer additional antiinfectives to a calf previously treated for BRD with efficacious antibiotics for an adequate period of time only adds expense and stress to a calf that has already been properly and adequately treated.

Calves that have developed clinical BRD must be treated for an adequate period of time to affect a complete recovery. Approved, efficacious antiinfectives should be placed in the treatment protocol, and it should be remembered that effective treatment requires antiinfective therapy to continue for a long time period enough to allow a sick calf to heal completely. This is an advantage of the longer acting antiinfectives; they reduce the stress and save labor associated with administering additional injections and help ensure compliance with prescribed treatment regimens. Duration of treatment and adequate time to recover are 2 factors important in consistently achieving a complete recovery. The concept of allowing adequate time for calves treated for BRD to respond to treatment with an antiinfective and achieve first-treatment success was evaluated in a study of 3 different posttreatment intervals after treatment of confirmed BRD (n = 750/250 head per treatment group) with tulathromycin.[15] The percentage of first-treatment success was identical regardless of whether retreatment was first allowed 7 days, 10 days, or 14 days posttulathromycin administration. This may indicate that many retreatments are either unnecessary or ineffective. Treatment success requires an adequate duration of therapy and time for the healing to occur.[12]

The most effective control of BRD-related losses is based on the following interventions:

1. Prearrival- or arrival-prevention opportunities should be maximized to reduce the BRD challenge in arriving groups.
2. An arrival antiinfective control should be used to reduce the incidence of BRD in groups.
3. First-treatment success after arrival should be prioritized. The outcome for those animals that fail to respond successfully to the first treatment is poor.[2] Typically, one-third to two-thirds of those animals that do not respond successfully to initial therapy are permanently affected or lost.

Established, effective treatment protocols should be followed until there is evidence that another antiinfective should be chosen based on information such as pathogen isolation, a difference in treatment response attributable only to antiinfective selection, and a clinical investigation by the herd veterinarian. Approved antiinfectives to treat individual sick animals should be incorporated into an evidence-based treatment protocol. Protocols established for each individual stocker operation should define a sick animal; designate when to treat, what antiinfective to treat with, how long the duration of therapy should be; and define when retreatment is indicated. In summary, prevention should be followed by control, and in those animals still requiring treatment, everything possible to achieve first-treatment success should be done.

INFORMATION MANAGEMENT

Management methods for BRD in an individual stocker operation can only be reliably improved by maintaining and evaluating records and analyzing the information generated. Arbitrarily and frequently changing vaccines and/or antiinfectives in an attempt to improve control of BRD in a stocker operation, rather than measuring results of established protocols and making changes based on evidence and data analysis, is an approach that frequently leads to inconsistent control of BRD and the inability to manage high-risk calves effectively and efficiently. Effective BRD control begins with established processing and treatment protocols. Processing and treatment records need to be a standard operating procedure, as do routine analysis of the records. Unusual BRD challenges need to be investigated with a records analysis as well.

Necropsies can be valuable in evaluating specific disease challenges if done early enough in an outbreak when the results can be used to plan some intervention, such as antiinfective control use, vaccination protocol changes, or biocontainment measures. This is especially true when an operation is in the process of receiving multiple groups of high-risk calves over a relatively short time period, as is often the case when stocker enterprises assemble calves in preparation for a flush in grazing availability. Necropsies must be performed timely on early mortalities to be of most value.

Effective, consistent BRD control in high-risk calves results from developing the discipline to measure, collect, and evaluate information to make management changes and to improve the health of stocker calves during the arrival period. H. James Harrington has been quoted often for stating that "Measurement is the first step that leads to control and eventually to improvement. If you can't measure something, you can't understand it. If you can't understand it, you can't control it. If you can't control it, you can't improve it." This statement is quite true for consistently and effectively controlling BRD in stocker operations. Inputs must be standardized with established protocols. Outcomes must be measured to begin the process of evaluating and understanding. Outcomes are measured by routinely collecting data on every load of calves, including morbidity, mortality, chronic rate, first-treatment success rate, and case fatality rate. Records are a must to investigate any disease challenge that occurs. The most useful records require individually identifying every animal processed as well as every animal that is treated. Evaluating the BRD control methods that are in use on an operation requires a record of every calf treated, when it was treated, what every calf was treated with, and the outcome of the treatment. Records evaluation allows educated management changes to address problems as well as to minimize the likelihood of a reoccurrence of that same challenge.

SUMMARY

The control of BRD in stocker calves begins with developing a sound system for receiving calves; keep it simple, be consistent, and stick to it until evidence based on data dictates a change. Develop a sound system for ensuring delivery of proper nutrition. Conscientiously work to control the movement of cattle into and within an operation to consequently control the pathogens in the operation. Establish protocols based on fundamentally sound practices for arrival processing and treating calves. The protocols should solidly support the foundational practices of prevention, control, and treatment of BRD. Finally, evaluate and manage the BRD control methods with information.

REFERENCES

1. Texas A&M. 1992–1997. Ranch-to-Rail—North/South summary reports. Texas Agricultural Extension Service, Texas A&M University, College Station, Texas.
2. Duff GC, Galyean ML. Board-invited review: recent advances in management of highly stressed, newly received feedlot cattle. J Anim Sci 2007;85:823–40. DOI: 10.2527/jas.2006-501.
3. Myers GH, Taylor RF. Ostertagiasis in cattle [review]. J Vet Diagn Invest 1989;1: 195–200.
4. Falkner TR. Biocontainment in high-risk commingled cattle: understanding and managing diseases likely to be present. In: Charting a course of success. Proceedings of the Missouri Veterinary Medical Association. 2005. p. 96–113.
5. Hessman BE, Fulton RW, Sjeklocha DB, et al. Evaluation of economic effects and the health and performance of the general cattle population after exposure to cattle persistently infected with bovine viral diarrhea virus in a starter feedlot. Am J Vet Res 2009;70(1):73–85.
6. Kirkpatrick JG, Step DL, Payton ME, et al. Effect of age at the time of vaccination on antibody titers and feedlot performance in beef calves. J Am Vet Med Assoc 2008;233(1):136–42.
7. Gómez-Muñozb MT, Canals-Caballero A, Almeria S, et al. Inhibition of bovine T lymphocyte responses by extracts of the stomach worm Ostertagia ostertagi. Vet Parasitol 2004;120(3):199–214.
8. Bretschneider G. Effects of age and method of castration on performance and stress response of beef male cattle: a review. Livest Prod Sci 2005;97:89–100.
9. Brazle F. How much do cutting bulls really cost? KSU Beef Stocker 2008 Field Day, October 2 2008.
10. Loneragan GH, Thomson DU, Montgomery DL, et al. Prevalence, outcome, and animal-health consequences of feedlot cattle persistently infected with bovine viral diarrhea virus. J Am Vet Med Assoc 2005;226(4):595–601.
11. Hessman B. Effects of bovine diarrhea virus (BVDV) persistently infected (PI) calves in the feedyard and management of PI calves after initial identification. In: Proceedings of BVD Control: The Future is Now Conference. Denver (CO), January 31, 2006.
12. Apley M. Strategic use of antibiotics in stocker operations. In: Proceedings of KSU Beef Conference. September 15, 2005. p. 123–32.
13. Wittum TE, Woollen NE, Perino LJ, et al. Relationships among treatment for respiratory tract disease, pulmonary lesions evident at slaughter, and rate of weight gain in feedlot cattle. J Am Vet Med Assoc 1996;209:814–8.
14. Gardner BA, Dolezal HG, Bryant LK, et al. Health of finishing steers: effects on performance, carcass traits, and meat tenderness. J Anim Sci 1999;77:3168–75.
15. Pfizer Animal Health Technical Bulletin: 7-, 10-, 14-Day PTI to Close. January 2007. DRX 06053. p. 1–6.

Control Methods for Bovine Respiratory Disease for Feedlot Cattle

T.A. Edwards, DVM

KEYWORDS

• Bovine • Bovine Respiratory Disease • Feedlot
• Control • Prevention • Morbidity • Mortality

Bovine Respiratory Disease (BRD) is the most devastating health problem of the beef industry. It remains the primary cause of morbidity (70%–80%) and mortality (40%–50%) in feedlots in the United States and continues to contribute to substantial losses in feedlot performance, health, and carcass quality.[1] As reported by the National Animal Health Monitoring System, the US Department of Agriculture Feedlot 1999 Study, 14.4% of cattle placed in feedlots developed BRD and treatment cost averaged $12.59.[2] This survey also indicated that death loss caused by BRD increased from 10.3 deaths per 1000 in 1994 to 14.2 deaths per 1000 in 1999.[3]

The finishing phase of beef cattle production in the United States is predominantly conducted in a confined-feedlot setting. Inventory of cattle can range from 100 head, up to 130,000 head within a single feedlot. According to the 2007 Census of Agriculture, the United States sold a total of 27,595,928 head of finished cattle. The following indicates the 2007 total sales of fed cattle for the top 10 states in the USA: Texas (5,742,350); Kansas (5,551,725); Nebraska (5,117,391); Iowa (2,319,313); Colorado (2,023,275); South Dakota (806,581); Oklahoma (766,139); California (744,262); Minnesota (703,091); and Idaho (534,839).[4]

Beef production standards follow established Beef Quality Assurance (BQA) guidelines and best management practices to assure the consumer is provided with the best protein source available. Controlling BRD among newly received cattle has been, and continues to be, the greatest challenge facing the feedlot industry. This multifactorial disease is the combined sum of viral and bacterial infectious agents, in conjunction with management, physiologic, and environmental factors. Together, these factors combine to suppress and overwhelm the immune system of susceptible cattle.

Although there have been aggressive advances in the technology of vaccine, antimicrobial, and antiinflammatory agents, these products are merely tools intended to

Midwest Feedlot Services, Inc, 5415 Summit Road, Kearney, NE 68845, USA
E-mail address: cowdoc@frontiernet.net

Vet Clin Food Anim 26 (2010) 273–284
doi:10.1016/j.cvfa.2010.03.005
0749-0720/10/$ – see front matter © 2010 Elsevier Inc. All rights reserved.

assist in the prevention and control of BRD. Despite these advances, morbidity and mortality rates among feedlots has not declined. We cannot overlook the affect that sound animal care and husbandry practices have on the health and performance of cattle. It is highly unlikely that control of BRD in the feedlot can be accomplished through an on-arrival vaccination program. Therefore, the initial effort for developing a competent immune system must be initiated at the cow-calf level and carried through each sector of the production chain.

The production of beef in a finishing feedlot is more than feeding cattle to an end point. There are many economic, health, nutritional, and animal welfare considerations that factor into the production of a safe and wholesome beef product. The beef industry is not necessarily the driver of production, but rather the consumer steers the direction through its demand for a diverse and high-quality product. In many cases, the cost of production at the producer level fluctuates greatly, whereas the end product exhibits minor changes. Progressively, pressure from special interest groups are pushing for greater restrictions on production practices that frequently lack scientifically based evidence, and compromises not only the economic efficiency of production but also the health and welfare of livestock. Judicious use of antimicrobials in controlling disease, coupled with science-based methods of tracking disease and antimicrobial resistance is a logical means of meeting the economical, quality, and safety needs within the ever-changing demands of the consumer.

Like any production business, raising cattle for beef has its input and output costs and assumes a level of production and market risk. To minimize risk and maximize production and profitability, cattle producers use breakeven projections to establish production and marketing goals. With respect to BRD, inexpensive cattle relative to current market prices may reflect the quality of the cattle, and therefore increase the risk for disease. Consequently, this purchasing strategy often leads to additional prevention and control tactics to assist in reducing the incidence of BRD.

UNDERSTANDING THE CAUSE OF BOVINE RESPIRATORY DISEASE

It should be understood that cattle are often exposed to many ubiquitous viral and bacterial pathogens throughout their lives. Many of the bacterial pathogens involved in BRD are normal inhabitants of the upper respiratory tract.[5] Depending on virulence and host susceptibility, BRD is typically manifested through a primary viral infection of the upper respiratory tract. Viral infections predispose cattle to secondary bacterial infections. The complex interaction between host and pathogen is a dynamic process and presents multiple challenges for the upper and lower respiratory systems. The innate and acquired immune systems are the initial responders and these defense mechanisms act to prevent adherence and migration of pathogens, and employ secretory antibodies against the invaders.

The most common scenario in the development of BRD involves the combination of an immunocompromised (stressed) calf, exposed to an immunosuppressive viral agent, such as bovine virus diarrhea virus (BVDV) or bovine herpesvirus-1 (infectious bovine rhinotracheitis virus [IBR]). The progressive nature in the development of BRD from the upper to the lower respiratory tract is typically established through primary viral infection. The ensuing viral immunosuppression results in a compromised innate immune system and mucociliary escalator. This condition allows commensal bacterial pathogens to migrate and colonize the lower respiratory track, resulting in pulmonary compromise, inflammation, and gross pathology.

PRIMARY PATHOGENS OF BOVINE RESPIRATORY DISEASE

Although there are many pathogens and host interactions recognized as potential causes of BRD, the scope of this discussion focuses on the most common recognized viral and bacterial pathogens of concern.

Viral pathogens associated with BRD and included in most vaccination protocols include: IBR, BVDV, parainfluenza-3 (PI3), and bovine respiratory syncytial virus.

The most common bacterial pathogens involved with the BRD complex include: *Mannheimia haemolytica* (formerly *Pasteurella haemolytica*); *Pasteurella multocida*; *Histophilus somni* (formerly *Haemophilus somnus*); and *Mycoplasma bovis*.

The viral and bacterial pathogens listed earlier are included in a variety of single or combination vaccines frequently used to immunize newly received cattle. Components of these vaccines are also available in modified live, killed, or combination formulations. Vaccination protocols are part of a comprehensive herd health program and designed to stimulate immunity upon arrival to the feedlot and reduce or control disease outbreaks.

STRESS AND RISK FACTORS THAT POTENTIATE BRD

Cattle arriving feedlots are sourced from a variety of outlets that include ranch direct, video and auction markets, and stocker and backgrounder operations. To compound matters, cattle originate from a wide range of geographic locations, breed types, in-weights, and immune status. Cattle arriving at the feedlot from multiple sources carry the added risk for contracting BRD because of pathogen exposure and disease susceptibility.

Development of a comprehensive herd health program within an individual feedlot is typically based on the type of cattle received or the level of risk associated with the cattle purchased. As the risk for morbidity and mortality increases, the intensity (labor) of disease control (drug costs) increases.

Wittum and Perino[6] reported that calves acquiring less than adequate colostrum shortly after birth had a 3.1 times greater chance of developing BRD at the feedlot. Prevention of BRD should ideally begin with sound husbandry management at the ranch and accompanied by pre-arrival vaccination and weaning programs. Further stimulation of the immune system will be reinforced through prescribed health programs at the feedlot. If immunity is not initiated before entry into the feedlot, it may be difficult to achieve protective immunity above early disease challenge, resulting in higher morbidity, mortality, and lost performance.

The nutritional status of cattle received at the feedlot is typically unknown. However, when cattle spend extended time in transit and are deprived of feed and water, a significant decrease in rumen fermentation and capacity occurs,[7] and can remain for several days after arrival. Research from Blecha and colleagues,[8] showed a negative effect on the immune system following the stress from weaning and transportation. Replenishing dehydration and nutritional imbalances may take several weeks. New cattle may not be familiar with concrete bunks or water tanks, and therefore it is extremely important to provide newly received cattle with a balanced and palatable receiving ration in combination with long-stem hay to attract them to the bunk.

The level of assigned risk can be designated to groups of cattle based on historical, animal or environmental factors.[9] At arrival, cattle with clinical evidence of BRD or a high potential for developing BRD shortly after arrival will be designated as high risk. The designated class of high risk will drive strategic management intervention programs for early prevention and therapy. Stress related activities, such as weaning, comingling, and transport have been implicated as primary contributors in the pathogenesis of BRD. These stressors are potentially additive and work synergistically to weaken the host defense mechanisms and promote development of disease.

DIAGNOSIS AND TREATMENT OF BOVINE RESPIRATORY DISEASE

As an industry, we rely on the pen rider (cowboy) or pen walker to identify cattle requiring antibiotic therapy or designated management intervention. Pens are checked daily, and among new or high-risk cattle, sometimes checked multiple times during the day. Early detection of a sick animal relies on the ability and experience of the pen rider to make an accurate diagnosis. Being a prey animal, cattle instinctively mask or hide the clinical signs of sickness as a means of self-preservation. For this reason, subclinical disease is difficult, if not impossible, to identify. Based on our subjective methods of disease identification, it is obvious that identifying sick cattle is not a science, but rather a learned skill or art.

A 469-head study[10] investigating the incidence of lungs lesions found that of 35% of cattle treated for BRD, only 72% had pulmonary lesions at slaughter. Of even greater interest, 68% of the untreated cattle had pulmonary lesions. Evaluation of feeding performance indicated that cattle with lung lesions (regardless of whether treated or non-treated) had a reduced average daily gain of 0.17 lb per head per day. This finding confirms that visual detection of BRD is less than accurate, and that performance and thus monetary losses caused by BRD are significant. Snowder and colleagues[11] reported that calves diagnosed with BRD had a significant reduction in average daily gain (ADG) ($P<.001$) compared with healthy cohorts.

With respect to clinical signs of BRD, the pen rider must closely observe the cattle for particular behavior patterns or visible signs of disease. Early clinical signs during the onset of BRD can be vague and pen riders make judgment calls based on instinct alone. Further evaluation and a final diagnosis can be accomplished once the animal is confined in the treatment chute. Clinical signs of BRD include, but are not limited to, depression, gaunt appearance, lethargy, labored or rapid respiration, nasal discharge, dry muzzle, drooping ear, and rough hair coat.[12]

Once an animal is identified with clinical signs of BRD and moved to the hospital, it will undergo further evaluation to confirm the diagnosis. Confirmation of BRD can be accomplished using several methods. Common procedures include the use of a stethoscope to determine pathologic lung sounds or the use of a rectal thermometer to determine core body temperature. It is common for cattle pulled for BRD to have a rectal temperature of 104°F or greater. As determined by the designated treatment protocol, the therapeutic regimen is administered and a hand-written or computer record of the product, dosage, route of administration, and withdrawal date is established. All products are US Food and Drug Administration (FDA) approved for beef cattle and administered within BQA guidelines.

Example of BRD treatment protocols

Diagnosis	Treatment	Dosage	Days Treated	Route	Withdrawal
Acute BRD	#1 Micotil	2.0 cc/cwt	d 1 only	SQ	42 d
	#2 Resflor Gold	6.0 cc/cwt	d 1 only	SQ	38 d
	#3 Baytril	3.0 cc/cwt	d 1, 2, 3	SQ	28 d

Following the prescribed treatment, and based on clinical impression score, the animal will either be placed in a hospital pen for further evaluation or returned to the home pen for recovery. Cattle admitted to the hospital will be observed daily for signs of recovery and fed a hospital ration with access to long-stem hay and water ad libitum. Cattle requiring daily or 48-hour therapies will be evaluated and retreated according to the therapeutic protocol. An animal that fails to respond to the initial therapy will be reevaluated, administered the next line of therapy, and returned to the hospital pen for further recovery and evaluation. A favorable response to first treatment should be 80% to 85%.

Evaluating therapeutic response is critical in determining if current treatment protocols are effective. This evaluation can be accomplished through weekly or monthly evaluation of morbidity and mortality records. The Case Fatality Rate (CFR) is a good means of determining the ability of the pen rider to identify and pull sick cattle effectively and provide feedback on treatment response. The CFR (for BRD) can be derived by dividing the number of BRD deaths by the number of cattle initially treated for BRD and multiplying by 100. An acceptable BRD CFR rate is between 6% and 10% and may vary based on type and risk of cattle. High-risk calves may reach a CFR in excess of 15%. CFR can also be calculated for all dead animals versus all pulls and is typically 10% to 15%.

In conjunction with evaluating CFR and treatment response records, necropsy assessment of lesions (or lack thereof) is a proven method for determining accuracy of diagnosis and lack of therapeutic response. Sometimes the best education comes from the humbling experiences of failure. Necropsy also provides an opportunity to collect and submit tissue samples to a diagnostic lab in an effort to identify pathology or pathogens associated with disease. Information gathered from necropsy can be vital in making future management decisions and recommendations. It is also an excellent opportunity for the veterinarian to educate feedlot personnel in disease processes and lesion identification.

PREVENTION AND CONTROL OF BOVINE RESPIRATORY DISEASE

The primary goal of a feedlot herd health program is to minimize the incidence and costs associated with morbidity and mortality (BRD and other diseases) through designated prevention and control programs, and thus maximize feeding performance and carcass value. The focus is to effectively minimize pathogen exposure, stimulate herd immunity, and manage risk factors that potentiate the spread of BRD. The first 45 days on feed has been identified as the most critical time in the development of BRD.[12] This time is frequently related to stressors associated with weaning, shipping, nutritional changes, and handling before or shortly after arriving at the feedlot.

Disease management and control can also be executed through the use of a feedlot biosecurity plan. An effective yet challenging means of disease control is to reduce exposure of pathogens to susceptible cattle, which involves stringent management practices in the area of sanitation. In particular, receiving and hospital pens, associated feed bunks, and water troughs should be frequently cleaned. Equipment used in manure management and dead stock removal should not be involved in the handling of feed sources.

Cattle fed in open-air pens are exposed to a range of environmental conditions that affect their health, performance, and well-being. Mud, snow, rain, dust, wind, and extreme temperatures can affect nutrient requirements necessary to regulate core body temperature. The thermal neutral zone for cattle is estimated to be between 23°F and 77°F. Providing protection or good management practices should be considered to help cattle cope with adverse weather conditions and minimize health and performance losses.

Management against heat stress would include overhead shade, sprinkler systems, and additional sources of drinking water. Protection from cold stress involves managing against accumulating mud, providing straw bedding, windbreaks, and protective shelters. Mud can be a problem in feedlots throughout the year. The National Research Council has reported that 4 to 8 in of mud will reduce feed intake by 5% to 15%, whereas mud depths of 12 to 24 in can result in a 15% to 30% reduction in feed intake.[13] Similarly, dust can cause environmental challenges in the feedlot. Within the feeding pens, increasing pen density or decreasing pen size relative to head count can manage dust control. Although more expensive to incorporate, sprinkler systems can be installed and provide dual control of dust and heat stress. Controlling dust within the feed alleys can be accomplished through direct water application from a water-dispensing wagon.

After establishing critical control points within the operation, standard operating procedures and good management practices can be developed to deal with threatening challenges. However, it should be understood that disease outbreaks could occur despite all precautions, because of the complex nature between animal, pathogen, environment, and management practices within a feedlot.

ANIMAL HUSBANDRY

Too often the industry relies on products or "management from a bottle" to provide improved animal health and feeding performance. Sometimes opportunities are overlooked to improve animal husbandry practices. As discussed earlier, stress has a negative impact on the host defense mechanisms, making cattle more vulnerable to pathogens of BRD. During times of physiologic and psychologic stress, cortisol levels increase and immune function declines. A correlation between hyper-excitable cattle and the affect in lost performance[14] and the negative impact on the immune response following vaccine administration has been demonstrated.[15] Castration of bull calves at the feedlot significantly reduces health and growth performance.[16]

Recognizing these consequences should alert us to improve the timing of stressful procedures and to employ better cattle handling techniques and improved facility designs, not just to improve cattle health and performance but also to address the growing concerns regarding animal welfare.

Low-stress cattle handling begins with an understanding of cattle behavior. Minimizing stress at the feedlot starts at the point of arrival, which includes avoiding whistling, loud vocalization, electric prods, and overcrowding in alleys or sorting pens. Cattle should always be handled in a quiet and calm manner. Providing good footing throughout all handling and working facilities will prevent slipping and falling, and in turn avoid costly musculoskeletal injuries.

A clean or bedded receiving pen (particularly during winter months) with a clean source of water, combined with fresh hay and feed will provide an environment conducive to post-shipment recovery. Receiving pens should be located away from and separate from the hospital pens to avoid pathogen exposure. Cattle should spend minimal time in the receiving pens, and following arrival processing procedures, moved to their assigned feeding pen. Again, handling during these procedures should be done in a calm and quiet manner.

The welfare of sick cattle in the hospital is a critical area for applying good animal husbandry practices. Veterinarians have an excellent opportunity to provide hands-on training with the cowboy and doctor crews to increase their knowledge in the areas of judicious antibiotic use, cattle handling, and disease recognition. Certainly the primary goal of the hospital is to provide therapeutic health care to sick cattle. Additional goals of the hospital are to reduce death loss, reduce repulls (cattle subsequently pulled and administered additional antimicrobial therapy) and chronic nonresponders, and minimize performance losses. Hospital pen capacity should be at least 2% of feedlot capacity and more if handling high-risk calves. Some basic guidelines for hospital pens are to provide: (1) 16 to 24 in of bunk space per animal, (2) 150 to 200 ft^2 per animal, (3) protection from extreme environmental conditions, and (4) combination of solid and dirt surface.

Once a sick animal enters the hospital and is administered the designated treatment protocol, daily evaluation of treatment response is the responsibility of the doctor crew. There are many types of hospital designs. Large capacity feedlots typically use a primary hospital facility in conjunction with multiple small satellite hospitals. Feedlots of smaller stature may use a single hospital facility with a three- to five-pen rotation system.

Nutrition plays an important role in the recovery process for hospitalized cattle. The challenge is to provide a palatable feed source to a calf with a depressed appetite. Feed intake is decreased by more than 50% in cattle with fever and respiratory disease,[17] so a sick calf would be expected to consume about 1.2% of its body weight in dry matter compared with 2.5% in a healthy calf.

Hospital rations should be formulated to have an elevated level of protein comprised of a blend of degradable and by-pass proteins. The energy of the diet should be elevated as well, but also reflect the general dietary energy level of the "home" pen. Hospital rations should provide 56 Mcal or greater to offset low feed intake with ample amount of consumed energy. The supplement should have higher levels of vitamins and trace minerals, including organic Zn and Cu.

(Sheri Bierman, and Sean Montgomery, Corn Belt Livestock Services, personal correspondence, 2010). Please refer to **Table 1** for suggested range of nutrients in hospital diets.[18]

Sick cattle that fail to respond following multiple therapeutic regimens are deemed chronic. Chronics are held in a long-term convalescent pen or turned out on a grass trap for extended recovery time and health and feed management. A chronic animal that recovers from illness and meets or exceeds pre-slaughter withdrawal time but fails to meet performance guidelines becomes eligible to be marketed for salvage as a "real-izer." Animals that become moribund or suffer from emergency conditions (fractures or terminal disease) are humanely euthanized in accordance with approved methods.

Table 1
Nutrient guide for hospital rations

Nutrient	Unit	Suggested Range
CP	lb/d	1.25–1.52
CP	%	13.5–14.5
NEg	Mcal/cwt	56–59 (higher roughage pens)
NEg	Mcal/cwt	60–63 (finisher type pens)
Cu	ppm	10–15
Fe	ppm	100–200
Zn	ppm	75–100
Iodine	ppm	0.3–0.6
Vitamin A	IU/lb	8500–13,000
Vitamin E	IU/lb	165–220

Abbreviation: NEg, net energy of gain.

IMMUNIZATION

Most calves are stress free and healthy when they leave the ranch. However, because of the stress of weaning, marketing, transportation, changes in environment, and other factors that lower disease resistance, the immune system is vulnerable to the development of respiratory disease. In many situations, vaccination and background history of newly received cattle is vague or unknown. Obtaining vaccination records from the source of origin can help determine potential inefficiencies within the immunization status.

Many industry-related programs exist that help develop the marketability of calves through pre-weaning and post-weaning vaccination programs. The Value Added Calf program addresses vaccination and management strategies that provide the calf an opportunity to build immunity during a time when stress and disease challenge is minimal.

Optimal vaccine response is related to providing an efficacious vaccine to an immunocompetent animal.[19] Immunity takes 2 to 3 weeks to develop, and may require multiple doses of vaccine to elicit protective immunity.[20] Administering a vaccine provides the immune system exposure to the antigen, but does not guarantee a positive immune response. Despite customary procedures for vaccinating cattle against BRD pathogens upon entering the feedlot, research data supporting its use is limited.[21] A literature review of scientifically valid field efficacy vaccine trials by Perino and Hunsaker found that modified-live BHV-1 (IBR) achieved equivocal results. Studies concerning efficacy of BVDV and PI3 vaccines lacked any reliable results, whereas BRSV vaccine studies showed efficacy was equivocal, lacking any negative impact on health.[21]

Upon entering the feedlot, timing of the initial vaccination may vary and is often determined by distance traveled, time in transit, or health and condition upon arrival. If cattle experience transit time of more than 12 hours, it may be beneficial to allow 1 hour of rest for every 1 hour of transit before administering the vaccination and processing protocols. A study conducted comparing on-arrival versus delayed (14 days) vaccination with a multivalent modified-live virus (MLV) vaccine showed improvement ($P \leq .05$) in daily body weight gain at day 0 to14 and day 0 to 42 in the delayed procedure.[22] This finding is in contrast to work done by Stokka and Edwards[23] that showed no detrimental effects in gain among high-stressed calves receiving multiple polyvalent MLV vaccines.

There are numerous viral vaccine products available in either MLV or killed antigen formulations. The most common viral antigens include BHV-1 (IBR); BVDV; PI3; and BRSV. Most products are now approved for subcutaneous administration.

Attributes for MLV vaccines include

- Strong, long-lasting immune response
- Requires fewer doses
- Less reliance on adjuvants
- Stimulates interferon production
- Stimulation of effector component of cell-meditated immunity
- Vaccine antigens closely resemble pathogenic organism
- Relatively inexpensive.

Attributes for Killed vaccines include

- Storage stability
- Longer shelf life

- Reduced likelihood of residual virulence or reversion of virulence
- Unlikely to contain contaminating organisms.

Common bacterial antigens used in commercially available vaccines for control of BRD include *Mannheimia haemolytica, Pasteurella multocida*; and *Histophilus somni*. These antigens can be used in a single antigen or combination product or included in a combined viral and bacterial vaccine. Diagnostic laboratories isolate other pathogens associated with BRD lesions including *Arcanobacterium pyogenes* and *Mycoplasma bovis*.

Feedlot studies have shown that cattle receiving a *Mannheimia haemolytica* bacterin-toxoid vaccine upon arrival, resulted in reduced morbidity, mortality, and relapse rates.[24,25] Bryant and colleagues[26] examined the effect of tilmicosin (Micotil) alone or in combination with *Mannheimia haemolytica* vaccine administered during initial feedlot processing and found reduced morbidity and mortality rates within the combination group compared with the tilmicosin alone.

Aside from the arrival vaccination protocol, high-risk or naïve calves may be scheduled for revaccination within 7 to 21 days of initial procedures. Because of the high level of stress, and thus a compromised immune system, the initial vaccine may be incapable of stimulating an effective response. The time between the initial vaccination and the booster may be sufficient in recovery from stressors and nutritional and metabolic imbalances. This time may allow the immune system to favorably respond to the additional vaccine exposure. In this circumstance, administering a second dose of viral vaccine may address two immunologic purposes: (1) initiate a booster effect among calves that favorably or somewhat responded to initial vaccine, and (2) provide repeated exposure to viral antigens among calves that lacked an initial immune response.

Revaccination is somewhat controversial and studies have shown mixed results within morbidity and mortality rates and feeding performance. Proving that revaccination provides a cause-and-effect response from the immune system, or the improvement in health was a time-associated function of natural recovery and positive immune response has been challenging.

METAPHYLAXIS

Metaphylaxis is the timely mass medication of a group of animals to eliminate or minimize an expected outbreak of disease. Prudent use of metaphylaxis in high-risk cattle has proven efficient and cost effective in controlling bacterial pathogens associated with BRD outbreaks. Studies have shown that florfenicol and tilmicosin phosphate effectively inhibit *Mannheimia haemolytica* from colonizing the nasopharynx, implying that pre-shipment administration should reduce early onset of acute BRD.[27,28] Lightweight, high-risk calves are the primary targets for metaphylaxis, although because of age and immunologic maturity, yearlings are less likely to receive metaphylactic therapy.

Although research has examined the effects of pre-arrival versus post-arrival use of metaphylaxis,[29] the most common time to administer metaphylaxis is during initial processing procedures, which is when stress and pathogen exposure in high-risk calves are high. Tilmicosin phosphate administered during arrival procedures improves ADG, dry matter intake and feed to gain performance.[30,31]

BRD metaphylaxis (mass medication) may also be used early (within 2–3 weeks) during the feeding period in a similar manner. A rule of thumb for mass treating a pen breaking with BRD is when a threshold of 10% of a pen is treated for 2 or 3 consecutive days or 25% or more of the calves are pulled and treated in a single day.

Table 2
Antimicrobials with approved label claim for metaphylaxis

Generic Name	Trade Name	Dosage	Route	Withdrawal
Injectable antimicrobials				
Ceftiofur crystalline free acid	Excede	6.6 mg/kg	SQ–ear	13 d
Florfenicol	Nuflor	40.0 mg/kg	SQ	38 d
Oxytetracycline	Tetradure 300	30.0 mg/kg	IM/SQ	28 d
Tilmicosin	Micotil	20.0 mg/kg	SQ	42 d
Tulathromycin	Draxxin	2.5 mg/kg	SQ	18 d
Feed grade antimicrobials				
Chlortetracycline –CTC	Aureomycin	10 mg/lb body wt/d	Feed	0 d
Chlortetracycline plus sulfamethazine	Aureo S 700	350 mg CTC/hd/d 350 mg SMZ/hd/d	Feed	7 d

Abbreviations: IM, intramuscular; SQ, subcutaneous.

Subclinical disease is difficult, if not impossible, to detect and the results can lead to costly health and performance losses. Selecting the appropriate metaphylactic drug is most often an economic decision based on research data or performance outcomes. Considerations should include: (1) cost of antibiotic, (2) expected reduction in morbidity and mortality, (3) expected gain performance, (4) cost of gain, and (5) sale price of cattle.

The use of orally medicated feeds for the treatment and control of BRD is also an approved form of metaphylaxis. Antimicrobial products approved for inclusion in feed or water are chlortetracycline (CTC) and chlortetracycline plus sulfamethazine (CTC + SMZ). These products are approved for the control of *Pasteurella* species susceptible to chlortetracycline. However, the challenge for a positive treatment response is to achieve adequate consumption levels sufficient to reach effective blood and tissue concentrations in animals with decreased feed and water intake.[32] More work is needed in the area of oral medicated feeds and delivery systems (**Table 2**).

SUMMARY

The cattle feeding industry has dealt with the challenges and consequences of bovine respiratory disease for decades. The knowledge and understanding about the dynamic relationship between host, environment, and pathogen has progressed steadily over the years. Despite the progress, vaccines and antibiotics are still relied upon as the standard methods of BRD prevention, control, and therapy. Success in building disease resistance begins with genetic selection and continues with colostrum management and reducing pathogen exposure. Purchasing single-source cattle with a history of pre- and post-weaning procedures will minimize pathogen exposure and enhance immunity. Using cattle-handling techniques and facilities that promote low stress will allow host immune defenses to remain effective against bacterial and viral colonization. Lastly, controlling BRD must be managed through a comprehensive herd health immunization and management program that effectively addresses disease challenges common to the operation.

REFERENCES

1. Smith RA. Impact of disease on feedlot performance: a review. J Anim Sci 1998; 76(1):272–4.

2. USDA. Part III: health management and biosecurity in US feedlots. 1999. Fort Collins (CO): USDA: APHIS:VS, CEAH, National Animal Health Monitoring System; 2000. #N336.1200.

3. Loneragan GH, Dargatz DA, Morley PS, et al. Trends in mortality ratios among cattle in US feedlot. J Am Vet Med Assoc 2001;219(8):1122–7.

4. USDA. National agriculture statistics service: total fed cattle sold 2007. Available at: http://www.beefmagazine.com. Accessed March 16, 2010.

5. Callan RJ, Garry FB. Biosecurity and bovine respiratory disease. Vet Clin North Am Food Anim Pract 2002;18(1):57–77.

6. Wittum TE, Perino LJ. Passive immune status at postpartum hour 24 and long-term health and performance of calves. Am J Vet Res 1995;56:1149–54.

7. Cole NA, Hutcheson DP. Influence of prefast feed intake on recovery from feed and water deprivation by beef steers. J Anim Sci 1985;60:772–80.

8. Blecha F, Boyles SL, Riley JG. Shipping suppresses lymphocyte blastogenic responses in Angus and Brahman × Angus feeder calves. J Anim Sci 1984;59: 576–83.

9. Thomson DU. Backgrounding beef cattle. Vet Clin North Am Food Anim Pract 2006;22(2):373–98.

10. Wittum TE, Woolen NE, Perino LJ, et al. Relationships among treatment for respiratory tract disease, pulmonary lesions evident at slaughter, and rate of weight gain in feedlot cattle. J Am Vet Med Assoc 1996;209(4):814–8.

11. Snowder GD, Van Vleck LD, Cundiff LV, et al. Bovine respiratory disease in feedlot cattle: environmental, genetic, and economic factors. J Anim Sci 2006;84(1): 1999–2008.

12. Edwards AJ. Respiratory diseases of feedlot cattle in the central USA. Bov Pract 1996;30:5–7.

13. National Research Council. Effect of environment on nutrient requirements of domestic animals. Washington, DC: National Academy Press; 1981.

14. Voisnet BD, Grandin T, Tatum TD, et al. Feedlot cattle with calm temperaments have greater average daily gains than cattle with excitable temperaments. J Anim Sci 1997;75:892–6.

15. Oliphint R, Burdick N, Laurenz J, et al. Relationship of temperament with immunization response and lymphocyte proliferation in Brahman bulls [abstract]. J Anim Sci 2006;84(Suppl 2):32.

16. Worrell MA, Clanton DC, Calkins CR. Effects of weight at castration on steer performance in the feedlot. J Anim Sci 1987;64:34.

17. Chirase NK, Hutcheson DP, Thompson GB. Feed intake, rectal temperature, and serum mineral concentrations of feedlot cattle fed zinc oxide or zinc methionine and challenged with infectious bovine Rhinotracheitis virus. J Anim Sci 1991; 69:4137–45.

18. National Research Council. Nutrient requirements of beef cattle, 7th edition. Washington, DC: National Academy Press, 1996.

19. Perino LJ. Immunology and prevention of bovine respiratory disease. Bovine Respiratory Disease, Sourcebook for the Veterinary Professional. Trenton (NJ): Veterinary Learning Systems Co, Inc 1996. p. 18–32.

20. Smith RA. Management practices to enhance calf value. Optimal health management for enhanced calf value. Proceedings of a symposium at the North American Veterinary Conference, Orlando, FL, 1997. p. 23–7.

21. Perino LJ, Hunsaker BD. A review of bovine respiratory diseases vaccine field efficacy. Bov Pract 1997;31(1):59–66.

22. Richeson JT, Beck PA, Gadberry MS, et al. Effect of an-arrival versus delayed modified live virus vaccination on health, performance, and serum infectious bovine Rhinotracheitis titers of newly receive beef calves. J Anim Sci 2008;86: 999–1005.

23. Stokka GL, Edwards AJ. Revaccination of stressed calves with a multiple polyvalent MLV vaccine. Agric Pract 1990;11:18–20.

24. Jim K, Guichon T, Shaw G. Protecting feedlot calves from pneumonic pasteurellosis. Vet Med 1988;83:1084–7.

25. MacGregor S, Smith D, Perino LJ, et al. An evaluation of the effectiveness of a commercial *Mannheimia (Pasteurella) haemolytica* vaccine in a commercial feedlot. Bov Pract 2003;37(1):78–82.

26. Bryant TC, Nichols JR, Adams JR, et al. Effect of tilmicosin alone or in combination with *Mannheimia haemolytica* toxoid administered at initial feedlot processing on morbidity and mortality of high-risk calves. Bov Pract 2008;42(1):50–4.

27. Frank GH, Briggs RE, Duff GC, et al. Effects of vaccination before transit and administration of florfenicol at time of arrival in a feedlot on the health of transported calves and detection of *Mannheimia haemolytica* in nasal secretions. Am J Vet Res 2002;63:251–6.

28. Frank GH, Duff GC. Effects of tilmicosin phosphate, administered before transport or at time of arrival, and feeding of chlortetracycline, after arrival in a feedlot, on *Mannheimia haemolytica* in nasal secretions of transported steers. Am J Vet Res 2000;61:1479–83.

29. McClary DG, Vogel GJ. Effect of timing of tilmicosin metaphylaxis on control of bovine respiratory disease an performance in feeder cattle. Bov Pract 1999; 33(2):155–61.

30. Duff GC, Walker DA, Malcolm-Callis KJ, et al. Effects of preshipping vs. arrival medication with tilmicosin phosphate and feeding chlortetracycline on health and performance of newly received beef cattle. J Anim Sci 2000;78(2):267–74.

31. Vogel GJ, Laudert SB, Zimmermann A, et al. Effects of tilmicosin on acute undifferentiated respiratory tract disease in newly arrived feedlot cattle. J Am Vet Med Assoc 1998;212:1919–24.

32. Buhman MJ, Perino LJ, Galyean ML, et al. Association between changes in eating and drinking behavior and respiratory tract disease in newly arrived calves at a feedlot. Am J Vet Res 2000;61(10):1163–9.

Metaphylactic Antimicrobial Therapy for Bovine Respiratory Disease in Stocker and Feedlot Cattle

Jason S. Nickell, DVM[a,b], Brad J. White, DVM, MS[c,*]

KEYWORDS

- Bovine respiratory disease • Metaphylaxis
- Antimicrobial • Cattle health

Bovine respiratory disease (BRD) is the most prevalent disease process experienced by stocker and feedlot cattle. BRD results in considerable economic loss from deleterious effects on cattle health and performance.[1–3] The BRD complex is a multifactorial syndrome influenced by host and environmental factors, pathogens, and management practices. The common pathogens of interest are composed of bacterial and viral components that tend to be ubiquitous within bovine populations.[4–7] Most bacterial organisms implicated in BRD have been shown to be normal inhabitants of the bovine upper respiratory tract.[8] Prevention and control of BRD in cattle relies on implementation of health and production strategies designed to reduce stress, generate immunity to pathogens, optimize nutrition, and minimize disease challenge.

One obstacle to the successful management of BRD in cattle populations is associated with the infrastructure of the beef industry. Calves progress through the production phases of cow-calf, stocker, and feedlot systems potentially changing ownership at any or all points in the production chain. These calf movements minimize the control that stocker or feedlot operators have over the BRD preventative strategy before arrival of the calves. The challenge for these operations is to manage calves on arrival with the anticipation that disease challenge may have already occurred in a given population. The beef production chain provides many opportunities for pathogens associated with BRD to invade the lower respiratory tract. Disease is induced

---

[a] Department of Diagnostic Medicine/Pathobiology, Kansas State University, J117 Mosier Hall, Manhattan, KS 66506-5706, USA
[b] Bayer Animal Health, Shawnee Mission, KS, USA
[c] Department of Clinical Sciences, Kansas State University, Q211 Mosier Hall, Manhattan, KS 66506-5706, USA
* Corresponding author.
E-mail address: bwhite@vet.k-state.edu

Vet Clin Food Anim 26 (2010) 285–301
doi:10.1016/j.cvfa.2010.04.006
0749-0720/10/$ – see front matter © 2010 Elsevier Inc. All rights reserved.

by various pathways, including increased stress leading to compromise of innate and acquired immunity (weaning, transport, and nutrition), instability in the endemic microbial population (due to commingling cattle from different sources), and elevated concentration of pathogen exposure (eg, cattle persistently infected with bovine viral diarrhea virus or cattle actively shedding herpes virus).[9–16]

Due to the challenges that BRD inflicts on management of stocker and feedlot cattle, many health, nutritional, and management practices are implemented in an attempt to minimize deleterious impacts of this disease. One particular management practice, metaphylactic antimicrobial administration at arrival, is commonly used to reduce the pulmonary bacterial pathogen load experienced by cattle populations. This practice entails the mass administration of an approved antimicrobial product to a population at risk of developing BRD with the intent to improve overall health and performance. The objective of this article is to (1) describe the practice of metaphylactic therapy, (2) review the veterinary literature regarding the impact of metaphylaxis on cattle health and performance, and (3) review the veterinary literature regarding individual antimicrobials currently labeled for metaphylactic administration for the control of BRD.

OVERVIEW OF METAPHYLAXIS

Metaphylactic antimicrobial therapy has been defined as the mass treatment of animal populations currently experiencing any level of disease before the onset of blatant illness.[17] Metaphylaxis can be considered as prevention and curative treatment because cattle arriving to a stocker or feedlot facility not only may be at risk of developing BRD but also currently experiencing various stages of the disease process.[17] This management tool is based on the concept of treating the entire population at a single point in time with the goal of decreasing pathogen burden in clinical and subclinical cases.

Treatment of the population is often preferable to selecting individuals for therapy due to the diagnostic challenges of identifying BRD in calves. Cattle are highly adept at concealing signs of sickness; thus, subjective assessment of sick cattle is highly variable. Animal caretakers potentially fail to identify all individuals experiencing clinical or subclinical disease. Objective measures, such as rectal temperature, respiratory rate, or even changes in white blood cell counts, could be used to identify clinically ill animals. A study monitoring these parameters after a *Mannheimia haemolytica* disease challenge indicated these variables were unreliable indicators of calf wellness state.[18] BRD is diagnosed in the feeding phase based on visual observation and general clinical signs of illness, including lack of rumen fill and apparent depression.[19,20]

BRD diagnosis based on clinical signs is inaccurate and has been estimated to provide diagnostic sensitivity and specificity values of only 61.8% and 62.8%, respectively.[21] The inability to accurately identify all clinical BRD cases during the feeding phase is further documented by several studies illustrating the presence of lung lesions at harvest in calves never treated for BRD.[2,22–24] Cattle possessing lung lesions at slaughter, 33% of the sample population, also displayed significantly reduced feed performance and inferior carcass characteristics compared with cattle without lung lesions.[22] These findings suggest that a large proportion of cattle afflicted with BRD are overlooked and subsequently fail to receive therapeutic BRD intervention.

This inability to diagnose afflicted individuals within a group is further illustrated by research comparing selective antimicrobial treatment at arrival with treatment of the entire population. Vogel and colleagues[25] displayed an improvement in health and performance in cattle administered mass metaphylactic tilmicosin therapy at arrival compared with cattle administered tilmicosin at arrival only when rectal temperatures exceeded 40°C (104°F). Another study observed no difference in health or performance in cattle receiving mass metaphylactic tilmicosin therapy compared with cattle administered the drug at arrival when possessing rectal temperatures greater than or equal to 39.7°C (103.5°F).[26] The results of these studies highlight the potential impact of treating subclinical cases and the role of reducing potential disease exposure to the entire population.

In many beef production systems, cattle are managed in cohoused populations (pens). Disease dynamics have the potential to have a significant impact on overall health outcomes. The goal of metaphylaxis is not only to reduce individual cases of BRD but also to reduce the risk of pen level disease. The rate of infectious pathogen spread in a population depends on 3 major factors: the contact rate between infected and susceptible animals, the duration of the infectious period, and the probability that a contact between infective and susceptible individuals leads to infection.[27] Treatment of the entire pen at arrival has the potential to reduce the number of animals infected with a susceptible bacterial pathogen, clinical or subclinical, reducing the disease challenge in the environment for noninfected animals and limiting disease spread. Metaphylactic tilmicosin administration has been shown to reduce the colonization rate of *M haemolytica* within the nasopharynx in cattle compared with negative controls.[28] The use of metaphylaxis as a population control measure provides a tool for operations receiving calves at high risk for disease and compensates for the inability to successfully discern the true health status of calves at arrival to a feeding operation.

IMPLEMENTATION AND TIMING OF METAPHYLACTIC PROGRAMS

The decision to metaphylactically administer any class of pharmaceutical products is based on clinical signs, expected illness rates in the group, and prior evidence of product efficacy. General guidelines that have an impact on the decision to administer metaphylactic treatment for BRD include (1) the clinical appearance of the cattle on arrival, (2) current (and expected) morbidity/mortality patterns, (3) feed consumption, (4) elevated body temperature, and (5) efficacy of products labeled for the control of BRD.[29] The decision for metaphylactic intervention is often determined at the time of cattle arrival. The decision must be made on limited data and a subjective prediction of the magnitude and timing of BRD in the group. The goal is to strategically implement metaphylactic therapy where it will provide optimum benefits.

Cattle characteristics and visual assessments are used to subjectively estimate the BRD risk for a specified population. The predicted level of BRD in a specific population of cattle is often divided into broad categories for the purposes of making preemptive health decisions on the group.[19,30,31] The population-wide characteristics of cattle classified as high risk for BRD include animals being of light weight, cattle from multiple origins, previous health history, and cattle experiencing long durations of travel before arrival at the stocker or feedlot facility.[32–37] Transient factors having an impact on the expected disease rate in groups of cattle include the time of year, weather,[30] and transit conditions.[38] These factors increase risk of respiratory disease in populations due to added stress and disease exposure. Limited tools are available to provide a quantitative estimate of risk of BRD within a population. Practitioners must use experience as well as known risk factors for the group to estimate the expected BRD risk for the population. This classification is then used to guide the metaphylactic decision.

In addition to estimating the overall magnitude of a potential BRD outbreak, the expected timing of peak disease incidence may influence the implementation of the metaphylaxis program. Plotting epidemic curves of the incidence rate of BRD has been advocated as a valuable method of evaluating population disease outbreaks.[39] Although most cases of BRD tend to occur in the first 45 days after arrival,[40] the timing of peak new case occurrence within a pen of animals can be highly variable due to the multifactorial nature of this disease complex. Evaluation of disease outbreaks in feed-yard settings has revealed there are distinct groupings of outbreak temporal patterns that have an impact on health and performance outcomes.[41] The timing of individual BRD cases within a group also has an impact on expected health and performance outcomes. This often modifies projected economic outcomes for groups of cattle.[42] Although there are currently no methods to predict the specific temporal disease pattern a group will display, the expected pattern of disease may influence the meta-phylaxis decision. **Fig. 1** displays morbidity patterns from 2 example pens of cattle. In this illustration, metaphylaxis at arrival may be a valuable tool to decrease the number of cases that occur early in the feeding phase (see **Fig. 1**A). The impact of metaphy-laxis when administered at arrival will not likely be the same on a group where disease occurs at a later time point (see **Fig. 1**B). If cattle are expected to be or become ill near arrival, metaphylaxis may decrease this population disease expression.

Metaphylaxis is most commonly administered within a few days of arrival at the feedlot. Prior research has evaluated the potential influence of administering the anti-microbial agent before arrival at the feedyard or later in the feeding period. Tilmicosin administered at arrival in one study was superior to preshipment injection and

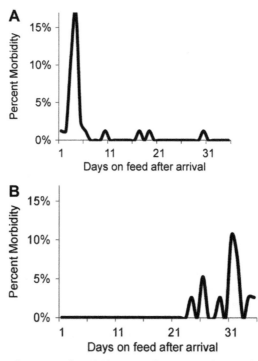

Fig. 1. Distribution of percent of morbidity cases for 2 example pens by days on feed after arrival. (*A*) Represents a pen with the majority of cases occurring early in the feeding phase whereas (*B*) displays pen with incidence rates higher after 3 weeks on feed.

a combination of preshipment and arrival medication.[43] Duff and colleagues[44] also observed an improvement in morbidity risk in cattle administered tilmicosin at arrival compared with cattle receiving the drug before shipment. Similar findings were reported by Frank and Duff,[28] who observed no difference in health outcomes in cattle administered metaphylactic tilmicosin before shipment or at arrival. Performance variables were not measured. Bremer and colleagues[45] observed a significant reduction in BRD morbidity in cattle administered ceftiofur crystalline free acid sterile suspension (CCFA-SS) at arrival compared with cattle receiving the drug on day 18 at revaccination, post arrival and compared with negative controls. Kreikemeier and colleagues[46] observed a significant reduction in ADG when processing, and metaphylaxis using tilmicosin or CTC was delayed until day 21 post arrival. These studies suggest that traditional timing of metaphylactic administration at arrival is ideal compared with other time points.

THE IMPACT OF METAPHYLAXIS ON CATTLE HEALTH AND PERFORMANCE

The immune system of cattle at high risk for BRD may be compromised and unable to adequately defend against the elevated microbial exposure experienced at this stage of the beef production chain. This increases risk of bacterial pneumonia. The goal of implementing a metaphylactic protocol is to address the bacterial pneumonia and decrease individual disease severity as well as population disease incidence rates.[47] Several studies have observed significant reductions in BRD morbidity and mortality along with significant increases in average daily gain (ADG) and feed efficiency (FE) when comparing cattle receiving metaphylactic antimicrobials with negative controls.[44,45,48–53] Van Donkersgoed[54] performed a meta-analysis on 107 field trials examining the efficacy of mass medication in feedlot cattle. These findings suggested that administering parenteral tilmicosin or long-acting oxytetracycline would significantly reduce BRD morbidity risk. A more recent meta-analysis comparing performance in feeder cattle subjected to conventional or organic methods indicated calves administered a metaphylactic antimicrobial on arrival gained 0.11 kg/d more compared with calves not receiving antimicrobial treatment.[55]

Metaphylactic treatment of cattle at arrival may reduce morbidity risk and increase performance. There is still a cost associated with administering the treatment to the population. The economic decision is influenced by the metaphylactic product selected, the expected reduction in disease risk if this pharmaceutical agent is applied at arrival, expenses associated with disease treatment in individual calves, and expected disease risk in the group if metaphylaxis is not given. The first 3 factors may vary by individual operation and the metaphylactic product selected, but by estimated values for each, the expected morbidity at which metaphylaxis is economically feasible can be determined.

Fig. 2 displays example scenarios based on estimated cost of metaphylaxis, percent reduction, and total health costs per head. Health costs in all scenarios are calculated using $92 per calf treated, which has been reported as an average difference in net return, including treatment cost and performance differences between sick and healthy individuals.[56] The metaphylactic agent cost in **Fig. 2**A is estimated at $10 per head and morbidity risk is expected to be reduced by 50% in the metaphylaxis group compared with not administering metaphylaxis.[48,51–53,57] Based on these estimates, applying metaphylaxis to the group is not economically efficient until the expected morbidity rate is at least 25% (see **Fig. 2**A). The cutoff expected morbidity necessary to justify metaphylaxis use increases to 40% if metaphylaxis cost is increased to $18 per head and the other variables are held constant (see **Fig. 2**B).

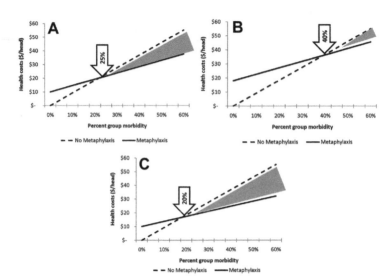

Fig. 2. Illustration of potential health costs ($/head) based on projected level of morbidity within a population and the potential change in morbidity based on metaphylaxis usage. Health costs are equal to the sum of metaphylaxis cost ($0 in nontreated group, cost of metaphylactic antimicrobial in metaphylaxis group) and estimated cost in medications and performance for each animal treated. Morbidity rates are estimated to be reduced on a percentage basis when comparing expected morbidity rates with no metaphylaxis to expected morbidity in the metaphylaxis-treated group. The block arrow on each graph designates the point beyond which total health costs per head become greater for the non-metaphylaxis group (representing an economic advantage to metaphylaxis). The shaded triangle represents the advantage in health costs per head for the metaphylaxis group compared with nonmetaphylaxis group at each estimated level of morbidity. (*A*) Comparisons based on estimated metaphylactic costs of $10 per head, estimated health costs for treated animals of $92 per head, and estimated percent reduction of morbidity (metaphylaxis vs no metaphylaxis) of 50%. (*B*) All estimates of variables held at same levels as in **Fig. 2**A, except metaphylactic cost per head moved to $18. (*C*) All estimates of variables held at same levels as in **Fig. 2**A, except estimated reduction in morbidity due to metaphylaxis increased to 60%.

If the baseline assumptions are maintained as in **Fig. 2**A, except that the expected reduction of morbidity due to metaphylaxis administration is increased to 60%, there is a slight decrease in the cutoff of expected morbidity necessary to economically justify metaphylaxis (see **Fig. 2**C). These are examples based on generic inputs, and the economic outcomes of metaphylaxis application in a specific set of cattle should be estimated based on the situation and most accurate estimates of the variables described previously.

Research illustrates the impact of metaphylactic protocols in reducing the risk of BRD with improved the feedlot performance. The decision to implement a metaphylactic program must be based on all available information to optimize the economical viability of the practice.

ANTIMICROBIAL DRUGS CURRENTLY APPROVED FOR CONTROL OF BRD IN CATTLE AT HIGH RISK FOR BRD

Many antimicrobial products are labeled for metaphylactic administration to aid in the control of BRD. The product selected for metaphylaxis in a specific operation or situation is dependent on the characteristics of the product and the expected efficacy and cost effectiveness. A complete list of currently approved antimicrobials labeled for metaphylactic administration is displayed in **Table 1**.

Ceftiofur

Original formulations of ceftiofur, ceftiofur sodium and ceftiofur hydrochloride (Naxcel and Excenel, respectively, Pfizer Animal Health, Kalamazoo, MI, USA), were designed and labeled for the treatment of BRD and also for the treatment of acute metritis and acute interdigital necrobacillosis. These drugs provided veterinarians and producers with a practical means of treating the aforementioned ailments while offering zero milk withdrawal and short meat withdrawals. In addition to not possessing a label for metaphylaxis, these products require multiple treatments to provide their intended effect, thereby requiring additional handling of the affected cattle and potentially affecting client compliance. A new formulation of ceftiofur, CCFA-SS (Excede, Pfizer Animal Health), has provided the beef and dairy industry with a product developed for single administration. Unlike its counterparts, this product is labeled for the treatment and control of BRD.

Efficacy as a metaphylactic agent is often reliant on the ability of the pharmaceutical agent to mitigate BRD in clinical cases. Early work with CCFA-SS illustrated that a 1-time subcutaneous (SC) injection (in the neck) to cattle experiencing BRD resulted in greater treatment success compared with negative controls and cattle receiving tilmicosin.[58] SC injection in the neck demonstrated drug residues exceeding the previously established tolerance for an extended time.[58] Subsequent studies revealed that SC administration of CCFA-SS in the posterior aspect of the ear was capable of efficacious drug delivery, removing concerns regarding the presence of tissue drug residues, and was tolerated with no adverse effects at injection site.[58,59] Two locations in the posterior aspect of the ear are currently approved for routes of SC injection: the middle third of the ear and the base of the ear. Inadvertent intraarticular injection of CCFA-SS should be avoided as it may cause acute death in the animal.

Table 1
Current antimicrobial drugs labeled for metaphylactic administration to cattle for control of BRD

Drug Name	Trade Name	Dose	Route of Administration	Meat Withdrawal (Days)
Ceftiofur	Excede	1.5 mL/100 lb	Posterior aspect of the ear	4
Chlortetracycline	Aureomycin	See product label[a]	Oral	48 Hours before slaughter
Chlortetracycline-sulfamethazine	AS-700	See product label	Oral	7
Florfenicol	Nuflor	6 mL/100 lb	SC	38
Oxytetracycline	Tetradure	4.5 mL/100 lb	IM or SC	28
Tilmicosin	Micotil	1.5 mL/100 lb	SC	28
Tulathromycin	Draxxin	1.1 mL/100 lb	SC	18

Abbreviations: IM, intramuscular; SC, subcutaneous.
 [a] This product is also available as a combination product with ionophore therapy.
 Data from Thomson DU, White BJ. Backgrounding beef cattle. Vet Clin North Am Food Anim Pract 2006;22(2):373–8.

Several clinical trials demonstrate metaphylactic efficacy of CCFA-SS at reducing BRD risk, modifying the time between arrival and first treatment for BRD, and increasing cattle performance. A reduced BRD morbidity risk compared with negative controls has been observed in calves treated metaphylactically with CCFA-SS.[57] CCFA-SS also illustrated lower cumulative incidence of BRD compared with negative controls, but BRD risk was equal to that of tilmicosin.[59] Encinias and colleagues[48] displayed a reduction in BRD morbidity and a significant reduction in second treatments in cattle receiving metaphylactic CCFA-SS compared with negative controls. CCFA-SS also may increase duration of time until first BRD treatment compared with negative controls in addition to modifying the risk for BRD.[59] Cattle treated with CCFA-SS at arrival also have increased ADG[57,59] and greater dry-matter intake[48] compared with negative controls, which may be related to the consistent reduction in BRD risk compared with negative controls.

Calves in the postweaning phase are commonly administered more than one product at the time of arrival to a feeding operation. One study illustrated a decreased BRD cumulative incidence in cattle receiving CCFA-SS alone or concurrently with a growth-promoting implant compared with negative controls.[60] Step and colleagues[61] illustrated that cattle administered CCFA-SS at arrival followed by tulathromycin 8 days later displayed reduced BRD morbidity risk compared with cattle treated with only CCFA-SS or tilmicosin. No differences in ADG were observed in the 3 treatment groups. Despite these findings, metaphylactic protocols that involve more than one parenteral antimicrobial are not typically practiced.

Chlortetracycline and Sulfamethazine

The administration of oral antimicrobials as metaphylactic therapy has been researched and used for decades.[44,49,62–67] Due to the timing of discovery and formulation for oral administration via feed, water, or oral bolus, oral delivery has been dominated by drugs such as tetracyclines, sulfonamides or a combination of drugs from the 2 classes of antimicrobials. From many viewpoints, metaphylactic application of oral antimicrobials provides a practical method of drug delivery by minimizing labor, human health risks (eg, tilmicosin), and cattle handling. Clinically ill cattle exhibit reduced feed intake and cattle inexperienced at eating from a bunk may not consume adequate amounts of feed to achieve a therapeutic dose.[47,68] Oral antimicrobials administered through drinking water may also reduce the palatability of the water.[29] This reduces the amount of drug delivered to the animal and may partially explain the variation when oral medications are used in control BRD in high-risk cattle not only reported in the literature but also observed in the clinical experience of the authors.

Although a large volume of research is available on the topic of oral metaphylaxis, a prior meta-analysis focused specifically on field trials evaluating metaphylactic protocols observed that a majority of the work on oral metaphylactic therapy contained several shortcomings. Shortcomings included lack of randomization, nonspecific case definitions, and minimal statistics casting doubt on the validity of the results.[54] This article focuses only on studies published since the publication of the meta-analysis and that incorporate the aforementioned attributes of clinical trials.

Gallo and Berg[49] observed that high-risk feeder cattle receiving an oral feed additive composed of chlortetracycline (CTC) and sulfamethazine displayed a significant decline in BRD morbidity, chronicity rates, and improved feed performance compared with negative controls. Kreikemeier and colleagues[46] also reported significant health and performance benefits in cattle fed CTC at 1 g/100 lb for 5 days beginning on day 1 as metaphylaxis compared with negative controls. Improvements in the CTC group were similar to cattle administered tilmicosin at arrival.

In contrast to these studies, Duff and colleagues[44] performed a 3 × 2 factorial study that evaluated the metaphylactic effect of oral CTC fed at 22 mg/kg from days 5 through 9 after arrival compared with that of tilmicosin in feeder calves during a 28-day receiving period. In this study, CTC failed to produce health and performance differences between cattle consuming oral CTC and that of negative controls. Frank and Duff[28] randomly allocated 349 feeder steers to receive either CTC fed at 22 mg/kg for the first 5 days post-arrival or to remain as negative controls. The investigators found no significant differences in health or performance effects between the 2 treatment groups.[28]

In addition to using CTC as the sole means of metaphylactic therapy, previous studies have evaluated the ability of CTC to complement a parenteral metaphylactic protocol. Duff and colleagues[44] displayed no added benefits to health or performance when feeding CTC at the rate (described previously) to cattle that had received tilmicosin for metaphylactic purposes at arrival compared with negative controls. These findings were similar to those of other investigators who also evaluated the combined effects of oral CTC metaphylactic therapy and tilmicosin.[28,46] Wallace[69] observed no additive effects when oral CTC was fed concurrently to high-risk stocker cattle previously administered metaphylactic tulathromycin at arrival. These data suggest that the addition of oral CTC therapy to existing parenteral metaphylactic protocols does not significantly alter health and performance.

Florfenicol

Florfenicol (Nuflor, Intervet/Schering-Plough Animal Health, Desoto, KS, USA) is currently labeled not only for the treatment of BRD but also for metaphylactic administration to cattle at high risk of the disease. In contrast to other antimicrobials labeled for metaphylactic BRD therapy, peer-reviewed data regarding the metaphylactic efficacy of florfenicol is minimal. In a study of 205 beef steers, cattle receiving metaphylactic florfenicol displayed a significant reduction in BRD morbidity, an increased interval between the time of arrival and incidence of BRD, and a reduction in *M haemolytica* colonization in the nasopharynx for 4 days post injection.[70]

Oxytetracycline

There are currently several injectable oxytetracycline products and formulations indicated for the treatment of many disease processes, such as BRD, foot rot, infectious bovine keratoconjunctivitis (pinkeye), and diphtheria. Many formulations are concentrated at 200 mg/mL of oxytetracycline and have displayed efficacy when administered as metaphylactic therapy to cattle at high risk for BRD.[53,63,67,71,72] Only one formulation, Tetradure (Merial, Duluth, GA, USA) (300 mg/mL [Tet 300]) is currently labeled for metaphylactic administration to cattle at high risk of BRD.[73] Like florfenicol, data evaluating the metaphylactic effects of this respective formulation of oxytetracycline are lacking and to the authors' knowledge no peer reviewed data are available that evaluates this oxytetracycline formulation to negative controls.

Tilmicosin

Efficacy of tilmicosin[74] (Micotil, Elanco, Greenfield, IN, USA) as a metaphylactic antimicrobial has been demonstrated by many research studies performed on high-risk cattle entering stocker or feedlot production systems. Compared with negative controls, cattle administered tilmicosin at arrival reduced cumulative incidence of morbidity and significantly improved ADG and FE during short (30–60 day) studies.[51,52] Galyean and colleagues[26] observed a significant decline in morbidity in cattle administered tilmicosin at arrival compared with negative control cattle but did not observe

Table 2
Summary of morbidity and mortality outcomes from published research comparing metaphylactic antimicrobials

Drug Comparison			Morbidity			Mortality		
Drug A	Drug B	Study	Drug A	Drug B	P Value	Drug A	Drug B	P Value
CTC	Tilmicosin	Hellwig et al 1998	47%	44%	≤0.05	NR	NR	NR
Florfenicol	Tulathromycin	Rooney et al 2005	NR	NR	NR	6.97	1.64%	≤0.05
Tilmicosin	Tulathromycin	Nickell et al 2008	68.1%	32.8%	≤0.05	13.5%	3.6%	≤0.05
		Booker et al 2007	14.0%	3.2%	≤0.05	4.9%	2.3%	≤0.05
		Godhino et al 2005	24.9%	14.6%	<0.01	NR	NR	NR
		Kilgore et al 2005	28.7%	13.2%	≤0.01	NR	NR	NR
		Rooney et al 2005	NR	NR	NR	5.0%	2.1%	0.09
		Van Donkersgoed et al 2008	13.0%	3.0%	<0.01	0.2%	0.04%	>0.05
Tilmicosin	Tet-300[a]	Schunict et al 2002	19.6%	22.6%	<0.02	1.4%	1.55%	>0.05
Tilmicosin	Tet-300	Booker et al 2007[b]	14.0%	17.0%	NR	1.88%	2.54%	NR
Tulathromycin	Tet-300	Booker et al 2007	3.42%	17.02%	<0.01	0.30%	2.54	<0.001
Tilmicosin	CCFA-SS[c]	Booker et al 2006	28.84%	27.96%	>0.05	10.93%	8.17	0.003
Tilmicosin	CCFA-SS	Step et al 2007	21.50%	23.50%	>0.05	NR	NR	NR

Abbreviation: NR, data not reported.
[a] Injectable Oxytetracycline (300 mg/mL).
[b] Contrasts between the respective drugs was not conducted.
[c] Based on a 7-day treatment moratorium.

Table 3
Summary of feed and gain performance outcomes from published research comparing metaphylactic antimicrobials

Drug Comparison			ADG (lb)			FE (lb)		
Drug A	Drug B	Study	Drug A	Drug B	P Value	Drug A	Drug B	P Value
CTC	Tilmicosin	Hellwig et al 1998	1.5	1.5	>0.05	NR	NR	NR
Florfenicol	Tulathromycin	Rooney et al 2005[a]	3.06	3.18	0.022	NR	NR	NR
Tilmicosin	Tulathromycin	Nickell et al 2008	2.00	2.50	≤0.05	7.10	5.90	≤0.05
		Booker et al 2007	2.58	2.64	≤0.05	6.80	6.94	≤0.05
		Godhino et al 2005	2.62	2.79	<0.01	NR	NR	NR
		Kilgore et al 2005	2.20	3.00	>0.05	NR	NR	NR
		Rooney et al 2005	3.36	3.37	>0.05	NR	NR	NR
		Van Donkersgoed et al 2008	2.87	2.87	>0.05	6.97	7.02	>0.05
Tilmicosin	Tet-300[b]	Schunict et al 2002	2.97	2.97	>0.05	6.45	6.43	>0.05
Tilmicosin	Tet-300	Booker et al 2007[c]	2.58	2.55	NR	6.80	6.92	NR
Tulathromycin	Tet-300	Booker et al 2007	2.64	2.55	<0.01	6.94	6.92	>0.05
Tilmicosin	CCFA-SS[d]	Booker et al 2006	2.71	2.76	>0.05	6.46	6.49	>0.05
Tilmicosin	CCFA-SS	Step et al 2007	2.42	2.45	>0.05	NR	NR	NR

Abbreviation: NR, data not reported.
[a] Results reported from only one study site (Idaho).
[b] Injectable oxytetracycline (300 mg/mL).
[c] Contrasts between the respective drugs was not conducted.
[d] Based on a 7-day treatment moratorium.

a difference in gain. In addition to health and performance impacts, cattle receiving metaphylactic tilmicosin were treated for BRD later in the feeding phase 21 days post arrival compared with control cattle 9 days post arrival.[51]

Many reports have displayed efficacious results for metaphylactic tilmicosin when cattle have been evaluated throughout the entire feeding period. Similar to the shorter-term studies, cattle administered tilmicosin at arrival display a significant reduction in the risk of morbidity and mortality compared with negative controls.[25,28,50,53] Metaphylactic administration of tilmicosin also increased the number of days until the first BRD treatment was indicated compared with nonmedicated cattle.[50] Several studies also observed improvement in ADG in cattle administered tilmicosin at arrival compared with negative controls.[25,50] Hot carcass weights tended to be greater in cattle administered tilmicosin at arrival compared with negative controls.[50]

These findings suggest that tilmicosin has repeatedly provided an improvement in health and performance when administered to cattle in stocker and feedlot systems compared with nonmedicated cattle. Tilmicosin is unique in that human exposure may result in death. Appropriate precautions should be practiced when handling this drug and all preventive measures should be exercised to avoid accidental exposure.[74] Tilmicosin has also shown to be fatal in cattle and sheep when injected intravenously and may be fatal in swine, nonhuman primates, horses, and goats.

Tulathromycin

Tulathromycin (Draxxin, Pfizer Animal Health) represents the most recent antimicrobial labeled for metaphylactic administration in cattle to control BRD. This drug, like tilmicosin, belongs to the macrolide class of antibiotics but provides a longer duration of therapeutic activity compared with tilmicosin.[75,76] Tulathromycin does not pose a human health threat.

When comparing tulathromycin with negative controls, Kilgore and colleagues[77] demonstrated that tulathromycin significantly reduced morbidity through day 14 compared with cattle administered saline on arrival to the feedlot. Godinho and colleagues[78] displayed similar results. Cattle administered tulathromycin in a metaphylactic manner were observed to be healthier during the 60-day study compared with cattle receiving tilmicosin or saline at arrival. Cattle administered metaphylactic tulathromycin also displayed a significant increase in ADG compared with the cattle in the saline group.[78]

HEALTH AND FEED PERFORMANCE COMPARISON BETWEEN METAPHYLACTIC ANTIMICROBIALS

Many clinical trials have been performed comparing metaphylactic agents by estimating their respective health and performance outcomes in stocker or feedlot cattle. **Tables 2** and **3** summarize the findings from several drug comparisons by listing common outcome parameters traditionally estimated in stocker/feedlot research studies. Outcome variables are sparingly estimated and infrequently encountered. Not all measured outcomes reported by individual investigators are listed in the tables. These data are not intended to promote individual metaphylactic protocols but were compiled as a tool that summarizes the available peer-reviewed data.

SUMMARY

Cattle entering stocker and feedlot production systems are subjected to many stressful events that can culminate in weakened of immune systems, nutritional concerns, and an elevated level of pathogen exposure, which can manifest as BRD. As a population, cattle may enter a stocker or feedlot facility possessing individuals experiencing different stages of BRD. Cattle are adept at concealing their true health status, reducing capabilities of recognizing sick cattle on arrival. The practice of metaphylaxis provides producers with a tool that has repeatedly been observed to reduce the negative health and performance effects induced by BRD. Veterinarians have the ability to use multiple antimicrobial products currently labeled for metaphylactic administration and have been demonstrated as efficacious in this capacity. The determination of which drug to implement is typically preceded by the perceived risk the cattle possess to developing BRD, prior experience, cost of the drug, and published literature. By improving overall health and feed performance, the practice of metaphylaxis provides veterinarians and producers with a tool to positively influence the economic viability of stocker and feedlot production systems.

REFERENCES

1. Smith RA. Impact of disease on feedlot performance: a review. J Anim Sci 1998; 76(1):272–4.
2. Wittum TE, Woollen NE, Perino LJ, et al. Relationships among treatment for respiratory tract disease, pulmonary lesions evident at slaughter, and rate of weight gain in feedlot cattle. J Am Vet Med Assoc 1996;209(4):814–8.
3. Larson RL. Effect of cattle disease on carcass traits. J Anim Sci. 2005;83(Suppl 13):E37–43.
4. Booker CW, Guichon PT, Jim GK, et al. Seroepidemiology of undifferentiated fever in feedlot calves in western Canada. Can Vet J 1999;40(1):40–8.
5. Martin SW, Bateman KG, Shewen PE, et al. The frequency, distribution and effects of antibodies, to seven putative respiratory pathogens, on respiratory disease and weight gain in feedlot calves in Ontario. Can J Vet Res 1989; 53(3):355–62.
6. Martin SW, Bateman KG, Shewen PE, et al. A group level analysis of the associations between antibodies to seven putative pathogens and respiratory disease and weight gain in Ontario feedlot calves. Can J Vet Res 1990;54(3):337–42.
7. Martin SW, Bohac JG. The association between serological titers in infectious bovine rhinotracheitis virus, bovine virus diarrhea virus, parainfluenza-3 virus, respiratory syncytial virus and treatment for respiratory disease in Ontario feedlot calves. Can J Vet Res 1986;50(3):351–8.
8. DeRosa DC, Mechor GD, Staats JJ, et al. Comparison of *Pasteurella* spp. simultaneously isolated from nasal and transtracheal swabs from cattle with clinical signs of bovine respiratory disease. J Clin Microbiol 2000;38(1):327–32.
9. Anderson NV, Youanes YD, Vestweber JG, et al. The effects of stressful exercise on leukocytes in cattle with experimental pneumonic pasteurellosis. Vet Res Commun 1991;15(3):189–204.
10. Arthington JD, Eichert SD, Kunkle WE, et al. Effect of transportation and commingling on the acute-phase protein response, growth, and feed intake of newly weaned beef calves. J Anim Sci 2003;81(5):1120–5.
11. Arthington JD, Spears JW, Miller DC. The effect of early weaning on feedlot performance and measures of stress in beef calves. J Anim Sci 2005;83(4): 933–9.
12. Cooke RF, Arthington JD, Austin BR, et al. Effects of acclimation to handling on performance, reproductive, and physiological responses of Brahman-crossbred heifers. J Anim Sci 2009;87(10):3403–12.

13. Carroll JA, Forsberg NE. Influence of stress and nutrition on cattle immunity. Vet Clin North Am Food Anim Pract 2007;23(1):105–49.
14. Cole NA, Camp TH, Rowe LD Jr, et al. Effect of transport on feeder calves. Am J Vet Res 1988;49(2):178–83.
15. Hessman BE, Fulton RW, Sjeklocha DB, et al. Evaluation of economic effects and the health and performance of the general cattle population after exposure to cattle persistently infected with bovine viral diarrhea virus in a starter feedlot. Am J Vet Res 2009;70(1):73–85.
16. Loneragan GH, Thomson DU, Montgomery DL, et al. Prevalence, outcome, and health consequences associated with persistent infection with bovine viral diarrhea virus in feedlot cattle. J Am Vet Med Assoc 2005;226(4):595–601.
17. Young C. Antimicrobial metaphylaxis for undifferentiated bovine respiratory disease. Compend Contin Educ Pract Vet 1995;17:133–42.
18. Hanzlicek GA, White BJ, Mosier DA, et al. Serial evaluation of physiological, pathological and behavioral changes related to disease progression of experimentally induced Mannheimia haemolytica pneumonia in feeder calves. Am J Vet Res 2010;71:359–69.
19. Lechtenberg KF, Smith RA, Stokka GL. Feedlot health and management. Vet Clin North Am Food Anim Pract 1998;14(2):177–97.
20. Smith RA, Stokka GL, Radostits OM, et al. Health and production management in beef feedlots. In: Radostits O, editor. Herd health: food animal production medicine. Philadelphia: WB Saunders Company; 2001. p. 592–5.
21. White BJ, Renter DG. Bayesian estimation of the performance of clinical observations and harvest lung scores for diagnosing bovine respiratory disease in postweaned beef calves. J Vet Diagn Invest 2009;21(4):446–53.
22. Gardner BA, Dolezal HG, Bryant LK, et al. Health of finishing steers: effects on performance, carcass traits, and meat tenderness. J Anim Sci 1999;77(12): 3168–75.
23. Thompson PN, Stone A, Schultheiss WA. Use of treatment records and lung lesion scoring to estimate the effect of respiratory disease on growth during early and late finishing periods in South African feedlot cattle. J Anim Sci 2006;84(2): 488–98.
24. Schneider MJ, Tait RG Jr, Busby WD, et al. An evaluation of bovine respiratory disease complex in feedlot cattle: impact on performance and carcass traits using treatment records and lung lesion scores. J Anim Sci 2009;87:1821–7.
25. Vogel GJ, Laudert SB, Zimmerman A, et al. Effects of tilmicosin on acute undifferentiated respiratory tract disease in newly arrived feedlot cattle. J Am Vet Med Assoc 1998;212:1919–24.
26. Galyean ML, Gunter SA, Malcolm-Callis KJ. Effects of arrival medication with tilmicosin phosphate on health and performance of newly received beef cattle. J Anim Sci 1995;73(5):1219–26.
27. Dietz K. The estimation of the basic reproduction number for infectious diseases. Stat Methods Med Res 1993;2(1):23–41.
28. Frank GH, Duff GC. Effects of tilmicosin phosphate, administered prior to transport or at time of arrival, and feeding of chlortetracycline, after arrival in a feedlot, on Mannheimia haemolytica in nasal secretions of transported steers. Am J Vet Res 2000;61(12):1479–83.
29. Pollreisz JH, Bechtol DT, Upson DW. Problems and practice in mass medication of beef cattle. Vet Clin North Am Food Anim Pract 1991;7(3):659–68.
30. Ribble CS, Meek AH, Janzen ED, et al. Effect of time of year, weather, and the pattern of auction market sales on fatal fibrinous pneumonia (shipping fever) in

calves in a large feedlot in Alberta (1985–1988). Can J Vet Res 1995;59(3): 167–72.

31. Smith RA, Stokka GL, Radostits OM, et al. Herd health: food animal production medicine. In: Radostits OM, editor. Health and production management in beef feedlots. 3rd edition. Philadelphia: WB Saunders Company; 2001. p. 592–5.

32. Sanderson MW, Dargatz DA, Wagner B. Risk factors for initial respiratory disease in United States' feedlots based on producer-collected daily morbiity counts. Can Vet J 2008;49:373–8.

33. Ribble CS, Meek AH, Shewen PE, et al. Effect of pretransit mixing on fatal fibrinous pneumonia in calves. J Am Vet Med Assoc 1995;207(5):616–9.

34. Snowder GD. Bovine respiratory disease in feedlot cattle: environmental, genetic, and economic factors. J Anim Sci 2006;84:1999–2008.

35. Loneragan GH. Feedlot mortalities: epidemiology, trends, classification. In: Academy of Veterinary Consultants Summer Meeting. Colorado Springs (CO), August 1–3, 2004. p. 34.

36. White BJ, McReynolds S, Goehl DR, et al. Effect of vaccination and weaning timing on backgrounding morbidity in preconditioned beef feeder calves. Bov Pract 2008;42(2):1–5.

37. APHIS, editor. USDA. Part III: health management and biosecurity in U.S. feedlots, 1999. Fort Collins (CO): National Health Monitoring System; 2000. p. 1–50.

38. White BJ, Blasi D, Vogel LC, et al. Associations of beef calf wellness and body weight gain with internal location in a truck during transportation. J Anim Sci 2009;87(12):4143–50.

39. Corbin MJ, Griffin D. Assessing performance of feedlot operations using epidemiology. Vet Clin North Am Food Anim Pract 2006;22(1):35–51.

40. Edwards A. Respiratory diseases of feedlot cattle in central USA. Bov Pract 1996; 30:5–7.

41. Babcock AH, Renter D, White BJ. Defining temporal distributions of respiratory disease events within pens of feedlot cattle and evaluating associations with health and performance outcomes. In: International Society for Veterinary Epidemiology and Economics Conference. Durban, South Africa, August 10–14, 2009.

42. Babcock AH, White BJ, Dritz SS, et al. Feedlot health and performance effects associated with the timing of respiratory disease treatment. J Anim Sci 2009; 87:314–27.

43. McClary D, Vogel G. Effect of timing of tilmicosin metaphylaxis on control of bovine respiratory diseases and performance in feeder cattle. Bov Pract 1999; 33(2):155–62.

44. Duff GC, Walker DA, Malcolm-Callis KJ, et al. Effects of preshipping vs. arrival medication with tilmicosin phosphate and feeding chlortetracycline on health and performance of newly received beef cattle. J Anim Sci 2000; 78(2):267–74.

45. Bremer VR, Vander Pol KJ, Griffin D, et al. Evaluation of excede given at either initial processing or revaccination on bovine respiratory disease and pasture vs. feedlot receiving systems. In: Animal science Department Nebraska Beef Cattle reports. University of Nebraska-Lincoln; 2007. p. 68–70 [Online].

46. Kreikemeier K, Stokka G, Marston T. Influence of delayed processing and mass medication with either chlortetracycline (CTC) or tilmicosin phosphate (Micotil) on health and growth of highly stressed calves. In: Proceedings of Kansas State University Cattle Feeders Day, 1996. p. 23.

47. Thomson DU, White BJ. Backgrounding beef cattle. Vet Clin North Am Food Anim Pract 2006;22(2):373–98.

48. Encinias AM, Walker DA, Murdock CW, et al. Effects of prophylactic administration of ceftiofur crystalline free acid on health and performance of newly received beef calves. Proc Western Section American Society of Animal Science 2006;57: 160–3.
49. Gallo GF, Berg JL. Efficacy of a feed-additive antibacterial combination for improving feedlot cattle performance and health. Can Vet J 1995;36(4):223–9.
50. Guthrie CA, Rogers KC, Christmas RA, et al. Efficacy of metaphylactic tilmicosin for controlling bovine respiratory disease in high-risk northern feeder calves. Bov Pract 2004;38(1):46–53.
51. Schumann FJ, Janzen ED, McKinnon JJ. Prophylactic tilmicosin medication of feedlot calves at arrival. Can Vet J 1990;31(4):285–8.
52. Schumann FJ, Janzen ED, McKinnon JJ. Prophylactic medication of feedlot calves with tilmicosin. Vet Rec 1991;128(12):278–80.
53. Morck DW, Merrill JK, Thorlakson BE, et al. Prophylactic efficacy of tilmicosin for bovine respiratory tract disease. J Am Vet Med Assoc 1993;202(2):273–7.
54. Van Donkersgoed J. Meta-analysis of field trials of antimicrobial mass medication for prophylaxis of bovine respiratory disease in feedlot cattle. Can Vet J 1992; 33(12):786–95.
55. Wileman BW, Thomson DU, Reinhardt CD, et al. Analysis of modern technologies commonly used in beef cattle production: conventional beef production versus nonconventional production using meta-analysis. J Anim Sci 2009;87(10): 3418–26.
56. McNeill JW, Paschal JC, McNeill MS, et al. Effect of morbidity on performance and profitability of feedlot steers. J Anim Sci 1996;74(Suppl 1):135.
57. Benton JR, Erickson GA, Klopfenstein TJ, et al. Effect of excede administered to calves at arrival in the feedlot on perofrmance and respiratory disease. In: Animal science Department Nebraska beef cattle reports. University of Nebraska-Lincoln, 2008 [Online].
58. Hibbard B, Robb EJ, Chester ST Jr, et al. Dose determination and confirmation of a long-acting formulation of ceftiofur (ceftiofur crystalline free acid) administered subcutaneously for the treatment of bovine respiratory disease. J Vet Pharmacol Ther 2002;25(3):175–80.
59. Hibbard B, Robb EJ, Chester ST Jr, et al. Dose determination and confirmation for ceftiofur crystalline-free acid administered in the posterior aspect of the ear for control and treatment of bovine respiratory disease. Vet Ther 2002;3(1): 22–30.
60. Hibbard B, Robb EJ, Apley MD, et al. Feedlot performance of steers treated concurrently with ceftiofur crystalline-free acid subcutaneously in the posterior aspect of the ear and a growth-promoting implant. Vet Ther 2002;3(3):252–61.
61. Step DL, Engelken T, Romano C, et al. Evaluation of three antimicrobial regimens used as metaphylaxis in stocker calves at high risk of developing bovine respiratory disease. Vet Ther 2007;8(2):136–47.
62. King NB, Edgington BH, Ferguson LC, et al. Preliminary results in the control and treatment of shipping fever complex in beef cattle. J Am Vet Med Assoc 1955; 127(943):320–3.
63. Bennett BW, Rupp GP, McCormick RM. Pre-shipment preventive medication of calves with liquamycin at weaning. Agri Pract 1983;4(6):6–10.
64. Perry TW, Beeson WM, Mohler MT, et al. Value of chlortetracycline and sulfamethazine for conditioning feeder cattle after transit. J Anim Sci 1971;32(1):137–40.
65. Lofgreen GP. Mass medication in reducing shipping fever-bovine respiratory disease complex in highly stressed calves. J Anim Sci 1983;56(3):529–36.

66. Lofgreen GP, Stinocher LH, Kiesling HE. Effects of dietary energy, free choice alfalfa hay and mass medication on calves subjected to marketing and shipping stresses. J Anim Sci 1980;50(4):590–6.
67. Gill DR, Smith RA, Hicks RB, et al. The effect of mass medication on health and performance of newly arrived stocker cattle. In: Animal science research report. Oklahoma Agricultural Experiment Station; 1986. p. 260–8.
68. Buhman MJ, Perino LJ, Galyean ML, et al. Association between changes in eating and drinking behaviors and respiratory tract disease in newly arrived calves at a feedlot. Am J Vet Res 2000;61(10):1163–8.
69. Wallace J. Concurrent metaphylaxis with chlortetracycline and tulathromycin on high-risk calves has no additive effects on cattle health and performance. In: Kansas State University Cattlemen's Day Report. Manhattan (KS), 2009. p. 5 [Online].
70. Frank GH, Briggs RE, Duff GC, et al. Effects of vaccination prior to transit and administration of florfenicol at time of arrival in a feedlot on the health of transported calves and detection of *Mannheimia haemolytica* in nasal secretions. Am J Vet Res 2002;63(2):251–6.
71. Peters AR. Use of a long-acting oxytetracycline preparation in respiratory disease in young beef bulls. Vet Rec 1985;116(12):321.
72. Janzen ED. Observations on the use of a long-acting oxytetracycline for in-contact prophylaxis of undifferentiated bovine respiratory disease in feedlot steers under Canadian conditions. Bov Pract 1980;15:87–90.
73. Tetradure 300 (oxytetracycline) injection. Product information. In: Federal Drug Administration: Merial, Ltd.
74. Micotil 300 injection (tilmicosin injection). Product information. In: Federal Drug Administration: Elanco Animal Health.
75. Draxxin (tulathromycin) injectable solution. Product information. In: Federal Drug Administration: Pfizer Animal Health.
76. Nowakowski MA, Inskeep PB, Risk JE, et al. Pharmacokinetics and lung tissue concentrations of tulathromycin, a new triamilide antibiotic, in cattle. Vet Ther 2004;5(1):60–74.
77. Kilgore WR, Spensley MS, Sun F, et al. Clinical effectiveness of tulathromycin, a novel triamilide antimicrobial, for the control of respiratory disease in cattle at high risk for developing bovine respiratory disease. Vet Ther 2005;6(2):136–42.
78. Godinho KS, Wolf RM, Sherington J, et al. Efficacy of tulathromycin in the treatment and prevention of natural outbreaks of bovine respiratory disease in European cattle. Vet Ther 2005;6(2):122–35.

Bovine Herpesvirus Type 1 (BHV-1) is an Important Cofactor in the Bovine Respiratory Disease Complex

Clinton Jones, PhD[a],*, Shafiqul Chowdhury, DVM, PhD[b]

KEYWORDS

- Bovine herpesvirus 1
- Bovine respiratory disease complex (BRDC) • Shipping fever
- Immune suppression • Latency • Vaccines

Infection of cattle by bovine herpesvirus 1 (BHV-1) can lead to upper respiratory tract disorders, conjunctivitis, genital disorders, and immune suppression. BHV-1–induced immune suppression initiates bovine respiratory disease complex (BRDC), which costs the US cattle industry more that a billion dollars each year. In addition, BHV-1 is an emerging virus in buffalo. The ability of BHV-1 to inhibit immune responses is crucial for the ability of BHV-1 to induce BRDC. BHV-1 encodes at least 3 proteins that can inhibit specific arms of the immune system: (1) the UL49.5 protein, (2) bICP0, and (3) glycoprotein G. Furthermore, BHV-1 can infect and induce high levels of apoptosis of CD4+ T cells, which also inhibit an efficient immune response. Following acute infection, BHV-1 establishes latency in sensory neurons of trigeminal ganglia (TG), and germinal centers of pharyngeal tonsil. Periodically BHV-1 reactivates from latency, virus is shed, and consequently virus transmission occurs. The latency-related gene is abundantly expressed in sensory neurons during latency and expression of a protein encoded by the latency-related gene is necessary for the

The laboratory of CJ is supported by 2 USDA grants (08-00891 and 09-01653), and, in part, a Public Health Service grant (1P20RR15635) to the Nebraska Center for Virology. The laboratory of SC is supported by 2 USDA grants (07-35204-05420 and 09-35204-05200).

[a] School of Veterinary and Biomedical Sciences, Nebraska Center for Virology, University of Nebraska, Lincoln, Fair Street at East Campus Loop, Lincoln, NE 68583-0905, USA
[b] Department of Pathobiological Sciences, School of Veterinary Medicine, Louisiana State University, Baton Rouge, LA 70803, USA
* Corresponding author.
E-mail address: cjones@unlnotes.unl.edu

latency-reactivation cycle. The ability of BHV-1 to enter permissive cells, infect sensory neurons, and promote virus spread from sensory neurons to mucosal surfaces following reactivation from latency is also regulated by several viral glycoproteins. BHV-1 modified live vaccines can be immunosuppressive as well as establish and reactivate from latency, which indicates that these strains can lead to BRDC in feedlots or cow-calf operations. This review summarizes the role that BHV-1 plays in BRDC.

DISEASE AND CLINICAL SIGNS INDUCED BY BHV-1

Bovine herpesvirus 1 (BHV-1) is an α-herpesvirinae subfamily member that causes significant economic losses to the cattle industry.[1] Three BHV-1 subtypes, BHV-1.1 (1), BHV-1.2a (2a), and BHV-1.2b (2b), have been identified based on antigenic and genomic analysis.[2] Subtype 1 virus isolates are the causative agent of infectious bovine rhinotracheitis (IBR), and are frequently found in the respiratory tract as well as in aborted fetuses. Subtype 1 strains are prevalent in Europe, North America, and South America. Subtype 2a is frequently associated with a broad range of clinical manifestations in the respiratory and genital tracts, such as IBR, infectious pustular vulvovaginitis (IPV), balanoposthitis (IPB), and abortions.[3] Subtype 2a is prevalent in Brazil, and was present in Europe before the 1970s.[3] Subtype 2b strains are associated with respiratory disease and IPV/IPB, but not abortion.[3,4] Subtype 2b strains are less pathogenic than subtype 1, and are frequently isolated in Australia or Europe, but not Brazil.[5]

In feedlot cattle, the respiratory form of BHV-1 is the most common (subtype 1 strains). In breeding cattle, abortions or genital infections tend to be more common. Genital infections can occur in bulls (IPB) and cows (IPV) within 1 to 3 days of mating or close contact with an infected animal. Transmission can also occur in the absence of visible lesions and through artificial insemination with semen from subclinically infected bulls.

The incubation period for the respiratory and genital forms of BHV-1 is 2 to 6 days.[6] Clinical signs of respiratory disease include high fever, anorexia, coughing, excessive salivation, nasal discharge, and conjunctivitis with lacrimal discharge, inflamed nares, and dyspneae if the larynx becomes occluded with purulent material. Nasal lesions consist of numerous clusters of grayish necrotic foci on the mucous membrane of septal mucosa. In the absence of bacterial pneumonia, recovery typically occurs 4 to 5 days after the onset of clinical signs. Abortions can occur at the same time as respiratory disease, but are also seen up to 100 days after infection, presumably the result of reactivation from latency.

With respect to genital infections, the first clinical signs are frequent urination, and a mild vaginal infection.[6] It is also common to observe swollen vulva or small papules followed by erosions and ulcers on the mucosal surface. In bulls, similar lesions occur on the penis and prepuce. If secondary bacterial infections occur, there may be inflammation of the uterus and transient infertility with purulent vaginal discharge for several weeks. In the absence of bacterial infections, animals usually recover within 2 weeks after infection. Regardless of the involvement of secondary bacterial infection, BHV-1 establishes lifelong latency following acute infection. Serologic testing and removal of infected animals has been used to eliminate BHV-1 from Austria, Denmark, and Switzerland.[7] In these countries, cattle populations are small and movement of cattle can be controlled. In the United States and many other countries, eradication will be difficult, perhaps impossible, and expensive.

BHV-1 IS AN EMERGING DISEASE IN BUFFALO

The seroprevalence of BHV-1 in bison raised on a ranch is 43.8%,[8] indicating that infection can readily occur in bison. Other studies have also found that BHV-1 is frequently present in buffalo in India.[9,10] BHV-1 can presumably be transmitted from buffalo to cattle and vice versa. Because more buffalo meat is being consumed each year in the United States and other nations, BHV-1 infections are having an effect on the emerging bison industry. It is not clear what the percentage of seropositive animals is due to vaccination or infection with virulent field strains. It is also not well established whether BHV-1 can be readily reactivated from latency in buffalo, as in cattle. It is clear that BHV-1 is widely disseminated in buffalo herds, suggesting that BHV-1 could induce BRDC in buffalo.

RELATIONSHIP BETWEEN BHV-1 AND BRDC

BRDC, also known as shipping fever, costs the US cattle industry at least $1 billion/y.[11–13] In addition to the clinical signs described earlier for BHV-1, BHV-1 can initiate BRDC by transiently suppressing the immune system of infected cattle.[6] BHV-1–induced immune suppression leads to secondary bacterial infections (eg, *Pasteurella haemolytica*, *Pasteurella multocida*, and *Histophilus somni*) that can cause pneumonia.[6] Increased susceptibility to secondary infection correlates with depressed cell-mediated immunity after BHV-1 infection.[14–17] CD8+ T cell recognition of infected cells is impaired by repressing expression of major histocompatibility complex class I and the transporter associated with antigen presentation.[18–20] CD4+ T cell function is impaired during acute infection of calves because BHV-1 infects CD4+ T cells and induces apoptosis.[21] Viral genes (UL49.5, bICP0, and gG) can inhibit specific immune responses in the absence of other viral genes. The ability of bICP0 to inhibit interferon (IFN)-dependent transcription is crucial for pathogenesis because BHV-1 does not grow in mice unless they lack IFN receptors.[22] The known viral genes that inhibit immune responses are discussed later.

UL49.5

The BHV-1 gene encoding the UL49.5 open reading frame (ORF), also known as glycoprotein N (gN), is present in the unique long region of the genome (**Fig. 1**). The UL49.5 ORF encodes a 96 amino acid protein with an apparent molecular mass of

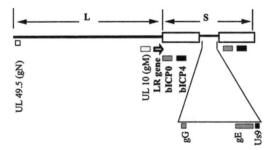

Fig. 1. Specific genes within the BHV-1 genome, showing the location of viral genes within the genome (bICP0, bICP4, gG, gE, Us9, UL49.5, UL10, and the latency related [LR] gene). The unique long (L) and unique short (S) regions of the genome are shown. The repeats are denoted by open rectangles. The bICP0 and bICP4 genes are in the repeats, and are thus present in 2 copies within the BHV-1 genome.

9 kDa.[23] The UL49.5 ORF contains a signal peptide (N terminal 22 amino acids), an extracellular domain of 32 amino acids, a transmembrane region of 25 amino acids, and a 17-amino-acid cytoplasmic tail.[23] The UL49.5 protein is expressed as a nonglycosylated type I membrane protein.[23,24]

All gN herpesvirus orthologs studied to date form complexes with glycoprotein M (gM), which is encoded by the UL10 ORF (see **Fig. 1** for location of gM).[25–27] gM is important for secondary envelopment because, in pseudorabies virus (PRV), secondary envelopment in the Golgi and subsequent egress requires gM, in the absence of gE.[28] The gN homologs encoded by PRV and BHV-1 inhibit transporter-associated antigen processing (TAP)–mediated transport of cytosolic peptides into ER, which consequently blocks the assembly of peptide-containing ternary major histocompatibility complex (MHC)-I complexes in vitro in virus-infected cells.[29,30] Furthermore, the BHV-1 gN targets the TAP complex for proteosomal degradation.[29] The TAP complex consists of a TAP1/TAP2 heterodimer, both of which are members of the ATP-binding cassette transporter superfamily.[31–33]

Peptide transport by TAP is a critical step in MHC class I antigen presentation.[29,34–36] In the absence of a functional TAP transporter, most MHC class I molecules are not loaded with peptides.[36] However, they are retained within the ER and ultimately directed for degradation by the proteasome.[36] Structurally, gM and TAPs are similar because they contain multiple membrane-spanning segments.[25,32] A gN mutant that lacks the cytoplasmic tail can still bind to the TAP complex and block peptide transport, but this mutant gN protein does not degrade TAP.[29] Recent results in our laboratory (Chowdhury, unpublished data) and others (Wiertz and colleagues) suggest that sequences within the gN luminal domain bind to TAP and block its peptide transport function. The ability of gN to inhibit TAP is hypothesized to prevent virus-infected cells from being killed by CD8+ T cells. Therefore, virulent field strains and modified live vaccine (MLV) viruses containing the intact gN will transiently immune suppress infected calves.

The bICP0 Protein Activates Viral Gene Expression and Inhibits the IFN Signaling Pathway

The bICP0 protein is the major transcriptional regulatory protein because it activates expression of all viral promoters,[37] and bICP0 mRNA is constitutively expressed during productive infection.[38] bICP0 contains a well-conserved C_3HC_4 zinc RING finger near its amino-terminus. Disruption of the bICP0 zinc RING finger prevents transactivation of a simple viral promoter,[39] and impairs the ability of bICP0 to simulate plaque formation.[40,41] The bICP0 protein also contains 2 transcriptional activation domains and a nuclear localization signal that is important for efficient transcriptional activation.[39] Unlike most transcription factors, bICP0 does not seem to directly bind to specific DNA sequences. However, bICP0 associates with chromatin remodeling enzymes,[42,43] suggesting that these interactions are necessary for activating viral transcription.

In the absence of other viral genes, bICP0 inhibits IFN signaling[44] by directly or indirectly reducing IFN regulatory factor 3 (IRF3) protein levels in human or bovine cells (**Fig. 2**).[45] In addition, bICP0 inhibits the ability of IRF7 to activate IFN-β promoter activity, but does not reduce IRF7 protein levels.[45] The C_3HC_4 zinc RING finger of bICP0[46] is an E3 ubiquitin ligase, suggesting that bICP0 degrades IRF3. IRF3 activation is an immediate early (IE) regulator of the IFN response (see **Fig. 1**), indicating that the ability of bICP0 to induce IRF3 degradation is important.[47–49]

Because IRF7 is more important to inhibiting viral infection when IRF3 versus IRF7 knockout mice are compared,[50] additional studies were performed to understand how

A IFN induction following virus infection

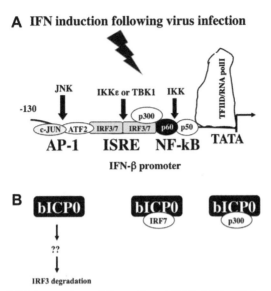

IFN-β promoter

Fig. 2. Activation of IFN-β promoter activity and how bICP0 inhibits IFN-β promoter activity. (*A*) The human IFN-β promoter necessary for inducing an IFN response to virus infection,[129–131] giving a summary of the signaling pathways that induce IFN-β promoter activity.[47,132–141] The IFN-β promoter contains 3 distinct transcription factor–binding sites, AP-1, the IFN response element (ISRE), and nuclear factor (NF)-κB. These transcription factor–binding sites are necessary for induction of the IFN response following virus infection. Induction of toll-like receptors can activate IRF3 and the transcription factor NF-κB, and consequently the IFN-β promoter is activated. Following virus infection, 2 cellular protein kinases, IKK-ε or TBK-1, phosphorylate serine residues at the C terminus of IRF3, which induces IRF3 homodimerization and nuclear translocation. Nuclear IRF3 associates with other transcriptional activators, resulting in direct binding and stimulation of IFN-β promoter activity. IRF3 also directly binds several consensus DNA-binding sites, including ISRE (IFN response elements), which stimulates transcription of IFN-stimulated genes in the absence of IFN. (*B*) The known steps by which bICP0 inhibits IFN-β promoter activity. For details, see text.

bICP0 inhibits the ability of IRF7 to transactivate the IFN-β promoter. bICP0 interacts with IRF7 or a complex containing IRF7,[51] and this interaction correlates with the ability of bICP0 to inhibit the ability of IRF7 to transactivate IFN-β promoter activity (see **Fig. 2B**). The ability of bICP0 to interact with a chromatin remodeling enzyme (p300- or p300-containing complexes)[43] may also interfere with IFN-β promoter activity because p300 is crucial for stimulating IFN-β promoter activity.

The Envelope Glycoprotein gG Interacts with Chemokines

BHV-1, BHV-5, and equine herpesvirus 1 encode glycoprotein G (gG) (see **Fig. 1** for location of gG), which is secreted from infected cells and can bind to a broad range of chemokines.[52] Chemokines are small proteins (8–10 kDa) that function as cytokines, and thus regulate trafficking and effector functions of leukocytes.[53] As such, chemokines are important regulators of inflammation and immune surveillance, and they have potent antiviral functions. Functionally, chemokines are divided into 2 groups: proinflammatory chemokines, which are inducible, and housekeeping chemokines, which are constitutively expressed. Activation of chemokine functions is dependent on selective recognition and activation of chemokine receptors.

Interactions between gG and chemokines block chemokine activity by preventing their interactions with specific receptors. Consequently, gG disrupts chemokine gradients, which control the local environment surrounding an infected cell. A BHV-1 gG deletion mutant was reported to have reduced virulence,[54] suggesting gG is a viral immune evasion gene. However, the exact role of gG in virulence requires additional studies because the gG mutant that was examined was not rescued, and expression of surrounding genes was not examined.

BHV-1 Infection Triggers Cytokine Expression that Increases the Detrimental Effect of Mannheimia haemolytica Leukotoxin

As noted earlier, respiratory infection with BHV-1 predisposes cattle to secondary bacterial pneumonia due to infections or colonization by bacteria including *Mannheimia haemolytica*. *M haemolytica* leukotoxin is the major factor that contributes to lung injury in bovine pneumonic pasteurellosis.[55] A recent study concluded that BHV-1 infection of bovine bronchial epithelial cells triggers cytokine expression, which subsequently promotes neutrophil recruitment to the lung.[56] As a result, the detrimental effects of *M haemolytica* leukotoxin are amplified.

IMMUNE RESPONSE TO BHV-1 FOLLOWING ACUTE INFECTION

Although BHV-1 can cause transient immunosuppression in cattle, a potent immune response eventually occurs during acute infection, which prevents systemic infection. With respect to BRDC, this implies that immunosuppression initiated by BHV-1 is short-lived.

The host immune response to BHV-1 infection includes innate and adaptive immune responses.[57] Innate immune responses include the antiviral action of IFN, alternative complement pathway, and local infiltration of lymphoid cells, macrophages, neutrophils, or natural killer (NK) cells, for example. Following BHV-1 infection, IFN-α and IFN-β are detectable in nasal secretions as little as 5 hours after infection, reaches a maximum level at 72 to 96 hours after infection, and can persist for up to 8 days after infection.[58] Soon after infection, IFN-α and IFN-β promote leukocyte migration, activate macrophages, and increase NK cell activity.[59–61] Activation of macrophages and increasing NK cell activity stimulates cytolytic activities against virus-infected cells.[57] NK cells are a diverse population of nonadherent effecter cells that lack T and B cell markers.[62] These cells require a long incubation period with the target cell for optimum lysis.[63] In addition, NK-like cytotoxicity is also associated with a population of CD3+ CD45+, Fc receptor-positive lymphocytes, which may represent a subset of γδ T cells.[64]

Adaptive or humoral immune responses lead to production of neutralizing antibodies that bind virus particles and inhibit productive infection. Envelope glycoproteins gB, gC, gD, and gH are the most potent inducers of virus-neutralizing antibodies.[65,66] Non-neutralizing antibody may also mediate the destruction of enveloped virus or cells expressing viral proteins on the cell membranes, and this process is referred to as antibody-mediated cell cytotoxcity.[67] Neutralizing and non-neutralizing antibodies produced against envelope proteins can inhibit virus infection by several distinct mechanisms: (1) membrane attack complex lysis of virus envelope and virus-infected cells mediated by antibody and complement, and (2) antibody-mediated cell cytotoxcity in which IgG interacts with Fc receptor–positive cells (macrophages), or (3) binding of C3b to IgM mediates binding to C3b receptor–positive cells (lymphocytes, macrophages). In all cases, virus-infected cells are lysed.[57,68–71] Production of virus-neutralizing and non-neutralizing antibodies (IgG) can be detected

8 to 12 days after infection.[57] Local/mucosal immunity depends on secreted neutralizing antibodies (IgA molecules) and systemic humoral immunity depends on IgG.

Cell-mediated immune (CMI) responses play an important role in killing virus-infected cells that express viral antigens on the cell surface.[72] A CD8+ cytotoxic T-lymphocyte (CTL) response is an important defense against BHV-1 because cell-to-cell spread in upper respiratory epithelium occurs before hematogenous spread.[72] Cytotoxic and proliferative T-lymphocyte responses are detected in circulating blood approximately 8 days after infection. CTL responses are induced by gB and gD DNA vaccines in mice.[73,74] gC and gD have been identified as targets for CTL responses in cattle,[75] and gB DNA vaccines elicit a CTL response in cattle.[74] Other structural and nonstructural viral proteins may also play a role in CMI response because only a limited number of BHV-1 proteins have been evaluated for CTL activity.[72] In addition to destruction of infected cells, T lymphocytes release several lymphokines that modulate specific and nonspecific immune responses. For example, IFN-γ and other factors that further activate macrophages[76] are produced. BHV-1 proteins (gB-, gC-, gD-, and VP8) are recognized by CD4+ T helper cells from immune cattle.[77] Cells expressing gB, gC, or gD on their membranes have also been identified as targets for CD4+ T cells.[78,79] CD4+ T cells are important for the development of antibody response and for developing effective CD8+ T-cell memory.[80,81] Thus, CD4+ T cells, CD8+ T cells, and antibodies are required for long-term protection.

THE BHV-1 LATENCY-REACTIVATION CYCLE OF BHV-1
Acute Infection Leads to High Levels of Virus Production

BRDC is not necessarily associated with acute BHV-1 infection. Although this clearly indicates that additional cofactors exist for developing BRDC, the ability of BHV-1 to reactivate from latency can also induce BRDC. Thus, the latency-reactivation cycle complicates the control of BRDC.

Acute BHV-1 infection is initiated on mucosal surfaces and results in high levels of programmed cell death.[21] Infection of permissive cells[82] with BHV-1 also leads to rapid cell death, in part due to apoptosis. Viral gene expression is temporally regulated in 3 distinct phases: IE, early (E), or late (L). IE gene expression is stimulated by a virion component, α-TIF.[83] Two IE transcription units exist: IE transcription unit 1 (IEtu1) and IEtu2 (see **Fig. 1A**). IEtu1 encodes 2 proteins, bICP0 and bICP4, which are activators of transcription. IEtu2 encodes a protein called bICP22. In general, IE proteins activate E gene expression, and then viral DNA replication occurs. L gene expression is also activated by bICP0, culminating in virion assembly and release. As discussed earlier, bICP0 is important for productive infection because it transcriptionally activates all viral promoters, and is expressed at high levels throughout infection.[38,84,85] Acute infection leads to high levels of virus production and secretion in ocular, oral, or nasal cavities. If acute infection is initiated in the genital tract, virus shedding can be readily detected in genital tissues. Regardless of the site of infection, virus shedding lasts for 7 to 10 days after infection.[86,87]

Summary of the Latency-Reactivation Cycle in Cattle

Viral particles enter the peripheral nervous system via cell-to-cell spread. If infection is initiated via the oral cavity, nasal cavity, or ocular orifice, the primary site for latency is sensory neurons within trigeminal ganglia (TG). High levels of viral gene expression[88] or infectious virus[89] are detected in TG from 1 to 6 days after infection (**Fig. 3** gives a summary of the latency-reactivation cycle of BHV-1). Viral gene expression and detection of infectious virus is subsequently extinguished, but viral genomes are

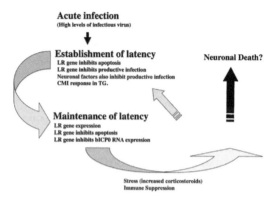

Fig. 3. Summary of BHV-1 latency-reactivation cycle. For details, see text.

detected in TG (establishment of latency). In contrast to productive infection in cultured cells, a significant number of infected neurons survive, and these neurons harbor latent genomes. A hallmark of latency is the abundant level of transcription that occurs from the latency-related (LR) gene.[86,87,90] It seems that the LR transcript is the first viral transcript expressed in infected neurons,[91] suggesting that LR gene products play a pivotal role in programming the outcome of virus infection in sensory neurons. Support for this prediction comes from the finding that LR gene products promote establishment of latency by inhibiting apoptosis[92,93] and viral gene expression.[94,95] During maintenance of latency, infectious virus is not detected using standard virological methods, but the LR gene is abundantly expressed.

Increased corticosteroid levels (stress) or immune suppression can initiate reactivation from latency. The stress associated with moving cattle from one location to another is an obvious stimulus that can trigger reactivation from latency and BRDC. During reactivation from latency, 3 significant events occur: (1) productive viral gene expression is readily detected in sensory neurons, (2) LR gene expression decreases, and (3) infectious virus is secreted from ocular and nasal cavities.[86,87,90] Administration of dexamethasone to calves or rabbits latently infected with BHV-1 reproducibly leads to activation of viral gene expression and reactivation from latency.[86,87,89,90,96,97] Although many latently infected neurons do not produce infectious virus, higher numbers of neurons express lytic viral genes,[97] indicating that virus-producing neurons are rare. For a summary of the steps involved in the latency-reactivation cycle, see **Fig. 3**.

Non-Neural Sites of Latency Persistence in Cattle

Although establishment of latency in ganglionic neurons is the main site of BHV-1 latency, viral DNA is present in tonsils,[98] peripheral blood cells,[99] lymph nodes, and spleen of latently infected calves, even when infectious virus is not detected.[100] PRV,[101,102] equine herpesvirus type 4,[103] and canine herpesvirus type 1[104] DNA are also detected in lymphoid tissue during latency. It is not yet known which non-neural cell types are latently infected with BHV-1, and whether viral genes are expressed in these latently infected cells. In contrast to latency in sensory neurons, LR-RNA is not abundantly expressed in latently infected lymphoid tissue.[98] Infectious virus can be detected when germinal centers from tonsil of latently infected calves are explanted,[105] adding support to the concept that BHV-1 establishes a latent or persistent infection in cells of lymphoid origin.

Proteins Encoded by the LR Gene are Necessary for the Latency-Reactivation Cycle

As discussed earlier, LR-RNA is abundantly transcribed in latently infected neurons,[97,106,107] and is antisense relative to the bICP0 gene. The LR gene has 2 ORFs (ORF1 and ORF2). A peptide antibody directed against ORF2 recognizes a protein encoded by the LR gene.[108–110] LR gene products inhibit cell proliferation, bICP0 RNA expression,[94,95,111] and apoptosis.[92] LR protein expression (ORF2) is necessary for inhibiting apoptosis,[92,112] but not cell growth[113] or bICP0 expression.[94,95,111]

A mutant BHV-1 strain with 3 stop codons at the N terminus of ORF2[114] does not express ORF2 following infection of bovine cells.[109] Calves infected with the LR mutant virus exhibit diminished clinical signs and reduced shedding of infectious virus from the eye, TG, or tonsil.[89,105,114] The LR mutant virus does not reactivate from latency following treatment with dexamethasone, whereas all calves latently infected with wild-type virus or the LR rescued virus shed infectious virus following dexamethasone treatment.[89] Thus, expression of wild-type LR gene products is necessary for the latency-reactivation cycle in calves. The authors believe that LR gene products, including LR proteins, directly regulate the establishment and maintenance of latency. It seems unlikely that LR gene products directly stimulate reactivation from latency because dexamethasone reduces LR-RNA levels.[97] LR gene products are predicted to promote neuronal survival following infection, thus increasing the number of neurons that can support reactivation for latency.

BHV-1 VACCINES

Many commercially available vaccines directed against BHV-1 can cause disease in small calves, partly because these vaccines are immunosuppressive. Consequently, certain vaccines have the potential to induce BRDC in small calves. The current status of BHV-1 vaccines and how they can be improved are discussed in the following paragraphs.

Commercially Available Vaccines

Commercially available vaccines directed against BHV-1 consist of an MLV or killed whole virus (KV).[115] In many cases MLVs are attenuated by serial passage in tissue culture. KV vaccines are usually produced by chemical treatments, such as formaldehyde, β-propiolactone, or binary ethyleneimine. MLVs generally induce humoral and cellular immune response because virus replication in infected cells leads to presentation of viral antigen on MHC class I$^+$ and II$^+$ molecules. Safety is a concern for MLVs because these strains can establish latency and, on reactivation from latency, can be transmitted to pregnant cows, which can lead to abortion. MLVs can also be pathogenic in small calves because their immune systems are not fully developed, and most MLVs can be immunosuppressive. KV vaccines are usually safe but they are not as efficacious because they usually produce only humoral immunity but no cellular immune responses. In addition, KV vaccines always require more than 1 injection to achieve acceptable neutralizing antibody levels. In the case of formaldehyde-inactivated KV, antigens may also be denatured, which may affect the immunogenicity of vaccine preparations. KV also requires suitable adjuvant formulations, and some adjuvants may induce injection-site reactions.

Commercially available BHV-1 vaccines are primarily evaluated on induction of neutralizing antibodies and the duration, as well as the level of virus shedding following challenge of vaccinated animals. As discussed earlier, the CMI response against the virus is important to prevent cell-to-cell spread of the virus. Therefore, a direct measure of CMI directed against a vaccine virus is important. Traditionally, IFN-γ levels in vaccinated calves have been an indicator of cellular immune responses. However, a recent study found that there is an increase in CD25 by CD4+, CD8+, and γδT lymphocytes from a BHV-1 MLV-vaccinated group.[116] Therefore, increased expression of CD25, in addition to IFN-γ production by T cells after vaccination, seems to be a useful cellular immunity marker.[72]

Development of Genetically Engineered Gene-Deleted BHV-1 Vaccines

During the last 10 to 15 years, the usefulness of genetically engineered gene-deleted vaccines has become increasingly apparent because they can be attenuated and serologically distinguished from wild-type field strains.[115] Numerous viral mutants (gC-, gE-, gG-, and Us9-deleted;[54,117,118] thymidine kinase [TK]–deleted;[119,120] and LR gene mutant virus[89]) have been constructed and their in vivo pathogenic properties, reactivation properties, and immunogenicity analyzed. Based on recent studies, gE- and Us9-deleted viruses were safe in calves because they do not reactivate from latency and they are highly attenuated (see Fig. 1 for location of gE and Us9 genes).[54,117,118,121,122] Studies with gC, gG, or TK-deleted viruses showed that they reactivate from latency or they retain some degree of virulence.[54,120,121] Studies with an LR mutant virus showed that the virus does not reactivate from latency and has reduced pathogenicity in calves.[89] Therefore, considering the virulence and reactivation properties of gene-deleted vaccine strains, gE, Us9-deleted, or the LR mutant virus have the potential to be safer vaccine candidates. Comparative vaccine efficacy studies showed that, relative to gC- and gG-deleted viruses, gE-deleted virus is less efficacious.[54] However, the gE-deleted vaccine has been used successfully to eradicate IBR from several European countries. Although the gE-deleted marker vaccine is not as efficacious as others noted earlier, it will be used until a better genetically engineered vaccine is developed.

Recent efforts to improve the IBR marker vaccine are directed to deleting viral gene sequences that are immunosuppressive. As noted earlier, gN inhibits TAP and downregulates MHC-I antigen presentation. Therefore, a vaccine virus lacking the gN TAP-binding domain may stimulate better cellular immune responses. Our recent studies show that a gE cytoplasmic tail truncated virus is attenuated in calves infected with the virus similarly to the entire gE ORF-deleted virus. Notably, like the gE-deleted virus, the gE cytoplasmic tail truncated virus does not reactivate from latency.[122] Because the cytoplasmic tail–specific amino acid sequences generate antibodies that immunoprecipitate gE, antibodies specific to the cytoplasmic tail sequence may serve as serologic markers to distinguish vaccinated versus infected calves.[123,124] Furthermore, the Us9 gene is located immediately downstream of the gE cytoplasmic tail (see Fig. 1), so a recombinant BHV-1 can be constructed in which the gE cytoplasmic tail and the Us9 coding regions are deleted. A vaccine virus that lacks US9, the cytoplasmic tail of gE, and gN TAP-binding domain may be a superior vaccine candidate because (1) it should stimulate BHV-1–specific CMI responses more efficiently, (2) it will incorporate a serologic marker, and (3) it should not be pathogenic. Concerns have been raised about recombination occurring between 2 vaccine strains, which could lead to the presence of virulent viral strains in vaccinated herds.[125] Although it is clear that recombination can occur, the process requires that both viruses must replicate at the same time in the same cell of an infected calf.

Problems Associated with Current Modified Live BHV-1 Vaccines and BHV-1 Eradication Effort

There has recently been an apparent increase in IBR outbreaks in vaccinated feedlot cattle (commonly referred to as vaccine outbreaks).[126,127] Many of these vaccine outbreaks occur in feedlots that have used several different BHV-1 MLVs without sero-logic markers, suggesting that they are not vaccine specific. Because the vaccines used in the feedlots did not have any serologic marker, it is difficult to determine by serology whether an animal is infected with an MLV or field strain. It is also possible that recombination between MLV strains could lead to a virus with increased patho-genic potential. Thus, determining the source of origin from a particular vaccine break is not possible, nor is it possible to test whether these outbreaks were due to changes in the vaccine strain. The emergence of a new IBR strain that is not covered by existing MLVs would also lead to clinical outbreaks in herds in which vaccination has occurred. A study investigating several isolates from such outbreaks determined that at least 1 such isolate had mutations within sequences comprising the gD-specific neutralizing epitope.[127]

In several European countries (Austria, Denmark, Finland, Norway, Sweden, Switzerland), IBR has presumably been eradicated by the use of gE marker vaccines. In these countries, until recently, cattle were no longer vaccinated against IBR (see later discussion). In several other EU countries, including Germany, The Netherlands, and the United Kingdom, the same strategy has been in use to eradicate the disease. However, IBR-free status for these countries has not yet been possible. Recently, new IBR cases have been recorded in several supposedly IBR-free countries. One such outbreak in Switzerland was tracked back to the importation of latently infected animals.[128] Previously, importation of BHV-1–positive semen was shown to be the cause of IBR outbreaks.[128]

Because the severity of IBR disease in immunologically naïve animals is more pronounced, outbreak of a virulent IBR could have severe consequences. Therefore, IBR-free countries are endangered as long as IBR eradication is not a common goal within countries that are involved in cattle trade and production of semen for artificial insemination. Currently, in these countries, vaccination with gE-deleted marker vaccine is again being allowed. Identification and characterization of the new isolates by a clustering system using DNA restriction profiles with HpaI, HindIII, SfiI, and PstI are being pursued. Strict import regulation, regular immunologic surveillance, tracing the source of an IBR outbreak, and a continued vaccine program will be necessary to control the disease.

SUMMARY

BRDC is the primary disease of cattle in the United States. Although it is recognized as being a multifactorial disorder, BHV-1 is known to play an important role in BRDC. The ability of BHV-1 to inhibit the immune system plays a role in allowing opportunistic bacterial infections to induce clinical disease. Furthermore, the tissue damage caused by BHV-1 acute infection also makes it possible for bacterial infections to spread throughout the upper respiratory tract. The ability of BHV-1 to establish a latent infec-tion in sensory neurons confounds treatment of BHV-1 related diseases. Development of vaccine strains that are not immunosuppressive and do not reactivate from latency would help to eliminate the clinical disorders caused directly and indirectly by BHV-1.

REFERENCES

1. Turin L, Russo S, Poli G. BHV-1: new molecular approaches to control a common and widespread infection. Mol Med 1999;5:261–84.
2. Metzler AE, Matile H, Gasman U, et al. European isolates of bovine herpesvirus 1: a comparison of restriction endonuclease sites, polypeptides and reactivity with monoclonal antibodies. Arch Virol 1985;85:57–69.

3. van Oirschot JT. Bovine herpesvirus in semen of bulls and the risk of transmission: a brief overview. Vet Q 1995;17:29–33.
4. D'Arce RCF, Almedia RS, Silva TC, et al. Restriction endonucleases and monoclonal antibody analysis of Brazilian isolates of bovine herpesvirus 1 and 5. Vet Microbiol 2002;88:315–34.
5. Edwards S, White H, Nixon P. A study of the predominant genotypes of bovine herpesvirus 1 isolated in the U.K. Vet Microbiol 1990;22:213–23.
6. Yates WD. A review of infectious bovine rhinotracheitis, shipping fever pneumonia, and viral-bacterial synergism in respiratory disease of cattle. Can J Comp Med 1982;46:225–63.
7. Ackermann M, Engels M. Pro and contra IBR-eradication. Vet Microbiol 2005; 113:293–302.
8. Sausker EA, Dyer NW. Seroprevalence of OHV-2, BVDV, BHV-1, and BRSV in ranch-raised bison (Bison bison). J Vet Diagn Invest 2002;14:68–70.
9. Lata J, Kanani AN, Patel TJ, et al. Seroprevalence of bovine herpesvirus 1 (BHV-1) in Indian breeding bulls of Gujarat. Buffalo Bull 2008;27:165–9.
10. Malmurugan S, Raja A, Saravanabava K, et al. Seroprevalence and infectious bovine rhinotracheitis in cattle and buffaloes using Avidin-Biotin ELISA. Cheiron 2004;33:146–9.
11. NASS. Agricultural statistics board. Washington, DC: US Department of Agriculture; 1996.
12. Bowland SL, Shewen PE. Bovine respiratory disease: commercial vaccines currently available in Canada. Can Vet J 2000;41(1):33–48.
13. Tikoo SK, Campos M, Babiuk LA. Bovine herpesvirus 1 (BHV-1): biology, pathogenesis, and control. Adv Virus Res 1995;45:191–223.
14. Carter JJ, Weinberg AD, Pollard A, et al. Inhibition of T-lymphocyte mitogenic responses and effects on cell functions by bovine herpesvirus 1. J Virol 1989; 63(4):1525–30.
15. Griebel P, Ohmann HB, Lawmann MJ, et al. The interaction between bovine herpesvirus type 1 and activated bovine T lymphocytes. J Gen Virol 1990; 71(Pt 2):369–77.
16. Griebel P, Qualtiere L, Davis WC, et al. T lymphocyte population dynamics and function following a primary bovine herpesvirus type-1 infection. Viral Immunol 1987;1(4):287–304.
17. Griebel PJ, Qualtiere L, Davis WC, et al. Bovine peripheral blood leukocyte subpopulation dynamics following a primary bovine herpesvirus-1 infection. Viral Immunol 1987;1(4):267–86.
18. Nataraj C, Eidmann S, Hariharan MJ, et al. Bovine herpesvirus 1 downregulates the expression of bovine MHC class I molecules. Viral Immunol 1997;10(1): 21–34.
19. Hariharan MJ, Nataraj C, Srikumaran S. Down regulation of murine MHC class I expression by bovine herpesvirus 1. Viral Immunol 1993;6(4):273–84.
20. Hinkley S, Hill AB, Srikumaran S. Bovine herpesvirus-1 infection affects the peptide transport activity in bovine cells. Virus Res 1998;53(1):91–6.
21. Winkler MT, Doster A, Jones C. Bovine herpesvirus 1 can infect CD4(+) T lymphocytes and induce programmed cell death during acute infection of cattle. J Virol 1999;73(10):8657–68.
22. Abril C, Engels M, Limman A, et al. Both viral and host factors contribute to neurovirulence of bovine herpesvirus 1 and 5 in interferon receptor-deficient mice. J Virol 2004;78(7):3644–53.

23. Liang X, Tang M, Manns B, et al. Identification and deletion mutagenesis of the bovine herpesvirus 1 dUTPase gene and a gene homologous to herpes simplex virus UL49.5. Virology 1993;195:42–50.
24. Liang X, Chow B, Raggo C, et al. Bovine herpesvirus 1 UL49.5 homolog gene encodes a novel viral envelope protein that forms a disulfide-linked complex with a second virion structural protein. J Virol 1996;70:1448–54.
25. Wu SX, Zhu XP, Letchworth GJ. Bovine herpesvirus 1 glycoprotein M forms a disulfide-linked heterodimer with the U(L)49.5 protein. J Virol 1998;72: 3029–36.
26. Jöns A, Dijkstra JM, Mettenleiter TC. Glycoproteins M and N of pseudorabies virus form a disulfide-linked complex. J Virol 1998;72:550–7.
27. Rudolph J, Seyboldt C, Granzow H, et al. The gene 10 (UL49.5) product of equine herpesvirus 1 is necessary and sufficient for functional processing of glycoprotein M. J Virol 2002;76:2952–63.
28. Brack AR, Dijkstra JM, Granzow H, et al. Inhibition of virion maturation by simultaneous deletion of glycoproteins E, I, and M of pseudorabies virus. J Virol 1999; 73:5364–72.
29. Koppers-Lalic D, Reits EA, Ressing ME, et al. Varicelloviruses avoid T cell recognition by UL49.5-mediated inactivation of the transporter associated with antigen processing. Proc Natl Acad Sci U S A 2005;102:5144–9.
30. Lipińska AD, Koppers-Lalic D, Rychlowski M, et al. Bovine herpesvirus 1 UL49.5 protein inhibits the transporter associated with antigen processing despite complex formation with glycoprotein M. J Virol 2006;81:5822–32.
31. Androlewicz MJ, Anderson KS, Cresswell P. Evidence that transporters associated with antigen processing translocate a major histocompatibility complex class I-binding peptide into the endoplasmic reticulum in an ATP-dependent manner. Proc Natl Acad Sci U S A 1993;90:9130–4.
32. Koch J, Gruntrum R, Heintke S, et al. Functional dissection of the transmembrane domains of the transporter associated with antigen processing (TAP). J Biol Chem 2004;279:10142–7.
33. van Endert PM, Saveanu L, Hewitt EW, et al. Powering the peptide pump: TAP crosstalk with energetic nucleotides. Trends Biochem Sci 2002;27:454–61.
34. Ahn K, Meyer TH, Uebel S, et al. Molecular mechanism and species specificity of TAP inhibition by herpes simplex virus ICP47. EMBO J 1996;15:3247–55.
35. Ambagala AP, Gopinath RS, Srikumaran S. Peptide transport activity of the transporter associated with antigen processing (TAP) is inhibited by an early protein of equine herpesvirus-1. J Gen Virol 2004;66:2383–94.
36. Hughes EA, Hammond C, Cresswell P. Misfolded major histocompatibility complex class I heavy chains are translocated into the cytoplasm and degraded by the proteosome. Proc Natl Acad Sci U S A 1997;94:1896–901.
37. Everett RD. ICP0, a regulator of herpes simplex virus during lytic and latent infection. Bioessays 2000;22(8):761–70.
38. Fraefel C, Zeng J, Coffat Y, et al. Identification and zinc dependence of the bovine herpesvirus 1 transactivator protein BICP0. J Virol 1994;68(5): 3154–62.
39. Zhang Y, Jones C. Identification of functional domains within the bICP0 protein encoded by BHV-1. J Gen Virol 2005;86:879–86.
40. Inman M, Zhang Y, Geiser V, et al. The zinc ring finger in the bICP0 protein encoded by bovine herpes virus-1 mediates toxicity and activates productive infection. J Gen Virol 2001;82:483–92.

41. Geiser V, Jones C. Stimulation of bovine herpesvirus 1 productive infection by the adenovirus E1A gene and a cell cycle regulatory gene, E2F-4. J Gen Virol 2003;84:929–38.
42. Zhang Y, Jones C. The bovine herpesvirus 1 immediate-early protein (bICP0) associates with histone deacetylase 1 to activate transcription. J Virol 2001; 75(20):9571–8.
43. Zhang Y, Jiang Y, Zhou J, et al. The bovine herpes virus 1 (BHV-1) immediate early protein (bICP0) interacts with the histone acetyltransferase p300, and these interactions correlate with stimulation of gC promoter activity. J Gen Virol 2006;87:1843–51.
44. Henderson G, Zhang Y, Jones C. The bovine herpesvirus 1 gene encoding infected cell protein 0 (bICP0) can inhibit interferon-dependent transcription in the absence of other viral genes. J Gen Virol 2005;86:2697–702.
45. Saira K, Zhou Y, Jones C. The infected cell protein 0 encoded by bovine herpesvirus 1 (bICP0) induces degradation of interferon response factor 3 (IRF3), and consequently inhibits beta interferon promoter activity. J Virol 2007;81:3077–86.
46. Dia L, Zhang B, Fan J, et al. Herpes virus proteins ICP0 and BICP0 can activate NF-kB by catalyzing IkBa ubiquitination. Cell Signal 2005;17:217–29.
47. Yoneyama M, Suhara W, Fukuhara M, et al. Direct triggering of the type 1 interferon system by virus infection: activation of a transcription factors containing IRF-3 and CBP/p300. EMBO J 1998;17:1087–95.
48. Sato M, Taniguchi T, Tanaka N. The interferon system and interferon regulatory factor transcription factors-studies from gene knockout mice. Cytokine Growth Factor Rev 2001;12:133–42.
49. Yuang Y, Lowther W, Kellum M, et al. Primary activation of interferon A and interferon B gene transcription by interferon regulatory factor 3. Proc Natl Acad Sci U S A 1998;95:9837–42.
50. Honda K, Yanai H, Negishi H, et al. IRF-7 is the master regulator of type-I interferon-dependent immune responses. Nature 2005;434:772–7.
51. Saira K, Jones C. The infected cell protein 0 encoded by bovine herpesvirus 1 (bICP0) associates with interferon regulatory factor 7 (IRF7), and consequently inhibits beta interferon promoter activity. J Virol 2009;83:3977–81.
52. Bryant NA, Davis-Poynter N, Vanderplasschen A, et al. Glycoprotein G isoforms from some alphaherpesvirus function as broad-spectrum chemokine binding proteins. EMBO J 2003;22:833–46.
53. Baggiolini M. Chemokines and leukocyte traffic. Nature 1998;392:565–8.
54. Kaashoek MJ, Fijsewijk FA, Ruuls RC, et al. Virulence, immunogenicity and reactivation of bovine herpesvirus 1 mutants with a deletion in the gC, gG, gI, gE, or in both the gI and gE gene. Vaccine 1998;16:802–9.
55. Jeyaseelan S, Sreevatson S, Maheswaran SK. Role of Mannheimia haemolytica leukotoxin in the pathogenesis of bovine pneumonic pasteurellosis. Anim Health Res Rev 2002;3:69–82.
56. Rivera-Rivas JJ, Kisiela D, Czuprynski CJ. Bovine herpesvirus type 1 infection of bovine bronchial epithelial cells increases neutrophil adhesion and activation. Vet Immunol Immunopathol 2009;131:167–76.
57. Rouse BT, Babiuk LA. Mechanism of recovery from herpesvirus infections. Can J Comp Med 1978;42:414–27.
58. Straub OC, Ahl R. Lokale interferonbildung beim rind nach intranasaler infektion mit avirulentm IBR-IPV-virus und deren wirkung auf eine anschliebende inkection mit maul und klauenseuche-virus. Zbl Vet Med B 1976;23:470–82.

59. Babiuk LA, Bielefeldt Ohamnn H, Gifford H, et al. Effect of bovine alpha 1 inter-feron on bovine herpesvirus type 1 induced respiratory disease. J Gen Virol 1985;66:2383–94.

60. Jensen J, Schulz RD. Bovine natural cell mediated cytotoxicity (NCMC): activation by cytokines. Vet Immunol Immunopathol 1990;24:113–29.

61. Lawman MJP, Gifford G, Gyongyossy-Issa M, et al. Activity of polymorphonu-clear (PMN) leukocytes during bovine herpesvirus-1 induced respiratory disease: effect of recombinant bovine interferon alpha I1. Antiviral Res 1987; 8:225–37.

62. Cook CB, Splitter GA. Characterization of bovine mononuclear cell population with natural cytotoxic activity against bovine herpesvirus-1 infected cells. Cell Immunol 1989;120:240–9.

63. Campos M, Rossi CR. Cytotoxicity of bovine lymphocytes after treatment with lymphokines. Am J Vet Res 1986;47:1524–8.

64. Amadori M, Archetti LL, Vernadi R, et al. Target recognition by bovine mononu-clear, MHC-untreated cytotoxic cells. Vet Microbiol 1992;33:383–92.

65. Marshall RL, Israel BA, Letchworth GJ. Monoclonal antibody analysis of bovine herpesvirus-1 glycoprotein antigenic areas relevant to natural infection. Virology 1988;165:338–47.

66. Van Drunen Littel-van den Hurk S, Babiuk LA. Polypeptide specificity of the anti-body response after primary and recurrent infection with bovine herpesvirus 1. J Clin Microbiol 1986;23:274–82. ˙

67. Van Drunen Littel-van den Hurk S, Tikoo SK, Liang X, et al. Bovine herpesvirus-1 vaccines. Immunol Cell Biol 1993;71:405–20.

68. Rouse BT, Wardley RC, Babiuk LA. Antibody dependent cell-mediated cytotox-icity in cows: comparison of effector cell activity against heterologous erythro-cytes and herpesvirus-infected bovine target cells. Infect Immun 1976;13: 1433–41.

69. Rouse BT, Grewal AS, Babiuk LA. Complement enhances antiviral antibody dependent cell toxicity. Nature 1977;266:456–8.

70. Rouse BT, Wardley RC, Babiuk LA. Enhancement of antibody dependent cell toxicity of herpesvirus infected cells by complement. Infect Immun 1977;18: 660–5.

71. Rouse BT, Babiuk LA. The direct antiviral cytotoxicity by bovine lymphocytes is not restricted by genetic incompatibility of lymphocytes and target cells. J Immunol 1977;118:618–24.

72. Van Drunen Littel-van den Hurk S. Cell-mediated immune responses induced by BHV-1: rational vaccine design. Expert Rev Vaccines 2007;6:369–80.

73. Deshpande MS, Ambagala TC, Hegde NR, et al. Induction of cytotoxic T-lymphocytes specific for bovine herpesvirus-1 by DNA immunization. Vaccine 2002;20:3744–51.

74. Huang Y, Babiuk LA, van Drunen Littel-van den Hurk S. Immunization with a bovine heprsvirus-1 glycoprotein B DNA vaccine induces cytotoxic T lympho-cyte responses in mice and cattle. J Gen Virol 2005;88:887–98.

75. Denis M, Slaoui M, Keil GM, et al. Identification of different target glycoproteins for bovine herpesvirus-1-specific cytotoxic T lymphocytes depending on the method of in vitro stimulation. Immunology 1993;78:7–13.

76. Campos M, Bielefeldt OH, Hutchings D, et al. Role of interferon gamma in inducing cytotoxicity of peripheral blood mononuclear leukocytes to bovine herpesvirus type 1 (BHV-1)-infected cells. Cell Immunol 1989;120:259–69.

77. Hutchings DL, van Drunen Littel-van den Hurk S, Babiuk LA. Lymphocyte proliferative responses to separated bovine herpesvirus 1 proteins in immune cattle. J Virol 1990;64:5114–22.
78. Leary TP, Splitter GA. Recombinant herpesviral proteins produced by cell-free translation provide a novel approach for the mapping of T lymphocyte epitopes. J Immunol 1990;145:718–23.
79. Tikoo SK, Campos M, Popowych YI, et al. Lymphocyte proliferative responses to recombinant bovine herpesvirus virus type 1 (BHV-1) glycoprotein gD (gIV) in immune cattle: identification of a T cell epitope. Viral Immunol 1995;8: 19–25.
80. Janssen EM, Lemmens EE, Wolfe T, et al. CD4$^+$ T cells are required for secondary expansion and memory in CD8$^+$ T lymphocytes. Nature 2003;421: 852–6.
81. Shedlock DJ, Shen H. Requirement for CD4 T cell help in generating functional CD8 T cell memory. Science 2003;300:337–9.
82. Devireddy LR, Jones C. Activation of caspases and p53 by bovine herpesvirus 1 infection results in programmed cell death and efficient virus release. J Virol 1999;73(5):3778–88.
83. Misra V, Walker S, Hayes S, et al. The bovine herpesvirus alpha gene trans-inducing factor activates transcription by mechanisms different from those of its herpes simplex virus type 1 counterpart VP16. J Virol 1995;69(9):5209–16.
84. Wirth UV, Vogt B, Schwyzer M. The three major immediate-early transcripts of bovine herpesvirus 1 arise from two divergent and spliced transcription units. J Virol 1991;65(1):195–205.
85. Wirth UV, Fraefel C, Vogt B, et al. Immediate-early RNA 2.9 and early RNA 2.6 of bovine herpesvirus 1 are 3' coterminal and encode a putative zinc finger transactivator protein. J Virol 1992;66(5):2763–72.
86. Jones C. Alphaherpesvirus latency: its role in disease and survival of the virus in nature. Adv Virus Res 1998;51:81–133.
87. Jones C. Herpes simplex virus type 1 and bovine herpesvirus 1 latency. Clin Microbiol Rev 2003;16:79–95.
88. Schang L, Jones C. Analysis of bovine herpesvirus 1 transcripts during a primary infection of trigeminal ganglia of cattle. J Virol 1997;71(9):6786–95.
89. Inman M, Lovato L, Doster A, et al. A mutation in the latency related gene of bovine herpesvirus 1 interferes with the latency-reactivation cycle of latency in calves. J Virol 2002;76:6771–9.
90. Jones C, Geiser V, Henderson G, et al. Functional analysis of bovine herpesvirus 1 (BHV-1) genes expressed during latency. Vet Microbiol 2006;113:199–210.
91. Devireddy LR, Jones C. Alternative splicing of the latency-related transcript of bovine herpesvirus 1 yields RNAs containing unique open reading frames. J Virol 1998;72(9):7294–301.
92. Ciacci-Zanella J, Stone M, Henderson G, et al. The latency-related gene of bovine herpesvirus 1 inhibits programmed cell death. J Virol 1999;73(12): 9734–40.
93. Henderson G, Perng GC, Nesburn A, et al. The latency related gene of bovine herpesvirus 1 can suppress caspase 3 and caspase 9 during productive infection. J Neurovirol 2004;10:64–70.
94. Bratanich AC, Hanson ND, Jones C. The latency-related gene of bovine herpesvirus 1 inhibits the activity of immediate-early transcription unit 1. Virology 1992; 191(2):988–91.

95. Geiser V, Inman M, Zhang Y, et al. The latency related (LR) gene of bovine herpes virus 1 (BHV-1) can inhibit the ability of bICP0 to activate productive infection. J Gen Virol 2002;83:2965–71.
96. Jones C, Newby TJ, Holt T, et al. Analysis of latency in cattle after inoculation with a temperature sensitive mutant of bovine herpesvirus 1 (RLB106). Vaccine 2000;18(27):3185–95.
97. Rock D, Lokensgard J, Lewis T, et al. Characterization of dexamethasone-induced reactivation of latent bovine herpesvirus 1. J Virol 1992;66(4):2484–90.
98. Winkler MT, Doster A, Jones C. Persistence and reactivation of bovine herpesvirus 1 in the tonsil of latently infected calves. J Virol 2000;74:5337–46.
99. Fuchs M, Hubert P, Detterer J, et al. Detection of bovine herpesvirus type 1 in blood from naturally infected cattle by using a sensitive PCR that discriminates between wild-type virus and virus lacking glycoprotein E. J Clin Microbiol 1999; 37(8):2498–507.
100. Mweene AS, Okazaki K, Kida H. Detection of viral genome in non-neural tissues of cattle experimentally infected with bovine herpesvirus 1. Jpn J Vet Res 1996; 44(3):165–74.
101. Cheung AK. Investigation of pseudorabies virus DNA and RNA in trigeminal ganglia and tonsil tissues of latently infected swine. Am J Vet Res 1995;56: 45–50.
102. Sabo A, Rajanci J. Latent pseudorabies virus infection in pigs. Acta Virologica 1976;20:208–14.
103. Borchers K, Wolfinger U, Ludwig H. Latency-associated transcript of equine herpesvirus 4 in trigeminal ganglia of naturally infected horses. J Gen Virol 1999;80:2165–71.
104. Miyoshi M, Ishii Y, Takiguchi M, et al. Detection of canine herpesvirus DNA in ganglionic neurons and the lymph node lymphocytes of latently infected dogs. J Vet Med Sci 1999;61:375–9.
105. Perez S, Inman M, Doster A, et al. Latency-related gene encoded by bovine herpesvirus 1 promotes virus growth and reactivation from latency in tonsils of infected calves. J Clin Microbiol 2005;43:393–401.
106. Kutish G, Mainprize T, Rock D. Characterization of the latency-related transcriptionally active region of the bovine herpesvirus 1 genome. J Virol 1990;64(12): 5730–7.
107. Rock DL, Beam SL, Mayfield JE. Mapping bovine herpesvirus type 1 latency-related RNA in trigeminal ganglia of latently infected rabbits. J Virol 1987; 61(12):3827–31.
108. Jiang Y, Hossain A, Winkler MT, et al. A protein encoded by the latency-related gene of bovine herpesvirus 1 is expressed in trigeminal ganglionic neurons of latently infected cattle and interacts with cyclin-dependent kinase 2 during productive infection. J Virol 1998;72(10):8133–42.
109. Jiang Y, Inman M, Zhang Y, et al. A mutation in the latency related gene of bovine herpesvirus 1 (BHV-1) inhibits protein expression of a protein from open reading frame 2 (ORF-2) and an adjacent reading frame during productive infection. J Virol 2004;78:3184–9.
110. Hossain A, Schang LM, Jones C. Identification of gene products encoded by the latency-related gene of bovine herpesvirus 1. J Virol 1995;69(9):5345–52.
111. Schang LM, Hossain A, Jones C. The latency-related gene of bovine herpesvirus 1 encodes a product which inhibits cell cycle progression. J Virol 1996; 70(6):3807–14.

112. Shen W, Jones C. Open reading frame 2 encoded by the latency related gene of bovine herpesvirus 1 has anti-apoptosis activity in transiently transfected neuro-blastoma cells. J Virol 2008;82:10940–5.
113. Geiser V, Jones C. The latency related gene encoded by bovine herpesvirus 1 encodes a small regulatory RNA that inhibits cell growth. J Neurovirol 2005;11: 563–70.
114. Inman M, Lovato L, Doster A, et al. A mutation in the latency-related gene of bovine herpesvirus 1 leads to impaired ocular shedding in acutely infected calves. J Virol 2001;75:8507–15.
115. Van Drunen Littel-van den Hurk S. Rationale and perspectives on the success of vaccination against bovine herpesvirus-1. Vet Microbiol 2005;113:275–82.
116. Endsley JJ, Quade MJ, Terhaar B, et al. BHV-1 specific CD4$^+$, CD8$^+$, and $\gamma\delta$ T cells in calves vaccinated with one dose of a modified live BHV-1 vaccine. Viral Immunol 2002;15:385–93.
117. Butchi NB, Jones C, Perez S, et al. Envelope protein Us9 is required for the anterograde transport of bovine herpesvirus-1 (BHV-1) from trigeminal ganglia to nose and eye upon reactivation. J Neurovirol 2007;13:384–8.
118. Chowdhury SI, Ross CS, Lee BJ, et al. Construction and characterization of a glycoprotein E gene-deleted bovine herpesvirus type 1 recombinant. Am J Vet Res 1999;60:227–32.
119. Chowdhury SI. Construction and characterization of an attenuated bovine herpesvirus type 1 (BHV-1) recombinant virus. Vet Microbiol 1996;52:13–23.
120. Kaashoek MJ, van Engelenburg FA, Moerman A, et al. Virulence and immuno-genicity in calves of thymidine kinase- and glycoprotein E-negative bovine herpesvirus 1 mutants. Vet Microbiol 1996;48:143–53.
121. Kaashoek MJ, Rijsewijk FA, Oirschot JT. Persistence of antibodies against bovine herpesvirus 1 and virus reactivation two to three years after infection. Vet Microbiol 1996;53(1–2):103–10.
122. Liu Z, Coats C, Jones C, Chowdhury SI. Construction and characterization of BHV-1 glycoprotein E (gE) cytoplasmic tail truncated and Us9 acidic domain deleted mutants. 32nd International Herpesvirus Workshop, Ashville, NC; 2007. 3.36.
123. Chowdhury SI, Lee BJ, Ozkul A, et al. Bovine Herpesvirus type-5 (BHV-5) glyco-protein E (gE) is important for neuroinvasiveness and neurovirulence in the olfactory pathway of the rabbit. J Virol 2000;74:2094–106.
124. Whitbeck JC, Knapp AC, Enquist LW, et al. Synthesis, processing, and oligo-merization of the bovine herpes virus 1 gE and gI membrane proteins. J Virol 1996;70:7878–84.
125. Thriy E, Muylkens B, Meurens F, et al. Recombination in the alphaherpesvirus bovine herpesvirus 1. Vet Microbiol 2005;113:171–7.
126. Ellis J, Waldner C, Rhodes C, et al. Longevity of protective immunity to experi-mental bovine herpesvirus-1 infection following inoculation with a combination modified-live virus vaccine in beef calves. J Am Vet Med Assoc 2005;227: 123–8.
127. Van Drunen Littel-van den Hurk S, Myers D, Doig PA, et al. Identification of a mutant bovine herpesvirus-1 (BHV-1) in post-arrival outbreaks of IBR in feedlot calves and protection with conventional vaccination. Can J Vet Res 2001;65: 81–8.
128. Ackermann M, Engels M. Pro and contra IBR-eradication. Vet Microbiol 2006; 113:293–302.

129. Katze MG, Heng Y, Gale M. Viruses and interferon: fight for supremacy. Nat Rev Immunol 2002;2:675–86.
130. Levy DE, Darnell JE Jr. Stats: transcriptional control and biological impact. Nat Rev Mol Cell Biol 2002;3:651–62.
131. Aaronson DS, Horvath CM. A road map for those who don't know JAK-STAT. Science 2002;296:1653–5.
132. Alexopoulou L, Holt AC, Medzhitov R, et al. Recognition of double-stranded RNA and activation of NF-kappaB by Toll-like receptor 3. Nature 2001;413: 732–8.
133. Doyle S, Vaidya S, O'Connell R, et al. IRF3 mediates a TLR3/TLR4-specific antiviral gene program. Immunity 2002;17:251–63.
134. Fitzgerald KA, McWhirter SM, Faja KL, et al. IKKe and TBKI are essential components of the IRF3 signaling pathway. Nature 2003;4:491–6.
135. Sharma S, tenOever BR, Grandvaux N, et al. Triggering the interferon antiviral response through and IKK-related pathway. Science 2003;300:1148–51.
136. Wathelet MG, Lin CH, Parekh BS, et al. Virus infection induces the assembly of coordinately activated transcription factors on the IFN-b enhancer in vivo. Mol Cell 1998;1:507–18.
137. Guo J, Peters KL, Sen GC. Induction of the human protein P56 by interferon, double stranded RNA, or virus infection. Virology 2000;267:209–19.
138. Mossman KL, Macgregor PF, Rozmus JJ, et al. Herpes simplex virus triggers and then disarms a host antiviral response. J Virol 2001;75(2):750–8.
139. Perkins ND. Integrating cell-signalling pathways with NF-kB and IKK functions. Nat Rev Mol Cell Biol 2007;8:49–62.
140. Jaeschke A, Karasarides M, Ventura JJ, et al. JNK2 is a positive regulator of the cJun transcription factor. Mol Cell 2006;23:899–911.
141. Weaver BK, Kumar KP, Reich NC. Interferon regulatory factor 3 and CREB-binding protein/p300 are subunits of double-stranded RNA-activated transcription factor DRAF1. Mol Cell Biol 1998;18:1359–68.

Bovine Respiratory Syncytial Virus

Bruce W. Brodersen, DVM, MS, PhD

KEYWORDS
- Bovine respiratory syncytial virus • BRSV • BRSV diagnosis
- Bovine respiratory disease complex • BRD

Bovine respiratory syncytial virus (BRSV) is a major cause of respiratory disease and a major contributor to the bovine respiratory disease (BRD) complex. BRD costs can be estimated by the beef producer by identifying the direct and indirect costs associated with disease.[1] It has been estimated that BRD in the feedlot results in losses from $23.23 to $151.18 per animal compared with those who remain healthy.[2] Approximately 32 million head of cattle are killed in the United States each year, equating to more than a billion dollars in losses because of BRD. BRSV infects the upper and lower respiratory tract and is shed in nasal secretions. This virus is closely related to the human respiratory syncytial virus (HRSV).[3] The close relatedness of BRSV to HRSV has allowed researchers to use BRSV and HRSV seemingly interchangeably to elucidate the mechanisms by which these viruses induce disease. Unique to these viruses, attempted vaccine production using formalin-inactivated vaccine resulted in exacerbated disease when infants became exposed to HRSV.[4] Similarly, cattle vaccinated with formalin-inactivated virus had enhanced disease when inoculated with BRSV.[5] BRSV remains a factor in BRD despite the progress that has been made in elucidating the immunopathogenic mechanisms involved.

This article discusses various aspects of BRSV, its epidemiology, pathogenesis, diagnostic tests, and select topics on immunity and vaccination.

EPIDEMIOLOGY

BRSV was first identified in Europe in 1970.[6,7] It was later identified in the United States in 1974.[8,9] A serologic survey of Iowa cattle in the early 1970s indicated 81% of cattle from 43 herds had neutralizing antibody to BRSV.[3] It has long been known that BRSV can be responsible for outbreaks of respiratory disease.[10–14] Respiratory disease caused by BRSV has been reported in many areas and under different management systems in beef and dairy.[6,7,10–12] Incidence of BRSV seroconversion soon after an outbreak of respiratory tract disease had been reported to be as high as 45%.[12] Collins

The author has nothing to disclose.
Veterinary Diagnostic Center, School of Veterinary Medicine and Biomedical Sciences, University of Nebraska-Lincoln, 1900 North 42nd Street, Lincoln, NE 68506-0907, USA
E-mail address: bbrodersen1@unl.edu

and colleagues[14] reported seropositive rates of 95% in feedlot cattle associated with a lack of respiratory disease. In range cattle with a lack of respiratory disease, calves had a seropositive rate of 28%, yearlings, 49%, and cows on range, 70%.

Atypical interstitial pneumonia (AIP) is often seen in feedlot cattle, but BRSV was not detected in these situations by means of immunohistochemical[15] or fluorescent antibody[16] tests. One study suggests recent BRSV infections may be a predisposing factor, but not a cause of AIP.[17] It was stated that possible preexisting bronchiolitis obliterans may have been present as the result of BRSV disease and exacerbated the lesions of AIP. Causes of AIP are discussed in detail in another article by Alan R. Doster elsewhere in this issue for further exploration of this topic.

In addition to calves being reported as being infected, adult animals are susceptible to disease from BRSV.[18] Bull testing stations are at risk for BRSV.[19] The risk at bull testing stations is because animals are often from multiple sources, similar to feedlot situations. Sperm quality is reported to have been reduced as a result of BRSV infection.[20] Six months after outbreaks of BRSV while in quarantine, bulls had poorer sperm morphology than seronegative bulls. Reduced sperm morphology is believed to be the result of testicular fibrosis and not the result of fever during BRSV disease.[20,21]

Syncytial virus isolates were reported from other species and characterized, showing similarities among the isolates.[22] Other species have been shown to be infected by RSVs around the world.[23–27] An isolate of RSV from a field outbreak of respiratory disease in sheep was shown to cause disease when experimentally inoculated into sheep. This isolate of RSV was later shown to cause lower respiratory tract lesions when experimentally inoculated into calves and deer.[28] Experimental infection of sheep by BRSV resulted in mild fever with oculonasal secretions and lymphopenia.[29] Bovine RSV was recovered from nasal secretions on days 2 to 6 following experimental inoculation. Viral antigen was shown deep in the lungs 2 to 4 days after inoculation. That other species are infected by RSVs raises the possibility that other species may be factors in transmission of BRSV under certain conditions.

It is not well understood where BRSV resides in a population of cattle for the virus to survive. Persistently infected calves may exist and possible triggering mechanisms such as change in temperature may trigger shedding.[30] One study suggested circulation among seropositive cattle in subclinical infections is not a plausible mechanism for persistence of BRSV in dairy herds.[31] Identical viruses have been isolated within closed herds during outbreaks and isolates from recurrent infections, in closed herds, vary as much as 11% in sequence.[32] The most likely explanation for recurrent infections is that BRSV was reintroduced into the herd before new outbreaks. Continuous generation of mutant virus is believed to be a key adaptive strategy of RNA viruses. Despite genetic stability, BRSV genome is heterogeneous and there is low fidelity of their replication.[33]

PATHOGENESIS AND CLINICAL SIGNS

Experimental inoculation with BRSV has resulted in reproduction of disease of varying degrees of severity. Three of 5 calves developed fevers of 40°C with increase respiratory rates, anorexia, serous nasal discharge, dry muzzle, and malaise.[3] Virus was recoverable from a nasal swab on day 6 after inoculation. Calves developed fever on day 2 after inoculation and persisted until day 6, when the temperatures gradually declined.[34] Concentration of virus in nasal swabs peaked at 6 days after inoculation at a concentration of up to $3.8\log_{10}(TCID_{50})/mL$. Other studies have shown similar clinical responses, with body temperatures increasing to approximately 40°C, coughing, nasal discharge, and tachypnea ranging between days 3 and 9 after inoculation.[35–37] Virus is recoverable from lung up to about 8 days after inoculation.[38] Affected areas of lung as a result of uncomplicated BRSV infection are grossly red, depressed, and firm.[36,37] These lesions are located mainly in the cranioventral areas of lung and can involve scattered individual lobules.[37] In some cases, there can be emphysema in other (mainly caudodorsal) areas of the lung.[36,37] Gross lesions in natural infections match those of experimentally inoculated calves.[39] Natural infection can lead to lesions of cor pulmonale.[39] Microscopic lesions in experimental and natural infections both consist of bronchial and bronchiolar epithelial necrosis (**Fig. 1**). Multinucleated (syncytial) cells (see **Fig. 1**) are present associated with areas of bronchitis or bronchiolitis. Eosinophilic intracytoplasmic inclusion bodies are sometimes seen (**Fig. 2**) in epithelial cells in airways. Alveoli may become lined by hyaline membranes, which adds to the similarity in lesions between BRSV and AIP.[15,17]

DIAGNOSIS

A variety of tests have been used to identify BRSV in field specimens collected during outbreaks of respiratory disease. Initially, identification of the virus was by virus isolation and recognition of cytopathic effect in the cell culture. Isolation of the virus was then confirmed by neutralization assays with hyperimmune serum.[3] Virus isolation has always been considered time consuming and laborious for veterinary diagnostic laboratories. The BRSV is labile and virus isolation attempts are often thwarted because of that lability.[9] Fluorescent antibody testing was later shown to be a useful rapid test for identification of BRSV antigen in cell culture.[40] For several years, FATs on frozen tissue sections were commonly used in veterinary diagnostic laboratories. This procedure provided a quick method for identification of viral antigen in tissues and was traditionally followed up with virus isolation. Nonspecific immunofluorescence presented as a problem when examining nasopharyngeal material.[41] Positive fluorescence was limited to days 2 to 4 in lambs experimentally infected with BRSV.[29] Nonspecific fluorescence was regularly noted in interalveolar septae and in the cytoplasm of alveolar macrophages.[29] No positive fluorescence was seen in lungs from days 6 to 12 after inoculation. Fluorescent antibody testing on field samples lacks sensitivity and specificity and is not satisfactory under veterinary diagnostic laboratory conditions.[42] Several variables contribute to the low sensitivity and specificity of this test. Those include degree of autolysis, difficulty in visualizing the positive-staining

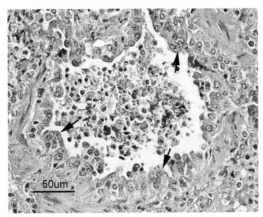

Fig. 1. Bronchiole lined by attenuated and necrotic epithelium. Note several syncytial cells (*arrows*).

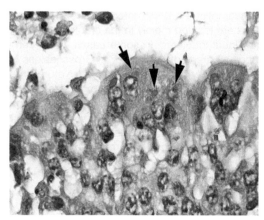

Fig. 2. Bronchiolar epithelium with intracytoplasmic inclusion bodies (*arrows*).

cell types, and stability of the sample and quenching of fluorescent signal on the stained slide over time.

Rapid detection of BRSV has been achieved by other means.[42] An antigen-capture enzyme immunoassay (EIA) developed for HRSV was shown to be sensitive and specific. Nasal samples and lung homogenates were useful in this test. However, the usefulness of this test never gained favor in veterinary diagnostic laboratories. A 1-step enzyme-linked immunosorbent assay (ELISA) test has recently been reported to be a reliable test for detecting BRSV in organ homogenates.[43] Comparison between the 1-step ELISA, an EIA, and an indirect immunofluoresence (IIF) test with reverse transcription polymerase chain reaction (RT-PCR) as the gold standard was reported. The 1-step ELISA was shown to have a sensitivity of 60% and specificity of 100% compared with RT-PCR. The EIA and IIF tests had a sensitivity of 47% each and specificities of 99% and 97%, respectively, when compared with the RT-PCR.

Immunohistochemistry (IHC) has an advantage over IIF in that there is a permanent stain that shows antigen that can be visualized by light microscopy in association with lesions (**Fig. 3**).[44,45] Visualization of viral antigen in association with the lesions makes IHC superior to IIF.[44] Formalin-fixed paraffin-embedded tissues are used for IHC. Formalin fixation addresses the problem of lability of the tissues and loss of antigen.[45] Fixation can result in masking the antigen of interest so that extra measures are needed to unmask the antigen for binding between antibody and antigen to occur.[46] No reports on the sensitivity of IHC for BRSV in field cases have been published.

RT-PCR and oligonucleotide hybridization of the RNA of the BRSV F protein was reported to add to the speed, sensitivity, and specificity of BRSV diagnostics.[47] This RT-PCR was tested against several isolates of BRSV and strains of HRSV subgroups A and B. The RT-PCR may be able to detect BRSV in nasal secretions longer than with ELISA-based tests because of the inhibitory effects of rising neutralizing antibody titers in nasal secretions.[48] Real-time (rt) RT-PCR developed to detect RNA of nucleoprotein has been shown to be more sensitive than conventional tests of IIF on nasal swab and bronchoalveolar lavage samples and IHC on formalin-fixed paraffin-embedded tissues.[49] The nucleoprotein was chosen because of the high conservation of the gene encoding this protein.[50] Availability of rapid results using rtRT-PCR may be useful in formulating vaccination plans in feedlots and on farms. Caution must be exercised if an intranasal vaccine is used, because rtRT-PCR can detect vaccine virus for as long as 14 days after vaccination.[51] A commercially available rtRT-PCR kit is available

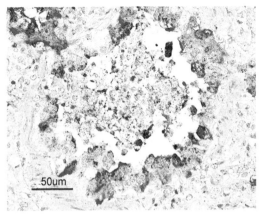

Fig. 3. Serial section of **Fig. 1.** Immunohistochemical stain for BRSV (positive staining is *red*).

and has been shown to be more sensitive than a direct fluorescent antibody test (FAT), which used a monoclonal antibody directed against the F protein.[52] Use of a commercially available test can lead to standardization of testing across laboratories.

IMMUNITY AND VACCINATION

Attempts at vaccination against RSV started with use of a formalin-inactivated vaccine.[4] The vaccine not only failed to prevent disease but induced an exaggerated clinical response to naturally occurring HRSV infection in younger vaccinees. It was concluded that the paradoxic effect of vaccination suggested antibody from vaccination plays a role in the pathogenesis of this disease. It was later believed formalin modified certain epitopes on the F and G proteins that are key to stimulation of a neutralizing antibody response.[53] A bovine model of vaccination with formalin-inactivated vaccine showed that IgG was produced, but was not neutralizing.[5] Further work reported the presence of virus-specific IgE and resultant release of histamine in nasopharyngeal secretions after HRSV infection.[54]

After initial inoculation of calves, a secretory humoral immune response is first detected as early as 8 days.[38] Bovine RSV-specific IgM and IgA appeared nearly simultaneously in serum and secretions. Serum IgG_1 was detected as early as 13 days after inoculation. Duration of presence of these antibodies varied with time, because IgA was present for as long as 3.5 months or longer. An age-dependent response was not seen when comparing 3- to 4-week-old calves with 5-month-old calves.[38] Comparison of antibody responses between colostrum-deprived calves and colostrum-fed calves revealed the colostrum-fed calves had suppressed local and systemic antibody responses. Virus was detected in equal amounts in lung lavage fluids from colostrum-deprived and colostrum-fed calves. This finding suggests there is not a clear protective effect by maternal antibody. No virus shedding was detected in either group of calves after reinoculation 3 months later.[38] A different study compared colostrum-deprived and colostrum-fed calves.[55] Colostrum-deprived calves had lower arterial oxygen tension and greater percentage of pneumonic lung compared with colostrum-fed calves. This finding indicates that there is a protective effect of maternal antibody. When calves with maternal antibodies were vaccinated with a commercial inactivated vaccine, there was a protective effect of vaccination based on clinical signs and virus shedding in nasal secretions.[56] Virus was detected in nasopharyngeal swab specimens from nonvaccinated calves up to day 9 after inoculation.[56] Clinical signs in nonvaccinated calves consisted of coughing for an average of 5.8 days after inoculation compared with 1 day for the vaccinates. Virus was not isolated from these specimens from vaccinated calves.[56]

A study was performed to determine if an inactivated BRSV vaccine induced the same antibody response compared with a modified live vaccine (MLV).[57] Calves that received the MLV developed a greater ratio of neutralizing antibody titer to change in BRSV-specific IgG antibody concentration compared with calves that received the inactivated virus vaccine. This work suggests certain inactivation processes can alter functionally important epitopes on BRSV envelope glycoproteins, leading to production of predominantly nonneutralizing antibodies in vaccinated cattle similar to what was postulated about the formalin-inactivated vaccine. Additional work agreed that vaccination with an inactivated vaccine resulted in less neutralizing antibody compared with IgG titers.[58] Vaccination with recombinant vaccinia virus expressing various individual proteins resulted in more F protein-induced neutralizing antibody production compared with G protein. Localized IgG1 and IgA antibodies were induced in the lung with F protein. Neutralizing antibodies were not detected in calves vaccinated with N protein.[59]

Bovine CD4+ T-cell epitopes are distributed predominantly on the F protein, allowing CD4+ cells to recognize F protein, similar to human CD4+ cells.[60] Infection by HRSV in human infant studies and in mouse models has shown that infection by HRSV induces production of a subset of cytokines that induces a CD4+ Th2 lymphocyte response.[61–63] These cytokines are interleukin 2 (IL-2), IL-4, and interferon gamma (IFN-γ). The result of a predominately Th2 response to HRSV infection is production of virus-specific IgE with resultant histamine release.[54] The pathogenesis of BRSV infection has been shown to result in virus-specific IgE and increased histamine release.[64] One of the cytokines that are part of the repertoire of Th2 lymphocytes is IL-4, which has been shown to be expressed early in infection with BRSV.[65] Similar to HRSV infection in humans, BRSV has been shown to induce IFN-γ.[66] Although vaccination with an inactivated vaccine did not induce high levels of neutralizing antibody, there appeared to be protection against challenge similar to that offered by vaccination with an MLV.[58]

Vaccination by inactivated vaccines continues to be a topic of interest. Different adjuvants have been used in attempts to create vaccines that generate high levels of neutralizing antibody and protect against natural infection and induce Th1 lymphocytes instead of Th2-type responses. A commercially available saponin-adjuvanted vaccine was tested to determine if it offered protection from experimental challenge or if there was enhancement of disease.[67] Similar to other inactivated vaccines, high levels of IgG were generated. Different to other inactivated vaccines, high levels of neutralizing antibodies were also produced. Vaccinated calves had no or minimal pneumonic changes compared with nonvaccinated controls, which had variable lung lesions. Two nonvaccinated animals were killed because they had severe respiratory disease. In a separate study, a modified version of formalin-inactivated vaccine was use.[68] The results of this study showed that vaccine composition plays a critical role in prevention of severe disease. Various preparations of inactivated vaccine can affect the immunologic outcome of an infection and high- dosage–inactivated BRSV can be prepared in such a way to circumvent BRSV-specific Th-2 response.

Nonstructural proteins NS1 and NS2 cooperate to antagonize IFN-α/β.[69] Following inoculation of calves with NS1 or NS2 deletion mutants low titers of virus were recovered from nasal swabs for 1 to 2 days compared with 6 to 7 days in calves infected with wild-type BRSV.[70] Further work showed the NS1 and NS2 proteins block

IFN-β by inhibition of one of the interferon gene promoters, IRF-3.[71] These gene-deleted mutants have been proposed as candidates for vaccine.

Vaccines containing DNA encoding either the F or N proteins have been have been shown to induce some level of protection in terms of priming of a memory response.[72,73] Vaccination with a vaccine containing DNA encoding for F protein resulted in priming for a BRSV-specific IgA response after challenge and offered nearly equal protection compared with prior BRSV infection. A second DNA vaccine that contained plasmids for F and N proteins offered data to support the ability of DNA vaccination to prime cell-mediated immunity in the face of high-titered maternally derived antibodies. Although not sufficient to ensure protection against clinical disease or viral excretion as a stand-alone vaccination strategy, priming immunity through DNA vaccination was proved to be an effective means of inducing cellular immunity for subsequent recall with an inactivated vaccine booster.[73] A study of a subunit vaccine based on nucleoprotein nanoparticles conferred partial clinical protection against BRSV challenge.[74] Vaccinated calves developed anti-N antibodies in blood and nasal secretions and N-specific cellular immunity in local lymph nodes. Nonvaccinated calves had moderate respiratory disease with local lung tissue consolidations. Lesions in the vaccinated calves were significantly reduced. Vaccinated calves had lower viral loads that the nonvaccinated control calves.

SUMMARY

BRSV has been recognized for 40 years. It remains a significant factor in BRD. This virus is spread by nasal secretions and may survive because of the heterogeneity of its genome and low fidelity in replication. Viral antigens and viral genome are easy to identify in field specimens by IHC and rtRT-PCR. The virus is labile and attempts at isolation in the laboratory from clinical specimens are often unrewarding. Because of the rapid turnaround time, rtRT-PCR is becoming more popular as a means of identifying BRSV in clinical cases. The immunopathogenesis of certain aspects of the disease revolves around subsets of CD4+ T lymphocytes and their stimulation of mediators of disease. Several vaccines are commercially available. New and more sophisticated vaccines with a molecular biologic approach in terms of use of DNA as part of the makeup are imminent.

REFERENCES

1. Jim K. Impact of bovine respiratory disease (BRD) from the perspective of the Canadian beef producer. Anim Health Res Rev 2009;10(2):109–10.
2. Smith RA. North American cattle marketing and bovine respiratory disease (BRD). Anim Health Res Rev 2009;10(2):105–8.
3. Smith MH, Frey ML, Dierks RE. Isolation, characterization, and pathogenicity studies of a bovine respiratory syncytial virus. Arch Virol 1975;47:237–47.
4. Kapikian AZ, Mitchell RH, Chanock RM, et al. An epidemiologic study of altered clinical reactivity to respiratory syncytial (RS) virus infection in children previously vaccinated with an inactivated RS virus vaccine. Am J Epidemiol 1969;89(4): 405–21.
5. Gershwin LJ, Schelegle ES, Gunther RA, et al. A bovine model of vaccine enhanced respiratory syncytial virus pathophysiology. Vaccine 1998;16(11–12): 1225–36.
6. Paccaud MF, Jacquier CL. A respiratory syncytial virus of bovine origin. Arch Gesamte Virusforsch 1970;30:327–42.

7. Wellemans G, Leunen J, Luchsinger E. Respiratory ailments of cattle: isolation of a virus (220/69) with serologic resemblance to the human respiratory syncytial virus. Ann Med Vet 1970;114:89–93.

8. Rosenquist BD. Isolation of respiratory syncytial virus from calves with acute respiratory disease. J Infect Dis 1974;130:177–82.

9. Smith MH, Frey ML, Dierks RE. Isolation and characterization of a bovine respiratory syncytial virus. Vet Rec 1974;94(25):599.

10. Baker JC, Ames TR, Markham RJ. Seroepizootiologic study of bovine respiratory syncytial virus in a dairy herd. Am J Vet Res 1986;47(2):240–5.

11. Baker JC, Ames TR, Werdin RE. Seroepizootiologic study of bovine respiratory syncytial virus in a beef herd. Am J Vet Res 1986;47(2):246–53.

12. Lehmkuhl HD, Gough PM. Investigation of causative agents of bovine respiratory tract disease in a beef cow-calf herd with an early weaning program. Am J Vet Res 1977;38(11):1717–20.

13. Bryson DG, McFerran JB, Ball HJ, et al. Observations on outbreaks of respiratory disease in calves associated with parainfluenza type 3 virus and respiratory syncytial virus infection. Vet Rec 1979;104(3):45–9.

14. Collins JK, Teegarden RM, MacVean DW, et al. Prevalence and specificity of antibodies to bovine respiratory syncytial virus in sera from feedlot and range cattle. Am J Vet Res 1988;49(8):1316–9.

15. Sorden SD, Kerr RW, Janzen ED. Interstitial pneumonia in feedlot cattle: concurrent lesions and lack of immunohistochemical evidence for bovine respiratory syncytial virus infection. J Vet Diagn Invest 2000;12(6):510–7.

16. Loneragan GH, Gould DH, Mason GL, et al. Association of 3-methyleneindolenine, a toxic metabolite of 3-methylindole, with acute interstitial pneumonia in feedlot cattle. Am J Vet Res 2001;62(10):1525–30.

17. Woolums AR, Mason GL, Hawkins LL, et al. Microbiologic findings in feedlot cattle with acute interstitial pneumonia. Am J Vet Res 2004;65(11):1525–32.

18. Harrison LR, Pursell AR. An epizootic of respiratory syncytial virus infection in a dairy herd. J Am Vet Med Assoc 1985;187(7):716–20.

19. Hägglund S, Hjort M, Graham DA, et al. A six-year study on respiratory viral infections in a bull testing facility. Vet J 2007;173(3):585–93.

20. Alm K, Koskinen E, Vahtiala S, et al. Acute BRSV infection in young AI bulls: effect on sperm quality. Reprod Domest Anim 2009;44(3):456–9.

21. Barth AD, Alisio L, Avilés M, et al. Fibrotic lesions in the testis of bulls and relationship to semen quality. Anim Reprod Sci 2008;106(3–4):274–88.

22. Trudel M, Nadon F, Simard C, et al. Comparison of caprin, human, and bovine strains of respiratory syncytial virus. Arch Virol 1989;107:141–9.

23. Frölich K, Hamblin C, Jung S, et al. Serologic surveillance for selected viral agents in captive and free-ranging populations of Arabian oryx (Oryx leucoryx) from Saudi Arabia and the United Arab Emirates. J Wildl Dis 2005;41(1):67–79.

24. Dunbar MR, Jessup DA, Evermann JF, et al. Seroprevalence of respiratory syncytial virus in free-ranging bighorn sheep. J Am Vet Med Assoc 1985; 187:1173–4.

25. Citterio CV, Luzzago C, Sala M, et al. Serological study of a population of alpine chamois (Rupicapra rupicapra) affected by an outbreak of respiratory disease. Vet Rec 2003;153:592–6.

26. Rivera H, Madewell BR, Ameghino E. Serologic survey of viral antibodies in the Peruvian alpaca (Lama pacos). Am J Vet Res 1987;48:189–91.

27. Sausker EA, Dyer NW. Seroprevalence of OHV-2, BVDV, BHV-1, and BRSV in ranch-raised bison (Bison bison). J Vet Diagn Invest 2002;14:68–70.

28. Bryson DG, Evermann JF, Liggitt HD, et al. Studies on the pathogenesis and inter-species transmission of respiratory syncytial virus isolated from sheep. Am J Vet Res 1988;49(8):1424–30.
29. Trigo FJ, Breeze RG, Evermann JF, et al. Pathogenesis of experimental bovine respiratory syncytial virus infection in sheep. Am J Vet Res 1984;45(8):1663–70.
30. Baker JC, Werdin RE, Ames TR, et al. Study on the etiologic role of bovine respiratory syncytial virus in pneumonia of dairy calves. J Am Vet Med Assoc 1986; 189:66–70.
31. De Jong MC, van der Poel WH, Kramps JA, et al. Quantitative investigation of population persistence and recurrent outbreaks of bovine respiratory syncytial virus on dairy farms. Am J Vet Res 1996;57(5):628–33.
32. Larsen LE, Tjørnehøj K, Viuff B. Extensive sequence divergence among bovine respiratory syncytial viruses isolated during recurrent outbreaks in closed herds. J Clin Microbiol 2000;38(11):4222–7.
33. Deplanche M, Lemaire M, Mirandette C, et al. In vivo evidence for quasispecies distributions in the bovine respiratory syncytial virus genome. J Gen Virol 2007; 88(Pt 4):1260–5.
34. Elazhary MA, Galina M, Roy RS, et al. Experimental infection of calves with bovine respiratory syncytial virus (Quebec strain). Can J Comp Med 1980;44(4):390–5.
35. Mohanty SB, Ingling AL, Lillie MG. Experimentally induced respiratory syncytial viral infection in calves. Am J Vet Res 1975;36(4 Pt1):417–9.
36. Bryson DG, McNulty MS, Logan EF, et al. Respiratory syncytial virus pneumonia in young calves: clinical and pathologic findings. Am J Vet Res 1983;44(9): 1648–55.
37. Castleman WL, Lay JC, Dubovi EJ, et al. Experimental bovine respiratory syncytial virus infection in conventional calves: light microscopic lesions, microbiology, and studies on lavaged lung cells. Am J Vet Res 1985;46(3):547–53.
38. Kimman TG, Westenbrink F, Schreuder BE, et al. Local and systemic antibody response to bovine respiratory syncytial virus infection and reinfection in calves with and without maternal antibodies. J Clin Microbiol 1987;25(6):1097–106.
39. Kimman TG, Straver PJ, Zimmer GM. Pathogenesis of naturally acquired bovine respiratory syncytial virus infection in calves: morphologic and serologic findings. Am J Vet Res 1989;50(5):684–93.
40. Rossi CR, Kiesel GK. Bovine respiratory syncytial virus infection of bovine embryonic lung cultures: a kinetic study by the fluorescent antibody technique. Am J Vet Res 1977;38(11):1901–4.
41. Thomas LH, Stott EJ. Diagnosis of respiratory syncytial virus infection in the bovine respiratory tract by immunofluorescence. Vet Rec 1981;108(20):432–5.
42. Osorio FA, Anderson GA, Sanders J, et al. Detection of bovine respiratory syncytial virus using a heterologous antigen-capture enzyme immunoassay. J Vet Diagn Invest 1989;1(3):210–4.
43. Quinting B, Robert B, Letellier C, et al. Development of a 1-step enzyme-linked immunosorbent assay for the rapid diagnosis of bovine respiratory syncytial virus in postmortem specimens. J Vet Diagn Invest 2007;19(3):238–43.
44. Bryson DG, Cush PF, McNulty MS, et al. An immunoperoxidase method of detecting respiratory syncytial virus antigens in paraffin sections of pneumonic bovine lung. Am J Vet Res 1988;49(7):1121–6.
45. Haines DM, Clark EG, Chelack BJ. The detection of bovine respiratory syncytial virus in formalin fixed bovine lung with commercially available monoclonal antibodies and avidin biotin complex immunohistochemistry. Can J Vet Res 1989; 53(3):366–8.

46. White AK, Hansen-Lardy L, Brodersen BW, et al. Enhanced immunohistochemical detection of infectious agents in formalin-fixed, paraffin-embedded tissues following heat-mediated antigen retrieval. J Vet Diagn Invest 1998;10(2):214–7.

47. Oberst RD, Hays MP, Hennessy KJ, et al. Identifying bovine respiratory syncytial virus by reverse transcription-polymerase chain reaction and oligonucleotide hybridizations. J Clin Microbiol 1993;31(5):1237–40.

48. West K, Bogdan J, Hamel A, et al. A comparison of diagnostic methods for the detection of bovine respiratory syncytial virus in experimental clinical specimens. Can J Vet Res 1998;62(4):245–50.

49. Willoughby K, Thomson K, Maley M, et al. Development of a real time reverse transcriptase polymerase chain reaction for the detection of bovine respiratory syncytial virus in clinical samples and its comparison with immunohistochemistry and immunofluorescence antibody testing. Vet Microbiol 2008;126(1–3):264–70.

50. Samal SK, Zamora M, McPhillips TH, et al. Molecular cloning and sequence analysis of bovine respiratory syncytial virus mRNA encoding the major nucleocapsid protein. Virology 1991;180(1):453–6.

51. Timsit E, Le Dréan E, Maingourd C, et al. Detection by real-time RT-PCR of a bovine respiratory syncytial virus vaccine in calves vaccinated intranasally. Vet Rec 2009;165(8):230–3.

52. Timsit E, Maingourd C, Le Dréan E, et al. Evaluation of a commercial real-time reverse transcription polymerase chain reaction kit for the diagnosis of Bovine respiratory syncytial virus infection. J Vet Diagn Invest 2010;22(2):238–41.

53. Prince GA, Jenson AB, Hemming VG, et al. Enhancement of respiratory syncytial virus pulmonary pathology in cotton rats by prior intramuscular inoculation of formalin-inactiva ted virus. J Virol 1986;57(3):721–8.

54. Welliver RC, Wong DT, Sun M, et al. The development of respiratory syncytial virus-specific IgE and the release of histamine in nasopharyngeal secretions after infection. N Engl J Med 1981;305(15):841–6.

55. Belknap EB, Baker JC, Patterson JS, et al. The role of passive immunity in bovine respiratory syncytial virus-infected calves. J Infect Dis 1991;163(3):470–6.

56. Patel JR, Didlick SA. Evaluation of efficacy of an inactivated vaccine against bovine respiratory syncytial virus in calves with maternal antibodies. Am J Vet Res 2004;65(4):417–21.

57. Ellis JA, Hassard LE, Morley PS. Bovine respiratory syncytial virus-specific immune responses in calves after inoculation with commercially available vaccines. J Am Vet Med Assoc 1995;206(3):354–61.

58. Ellis J, West K, Konoby C, et al. Efficacy of an inactivated respiratory syncytial virus vaccine in calves. J Am Vet Med Assoc 2001;218(12):1973–80.

59. Taylor G, Thomas LH, Furze JM, et al. Recombinant vaccinia viruses expressing the F, G or N, but not the M2, protein of bovine respiratory syncytial virus (BRSV) induce resistance to BRSV challenge in the calf and protect against the development of pneumonic lesions. J Gen Virol 1997;78(Pt 12):3195–206.

60. Fogg MH, Parsons KR, Thomas LH, et al. Identification of CD4+ T cell epitopes on the fusion (F) and attachment (G) proteins of bovine respiratory syncytial virus (BRSV). Vaccine 2001;19(23–24):3226–40.

61. Hussell T, Spender LC, Georgiou A, et al. Th1 and Th2 cytokine induction in pulmonary T cells during infection with respiratory syncytial virus. J Gen Virol 1996;77(Pt 10):2447–55.

62. Tang YW, Graham BS. Anti-IL-4 treatment at immunization modulates cytokine expression, reduces illness, and increases cytotoxic T lymphocyte activity in mice challenged with respiratory syncytial virus. J Clin Invest 1994;94(5):1953–8.

63. Román M, Calhoun WJ, Hinton KL, et al. Respiratory syncytial virus infection in infants is associated with predominant Th-2-like response. Am J Respir Crit Care Med 1997;156(1):190–5.

64. Stewart RS, Gershwin LJ. Role of IgE in the pathogenesis of bovine respiratory syncytial virus in sequential infections in vaccinated and nonvaccinated calves. Am J Vet Res 1989;50(3):349–55.

65. Gershwin LJ, Gunther RA, Anderson ML, et al. Bovine respiratory syncytial virus-specific IgE is associated with interleukin-2 and -4, and interferon-gamma expression in pulmonary lymph of experimentally infected calves. Am J Vet Res 2000;61(3):291–8.

66. West K, Petrie L, Konoby C, et al. The efficacy of modified-live bovine respiratory syncytial virus vaccines in experimentally infected calves. Vaccine 1999; 18(9–10):907–19.

67. Ellis JA, West KH, Waldner C, et al. Efficacy of a saponin-adjuvanted inactivated respiratory syncytial virus vaccine in calves. Can Vet J 2005;46(2):155–62.

68. Kalina WV, Woolums AR, Gershwin LJ. Formalin-inactivated bovine RSV vaccine influences antibody levels in bronchoalveolar lavage fluid and disease outcome in experimentally infected calves. Vaccine 2005;23(37):4625–30.

69. Schlender J, Bossert B, Buchholz U, et al. Bovine respiratory syncytial virus nonstructural proteins NS1 and NS2 cooperatively antagonize alpha/beta interferon-induced antiviral response. J Virol 2000;74(18):8234–42.

70. Valarcher JF, Furze J, Wyld S, et al. Role of alpha/beta interferons in the attenuation and immunogenicity of recombinant bovine respiratory syncytial viruses lacking NS proteins. J Virol 2003;77(15):8426–39.

71. Bossert B, Marozin S, Conzelmann KK. Nonstructural proteins NS1 and NS2 of bovine respiratory syncytial virus block activation of interferon regulatory factor 3. J Virol 2003;77(16):8661–8.

72. Taylor G, Bruce C, Barbet AF, et al. DNA vaccination against respiratory syncytial virus in young calves. Vaccine 2005;23(10):1242–50.

73. Hamers C, Juillard V, Fischer L. DNA vaccination against pseudorabies virus and bovine respiratory syncytial virus infections of young animals in the face of maternally derived immunity. J Comp Pathol 2007;137(Suppl 1):S35–41.

74. Riffault S, Meyer G, Deplanche M, et al. A new subunit vaccine based on nucleoprotein nanoparticles confers partial clinical and virological protection in calves against bovine respiratory syncytial virus. Vaccine 2010;28(21):3722–34.

The Contribution of Infections with Bovine Viral Diarrhea Viruses to Bovine Respiratory Disease

Julia Ridpath, PhD

KEYWORDS

• Bovine viral diarrhea viruses • Respiratory disease
• Persistent infection • Immunosuppression • Pathogen synergy

Although bovine viral diarrhea viruses are arguably the most researched of all viral pathogens associated with bovine respiratory disease (BRD), the impact of bovine viral diarrhea viruses (BVDV) on BRD is still unknown. This uncertainty is because the determination of total impact must factor in the contribution of acute, uncomplicated BVDV infections, impact of high incidence of respiratory disease in animals persistently infected with BVDV, impact of the immunosuppression that accompanies acute BVDV infections and predisposes animals to secondary infections, and impact of increased virulence of pathogens caused by synergy in coinfections. Adding to the complexity is the heterogeneity observed among BVDV strains that results in differences in genotype (species), biotype, and virulence. Because variation among BVDV strains underlies the complicated nature of these infections this article begins with a review of the factors that give rise to BVDV heterogeneity and then proceeds to the different ways in which BVDV infections contribute to BRD.

BASIS OF HETEROGENEITY OBSERVED AMONG BOVINE VIRAL DIARRHEA VIRUSES STRAINS
Size of Lipid Envelope Surrounding Virion is Variable

The term BVDV refers to a heterogeneous group of viruses that belong to two different species, BVDV1 and BVDV2, within the *pestivirus* genus of the Flavivirus family.[1,2] Similar to other Flaviviridae, the infectious viral particle consists of an outer lipid envelope surrounding an inner protein shell or capsid that contains the viral genome.

The author has nothing to disclose.
Ruminant Diseases and Immunology Research Unit, United States Department of Agriculture, Agricultural Research Service, National Animal Disease Center, 1920 Dayton Avenue, PO Box 70, Ames, IA 50010, USA
E-mail address: julia.ridpath@ars.usda.gov

Pestiviruses differ from other members of the Flaviviridae in that the lipid envelope that surrounds the virion is pleomorphic. The practical significance of the resulting variation in size of enveloped particles is that it precludes identification by electron microscopy in clinical samples. Further, this variation in size prevents the purification of the virus by standard techniques used in virology. This lack of purification means that the BVDV component of most killed and modified-live vaccines is not pure BVDV but a mixture of viral proteins and proteins derived from the cells in which the virus was propagated.

The Genome of Bovine Viral Diarrhea Viruses is a Single-Stranded RNA Prone to Mutation

The BVDV genome consists of a single strand of RNA about 12.3 Kb long. The genomic organization is the same as that of all pestiviruses. In the absence of insertions, the genome codes for one open reading frame (ORF) approximately 4000 codons long. The ORF is preceded and followed by 5′ and 3′ untranslated regions (UTR) of 360 to 390 nucleotides and 200 to 240 nucleotides, respectively. Much of the heterogeneity observed among BVDV is caused by the variability inherent in having a single-stranded RNA genome. Point mutations in this type of genome are introduced with each round of virus replication because there is no proofreading function associated with replication. The impact of this heterogeneity is observed as differences in genotype, biotype, and virulence. It is thought that the accumulation of point mutations over time resulted in the branching of BVDV into two genetically distinct species, now known as BVDV1 and BVDV2.[3,4] Although the first studies, segregating BVDV strains into two species, were based on comparison of the 5′ UTR, differences between BVDV1 and BVDV2 strains are found throughout the genome.[5,6] Antigenic differences, between the two species, are revealed in the laboratory by serum neutralization studies using polyclonal sera[7-11] and by monoclonal antibody binding studies.[4,12] These antigenic differences are also shown in nature by the birth of BVDV2 persistently infected animals to dams that had been vaccinated against BVDV1 strains.[4] The fact that cattle persistently infected with and immunotolerant of one species have a serologic response to vaccination with another BVDV species further demonstrates antigenic differences between the two species.[13] Although modified-live BVDV1 vaccines may induce antibodies against BVDV2 strains, the titers average one log less than titers against heterologous BVDV1 strains.[7-11] These observations led to the inclusion of both BVDV species in many BVDV vaccines.

Genomic Recombination that Result in Changes in Biotype

BVDV1 and BVDV2 strains may exist as one of two biotypes (cytopathic and non-cytopathic) based on their activity in cultured epithelial cells, with non-cytopathic BVDV predominating in nature.[14,15] Studies of proteins associated with BVDV replication in cultured cells reveal that cytopathic BVDV could be distinguished from non-cytopathic BVDV by the production of an extra nonstructural protein known as NS3.[16,17] This protein is the result of the cleavage of another nonstructural protein, NS2/3. Comparison of NS2/3 coding region of cytopathic and non-cytopathic BVDV revealed that genomes of most cytopathic viruses had under gone a recombinational event resulting in the introduction of a cleavage site into the NS2/3 protein.[18] The most commonly observed means of introducing this cleavage site was by insertion of host cell genetic sequences or duplicated BVDV genetic sequences inserted into the NS2-3 coding region.[19]

Exposure of cattle to viruses from either biotype may result in acute infection. In addition, infection of a bovine fetus before 125 days gestation to non-cytopathic, but not cytopathic, viruses may result in the establishment of a lifelong persistent infection.[20,21]

The prerequisite for such persistent BVDV infections appears to arise from specific B- and T-lymphocyte immunotolerance.[22,23] It is theorized that there is negative selection or downregulation of BVDV-specific B and T lymphocytes during ontogeny resulting in an absence of neutralizing and non-neutralizing antibodies and cell mediated immunity to the persistent BVDV.[24] The result is that viral proteins are accepted as self-antigens. Persistently infected animals (PIs) may appear normal or suffer from an array of congenital anomalies, including defects of the nervous system, eyes, skeletal system, and skin/hair (Table 1). In addition to these more noticeable defects, PIs are more likely than normal cattle to require treatment for respiratory tract disease and either become chronically ill or die.[25] The PI animal also has a high risk for succumbing to a highly fatal form of BVD called mucosal disease (BVD-MD). BVD-MD is the sequela of a persistent infection with non-cytopathic BVDV strain, followed by an acute concurrent infection with a cytopathic BVDV strain. The cytopathic BVDV inducing BVD-MD is most frequently derived from the non-cytopathic BVDV with which the PI animal is persistently infected.[26–29] Other sources for cytopathic BVDV include other cattle suffering from BVD-MD[30] and modified-live virus vaccines.[31–33] BVD-MD is invariably fatal. However, because the number of PI animals within a herd tends to be low, morbidity for BVD-MD also tends to be low. The major economic impact of PIs is not death caused by BVD-MD, but that these animals continually shed the virus and are the principal vector for introduction and maintenance of BVDV infections within cattle populations.[34]

Fetal exposure to BVDV after 125 days gestation, although not resulting in persistent infections, may give rise to many of the same congenital anomalies as persistent infection and there are reports that non-persistently infected cattle that were exposed to BVDV in utero have higher morbidity and mortality rates[35,36] and lower fertility rates[37] than cattle not exposed in utero.

BOVINE VIRAL DIARRHEA VIRUS INFECTIONS AND RESPIRATORY DISEASE

The contribution of BVDV infections to the development of clinical respiratory disease depends on several factors, including the virulence of the infecting BVDV strain, type of infection (acute or persistent), time of exposure (fetal or postnatal), and the

Table 1
Defects resulting from in utero exposure to BVDV

System/Tissue	Defect
Central nervous system	Cerebellar hypoplasia[74–81] Microencephaly, hydrocephalus, hydranencephaly[82] Hypomyelination[81,83–85]
Skeletal	Abnormal osteogenesis[86] Brachygnathism[87] Failure of limb development[87]
Eye	Optic neuritis[77,88] Cataracts[89] Retinal degeneration[77,90] Microphthalmia[91,92]
Endocrine	Thymic hypoplasia[93]
Skin/hair	Curly coat[94] Hypotrichosis/alopecia[95]

presence of secondary pathogens. It is not always possible to determine if clinical reports and surveys are describing outbreaks of respiratory disease in PIs or the contribution of BVDV to BRD in a herd as the result of acute infections. On the other hand, it is difficult to design studies of BVDV infections under controlled conditions that reproduce the numerous factors that contribute to the development of BRD.

IMPACT OF RESPIRATORY DISEASE IN PERSISTENTLY INFECTED ANIMALS

PIs are more likely to succumb to disease than their normal counterparts. Surveys of cattle entering feedlots in the United States indicate that although PIs represent less than 0.5% of the general population, they represent 2.5% to 5% of the cattle succumbing to fatal illnesses.[25,38] Because PIs have a higher rate of morbidity and mortality than the general population, a portion of the observed association of BVDV with BRD may be the result of PIs vulnerability to respiratory disease. In fact, in utero exposure to BVDV may predispose even non-PIs to BRD. A study by Barber and colleagues[35] detailing calf loss caused by disease in a dairy herd over a 3-year time span demonstrated that in utero exposure to BVDV results in a higher susceptibility to respiratory disease. In the first year of this study an outbreak of diarrhea among adult milking cows was traced to BVDV. Of 121 calves born that year, five died with mucosal disease-like symptoms and 21 (17%) died of pneumonia. Calf losses remained high the following 2 years with suppurative or fibrinous pneumonia as the leading cause of death. Testing results were not available for all animals dying of pneumonia, and data regarding animals that developed pneumonia but recovered was not included. BVDV was isolated from 36 animals examined with 12 being identified as persistently infected. In addition, the investigators looked at the relationship between the BVDV serologic status of cows and calf survival. It was observed that the death rate among calves born to BVDV seropositive cows was 22% (of these deaths 15/35 or 43% were caused by pneumonia), whereas the death rate among calves born to cows infected during pregnancy, based on serology, was 50% (of these 18/24 or 75% were caused by pneumonia). Based on this comparison, the investigators concluded that fetal exposure to BVDV, regardless of whether exposure resulted in persistent infection, reduced a calf's chance of survival and increased its risk for developing pneumonia. Further evidence that fetal exposure predisposes cattle to disease is provided by a study showing that calves born with titers against BVDV (indicating a fetal exposure) were twice as likely to develop serious illness.[36] Thus studies of association of pathogens with respiratory lesions, based on isolation or detection of pathogens currently present, may underestimate the contribution of BVDV fetal exposure to the development of BRD.

BOVINE VIRAL DIARRHEA VIRUS INFECTIONS AND THE DEVELOPMENT OF BOVINE RESPIRATORY DISEASE IN NORMAL CATTLE (CATTLE NOT EXPOSED IN UTERO)

Although PI and animals exposed in utero may make up a portion of respiratory disease cases, there are three lines of evidence showing that current acute-BVDV infections in cattle that were not exposed to BVDV in utero contribute to respiratory disease. One line of evidence is the detection of BVDV in lung lesions of acutely infected cattle. In a study of fatal BRD cases in Western Canada, 90 feedlot calves diagnosed at necropsy with BRD and nine control calves without BRD were examined for the presence of seven pathogens (BVDV, bovine herpesvirus-1, bovine respiratory syncytial virus [BRSV], parinfluenza-3 virus, *Mannheimia haemolytica* [MH], *Mycoplasma bovis*, and *Histophilus somni*) based on immunohistochemical (IHC) staining of lung tissue.[39] In addition, a distinction was made between persistent or acute infection with BVDV based on IHC staining of skin biopsy samples.[40] BVDV was detected in the lungs of 26 calves succumbing to BRD but not in the lungs of any control animals. Of the 26 BVDV-positive calves, three were determined to be PI indicating that acute BVDV infections were more prevalent than persistent infections in these BRD cases.

A second line of evidence is based on serologic data collected from cattle in feedlots. Several studies have reported that higher serum antibody titers against BVDV in cattle on arrival to feedlots reduced the risk for subsequent BRD,[41–44] and conversely, increases in BVDV titer after arrival were associated with an increased risk for BRD.[41,42,44]

The third line of evidence is illustrated by a study comparing calves exposed to BVDV after receiving colostrum from seronegative dams to calves exposed to BVDV after receiving colostrum from seropositive dams.[45] Calves exposed to BVDV soon after birth that received passive antibodies against BVDV via ingestion of colostrum were 28% less likely to develop respiratory disease than exposed calves that did not receive passive antibodies.

Thus it appears that fetal exposure to BVDV and acute postnatal BVDV infections contribute to BRD. The mechanism of this contribution is variably dependent on the type of infection (acute or persistent), virulence of viral strain, impact of immune suppression, and interaction with secondary pathogens as discussed later.

IMPACT OF UNCOMPLICATED ACUTE INFECTIONS

Acute BVDV infection is the term used to describe clinical or subclinical disease that occurs in non-persistently infected immunocompetent cattle following exposure to BVDV.[46] Exposure is typically via short range, large droplet aerosols, or direct contact with infected animals. Exposure results in the infection of the nasal mucosa. Although there can be transmission from acutely infected cattle, the most frequent vector is a PI animal. Infection spreads from the nasal mucosa to the draining lymph nodes and from there is transmitted to other tissues via circulating lymphoid cells. The incubation period is 5 to 7 days and viremia is typically less than 15 days[46] but may be longer depending on viral strain, stress levels, and presence of secondary pathogens. Although not the primary site of replication, controlled studies and field reports demonstrate that BVDV can establish infections in the respiratory tract of cattle.[47–50] Although these infections result in damage to the epithelial surfaces of the respiratory system[51] and depletion of lymphoid tissue associated with the respiratory tract,[50,52–54] it is estimated that 70% to 90% are subclinical.[55] Although some studies have demonstrated clinical respiratory disease resulting from acute, uncomplicated BVDV infections under controlled conditions,[56,57] a model system that reproducibly replicates BVDV-associated pneumonia has yet to be developed. This is problematic for the study of BVDV infections and for demonstrating the efficacy of vaccines in preventing BVDV infections of the respiratory system.[58]

Differences in virulence[53,59–65] and pneumopathogenicity[57] exist among BVDV strains. The length of viremia is longer and the amount of viral shed is greater following infection with highly virulent BVDV compared with infections with low virulence strains.[59,61,66] Transmission by acutely infected animals is significant and the sources of virus increase as the number of infected animals increases.[60] Thus management to control outbreaks of severe, acute BVD requires a different approach than that used for subclinical BVD.

Although acute BVDV infections may, in some situations, directly result in respiratory disease, the majority of evidence suggests that BVDV infections contribute to

BRD mainly as potentiators for secondary infections (**Table 2**). It is theorized that BVDV potentiation of BRD occurs by two different mechanisms, immunosuppression[67,68] and synergism,[69] as discussed later.

IMMUNOSUPPRESSION ASSOCIATED WITH BOVINE VIRAL DIARRHEA VIRUS INFECTION

The immunosuppression that accompanies acute BVDV infections results from a combination of outright lymphoid cell death[2,63,64] and reduced function in remaining lymphoid cells.[67] Although there are several reports in the literature detailing in vitro studies of cell death or immune cell dysfunction resulting from infection with cytopathic BVDV strains, cytopathology in cultured epithelial cells is not analogous to cell death resulting in immunosuppression in vivo. The cytopathic effects observed following the infection of epithelial cells in vitro with a cytopathic BVDV is not equivalent to lymphoid depletion observed following BVDV infection in vivo for several reasons. For one, nearly all field strains of BVDV are non-cytopathic. Cytopathic strains of BVDV are only rarely isolated and usually from cases of BVD-MD. Secondly, the cell death observed in vivo is in lymphoid cell populations, not epithelial cell populations. Further, it appears that cell death caused by cytopathic BVDV in vitro may occur by a different mechanism than cell death that occurs following infection with non-cytopathic BVDV.[70,71] Finally, the lymphoid depletion that is associated with BVDV infections in vivo results from a complex and intertwined response of the innate and acquired immune system that cannot be replicated in a culture flask.

Infection, with either high- and low-virulence BVDV, results in the reduction of circulating lymphocytes[59,63,64] and the depletion of lymphoid tissue.[50,54] The mechanism behind lymphoid depletion following acute BVDV infection is largely undefined. Comparison of high- and low-virulence BVDV strains has yielded some intriguing results. The difference in pathology between high- and low-virulence BVDV strains is in the extent of cell death or loss, with reduction of circulating lymphocytes and lymphoid depletion being significantly higher following infection with highly virulent BVDV. The mechanisms involved in the destruction of lymphoid tissue by

Table 2
Reported interaction of BVDV with secondary pathogens in the development of BRD

Pathogen type	Viral Pathogen	Interaction
Viral	BRSV[68,96–98]	Synergism resulting in increased pathogenesis/dissemination
	Infectious bovine rhinotracheitis virus[72,99–102]	Synergism resulting in increased pathogenesis/dissemination
	Parainfluenza-3 virus[102]	Synergism resulting in increased pathogenesis/dissemination
Bacterial	*Mycoplasma bovis*[103,104]	Synergism resulting in increased pathogenesis, immunosuppression resulting in increased opportunist infections and chronic infections
	Mannheimia haemolytica[39,56,57]	Synergism resulting in increased pathogenesis, immunosuppression resulting in increased opportunist infections

non-cytopathic BVDV strains are poorly understood. Decreased numbers of circulating lymphocytes may be the result of trafficking from blood into tissue, a reduction in leukogenesis, or outright death of cells. The high percentage of apoptotic or necrotic lymphocytes observed in animals infected with a high-virulence BVDV strain suggest that the reduction may be caused by cell death.[50,53] This in vivo observation is supported by the in vitro observation that infection of a cultured lymphoid cell line, with a high-virulence virus leads to cell death.[70] Although this mechanism of cell death has yet to be defined, it appears to be different than the mechanism that induces apoptosis in cells infected with cytopathic BVDV.[71]

In addition to reducing lymphoid cell numbers, BVDV infections impair the function of cells associated with both the acquired and innate immune systems (**Table 3**).[67] The interactions resulting in immune suppression are complex and it is difficult to design experimental models that reflect natural conditions. Stages in the innate immune response that are reported to be suppressed in response to BVDV infection include interferon production, phagocytosis, chemotaxis, and microbicidal killing. On the acquired immune side, changes, such as downregulation of MHC II and IL-2, suppress the T-helper cell response.

SYNERGISTIC EFFECTS

Synergy occurs when coinfection of two or more pathogens results in an enhanced pathogenesis or change in character of the pathogenesis. Synergistic effects have been reported between BVDV and several viral and bacterial pathogens that are associated with BRD (see **Table 3**). Once again, when reading through the literature it is necessary to differentiate between enhanced pathogenesis observed following infection of PIs and synergy observed following acute coinfection with BVDV and a secondary pathogen. Synergism may occur by several different routes depending on coinfecting pathogens and target tissues. One possible result of synergy is increased dissemination of pathogens in tissues. Viral dissemination of BVDV and BHV-1 were higher in concurrent infections than in single infections.[72] Dual infections

Table 3
Effects of BVDV that result in immunosuppression

Change	Effect	Impact
Decreased chemotaxis Decreased Fe, CD14, and complement receptor expression Decreased phagocytosis	Decreased neutrophil function	Decreased ability to fight off bacterial infections
Decrease in TNF-α production and increase in IL-1 inhibitors	Decreased inflammatory and T-cell cytokine production	Decreased innate and adaptive immune response
Decrease in IFN production	Decreased antiviral response	Decreased ability to fight off viral infections
Decrease in MHC II production	Decrease in antigen presentation	Reduction in capacity of adaptive immune response
Decrease in MHC I expression	Decrease in cytotoxic T-lymphocyte response	Increase in immune evasion and viral infection

Abbreviations: IFN, interferon; IL-1, interleukin-1; MHC, major histocompatibility complex; TNF, tumor necrosis factor.

may also combine to reduce immune cell function. Liu and Lehmkuhl demonstrated that coinfections of bovine alveolar macrophage (AM) with BVDV and BRSV produced a synergistic depression on AM functions. Although the mechanism of synergy may not be defined, indirect evidence may point to synergistic interaction. BVDV is frequently detected in diseased respiratory tract tissues in association with MH.[39,73] As it is difficult to reliably reproduce respiratory disease under controlled conditions in infections with BVDV or MH alone, a synergistic relationship (albeit currently undefined) is indicated.

SUMMARY

Although it is difficult to confirm by direct experimental evidence, several lines of research indicate that BVDV may be a pivotal component in BRD. This research includes the following examples. Some strains of BVDV may cause BRD following acute uncomplicated infections. Calves exposed to BVDV in utero have increased susceptibilities to BRD. Acute BVDV infections result in a broad spectrum immunosuppression that predisposes cattle to opportunistic infections of secondary respiratory pathogens. Finally, synergistic interaction of BVDV and other respiratory pathogens during coinfections results in more clinically severe respiratory disease.

REFERENCES

1. Thiel HJ, Collett MS, Gould EA, et al. Family *Flaviviridae*. In: Fauquet CM, Mayo MA, Maniloff J, et al, editors. Eighth report of the International Committee on taxonomy of viruses. San Diego (CA): Elsevier Academic Press; 2005. p. 981–98.
2. Ridpath JF. Bovine viral diarrhea virus. In: Mahy BWJ, Regenmortel MHV, editors. Encyclopedia of virology. Oxford (UK): Elsevier; 2008. p. 374–80.
3. Pellerin C, van den Hurk J, Lecomte J, et al. Identification of a new group of bovine viral diarrhea virus strains associated with severe outbreaks and high mortalities. Virology 1994;203(2):260–8.
4. Ridpath JF, Bolin SR, Dubovi EJ. Segregation of bovine viral diarrhea virus into genotypes. Virology 1994;205(1):66–74.
5. Ridpath JF, Bolin SR. The genomic sequence of a virulent bovine viral diarrhea virus (BVDV) from the type 2 genotype: detection of a large genomic insertion in a noncytopathic BVDV. Virology 1995;212(1):39–46.
6. Ridpath JF, Bolin SR. Comparison of the complete genomic sequence of the border disease virus, BD31, to other pestiviruses. Virus Res 1997;50(2):237–43.
7. Fulton RW, Purdy CW, Confer AW, et al. Bovine viral diarrhea viral infections in feeder calves with respiratory disease: interactions with Pasteurella spp., parainfluenza-3 virus, and bovine respiratory syncytial virus. Can J Vet Res 2000;64(3):151–9.
8. Chase CC, Chase SK, Fawcett L. Trends in the BVDV serological response in the Upper Midwest. Biologicals 2003;31(2):145–51.
9. Bolin SR, Ridpath JF. Prevalence of bovine viral diarrhea virus genotypes and antibody against those viral genotypes in fetal bovine serum. J Vet Diagn Invest 1998;10(2):135–9.
10. Fulton RW, Saliki JT, Burge LJ, et al. Neutralizing antibodies to type 1 and 2 bovine viral diarrhea viruses: detection by inhibition of viral cytopathology and infectivity by immunoperoxidase assay. Clin Diagn Lab Immunol 1997;4(3):380–3.

11. Fulton RW, Burge LJ. Bovine viral diarrhea virus types 1 and 2 antibody response in calves receiving modified live virus or inactivated vaccines. Vaccine 2000;19(2–3):264–74.
12. Deregt D, Bolin SR, van den Hurk J, et al. Mapping of a type 1-specific and a type-common epitope on the E2 (gp53) protein of bovine viral diarrhea virus with neutralization escape mutants. Virus Res 1998;53(1):81–90.
13. Fulton RW, Step DL, Ridpath JF, et al. Response of calves persistently infected with noncytopathic bovine viral diarrhea virus (BVDV) subtype 1b after vaccination with heterologous BVDV strains in modified live virus vaccines and Mannheimia haemolytica bacterin-toxoid. Vaccine 2003;21(21–22):2980–5.
14. Lee KM, Gillespie JH. Propagation of virus diarrhea virus of cattle in tissue culture. Am J Vet Res 1957;18:952–3.
15. Gillespie J, Baker J, McEntee K. A cytopathogenic strains of virus diarrhea virus. Cornell Vet 1960;50:73–9.
16. Pocock DH, Howard CJ, Clarke MC, et al. Variation in the intracellular polypeptide profiles from different isolates of bovine virus diarrhoea virus. Arch Virol 1987;94(1–2):43–53.
17. Donis RO, Dubovi EJ. Differences in virus-induced polypeptides in cells infected by cytopathic and noncytopathic biotypes of bovine virus diarrhea-mucosal disease virus. Virology 1987;158(1):168–73.
18. Meyers G, Tautz N, Stark R, et al. Rearrangement of viral sequences in cytopathogenic pestiviruses. Virology 1992;191(1):368–86.
19. Kummerer BM, Tautz N, Becher P, et al. The genetic basis for cytopathogenicity of pestiviruses. Vet Microbiol 2000;77(1–2):117–28.
20. Grooms DL. Reproductive consequences of infection with bovine viral diarrhea virus. Vet Clin North Am Food Anim Pract 2004;20(1):5–19.
21. Brock KV, Grooms DL, Givens MD. Reproductive disease and persistent infections. In: Goyal SM, Ridpath JF, editors. Bovine viral diarrhea virus: diagnosis, management and control. Ames (IA): Blackwell Publishing; 2005. p. 145–56.
22. Coria MF, McClurkin AW. Specific immune tolerance in an apparently healthy bull persistently infected with bovine viral diarrhea virus. J Am Vet Med Assoc 1978;172(4):449–51.
23. McClurkin AW, Littledike ET, Cutlip RC, et al. Production of cattle immunotolerant to bovine viral diarrhea virus. Can J Comp Med 1984;48(2):156–61.
24. Donis RO, Dubovi EJ. Molecular specificity of the antibody responses of cattle naturally and experimentally infected with cytopathic and noncytopathic bovine viral diarrhea virus biotypes. Am J Vet Res 1987;48(11):1549–54.
25. Loneragan GH, Thomson DU, Montgomery DL, et al. Prevalence, outcome, and health consequences associated with persistent infection with bovine viral diarrhea virus in feedlot cattle. J Am Vet Med Assoc 2005;226(4):595–601.
26. Brownlie J. Pathogenesis of mucosal disease and molecular aspects of bovine virus diarrhea virus. Vet Microbiol 1990;23(1–4):371–82.
27. Bolin SR. The pathogenesis of mucosal disease. Vet Clin North Am Food Anim Pract 1995;11(3):489–500.
28. Baker JC. The clinical manifestations of bovine viral diarrhea infection. Vet Clin North Am Food Anim Pract 1995;11(3):425–45.
29. Tautz N, Meyers G, Thiel HJ. Pathogenesis of mucosal disease, a deadly disease of cattle caused by a pestivirus. Clin Diagn Virol 1998;10(2–3):121–7.
30. Brownlie J, Clarke MC, Howard CJ. Experimental production of fatal mucosal disease in cattle. Vet Rec 1984;114(22):535–6.

31. Ridpath JF, Bolin SR. Delayed onset postvaccinal mucosal disease as a result of genetic recombination between genotype 1 and genotype 2 BVDV. Virology 1995;212(1):259–62.
32. Peter C, Tyler D, Ramsey F. Characteristics of a condition following vaccination with bovine virus diarrhea vaccine. J Am Vet Med Assoc 1967;150:46–52.
33. McKercher M, Saito J, Crenshaw G. Complications following vaccination with a combined viral diarrhea-infectious bovine rhinotracheitis vaccine. J Am Vet Med Assoc 1968;152:1621–4.
34. Hessman BE, Fulton RW, Sjeklocha DB, et al. Evaluation of economic effects and the health and performance of the general cattle population after exposure to cattle persistently infected with bovine viral diarrhea virus in a starter feedlot. Am J Vet Res 2009;70(1):73–85.
35. Barber DM, Nettleton PF, Herring JA. Disease in a dairy herd associated with the introduction and spread of bovine virus diarrhoea virus. Vet Rec 1985;117(18):459–64.
36. Munoz-Zanzi CA, Hietala SK, Thurmond MC, et al. Quantification, risk factors, and health impact of natural congenital infection with bovine viral diarrhea virus in dairy calves. Am J Vet Res 2003;64(3):358–65.
37. Munoz-Zanzi CA, Thurmond MC, Hietala SK. Effect of bovine viral diarrhea virus infection on fertility of dairy heifers. Theriogenology 2004;61(6):1085–99.
38. Fulton RW, Blood KS, Panciera RJ, et al. Lung pathology and infectious agents in fatal feedlot pneumonias and relationship with mortality, disease onset, and treatments. J Vet Diagn Invest 2009;21(4):464–77.
39. Booker CW, Abutarbush SM, Morley PS, et al. Microbiological and histopathological findings in cases of fatal bovine respiratory disease of feedlot cattle in Western Canada. Can Vet J 2008;49(5):473–81.
40. Njaa BL, Clark EG, Janzen E, et al. Diagnosis of persistent bovine viral diarrhea virus infection by immunohistochemical staining of formalin-fixed skin biopsy specimens. J Vet Diagn Invest 2000;12(5):393–9.
41. Martin SW, Nagy E, Armstrong D, et al. The associations of viral and mycoplasmal antibody titers with respiratory disease and weight gain in feedlot calves. Can Vet J 1999;40(8):560–7 70.
42. O'Connor A, Martin SW, Nagy E, et al. The relationship between the occurrence of undifferentiated bovine respiratory disease and titer changes to bovine coronavirus and bovine viral diarrhea virus in 3 Ontario feedlots. Can J Vet Res 2001;65(3):137–42.
43. Durham PJ, Hassard LE, Van Donkersgoed J. Serological studies of infectious bovine rhinotracheitis, parainfluenza 3, bovine viral diarrhea, and bovine respiratory syncytial viruses in calves following entry to a bull test station. Can Vet J 1991;32(7):427–9.
44. Fulton RW, Cook BJ, Step DL, et al. Evaluation of health status of calves and the impact on feedlot performance: assessment of a retained ownership program for postweaning calves. Can J Vet Res 2002;66(3):173–80.
45. Moerman A, Straver PJ, de Jong MC, et al. Clinical consequences of a bovine virus diarrhoea virus infection in a dairy herd: a longitudinal study. Vet Q 1994;16(2):115–9.
46. Evermann JF, Barrington GM. Clinical features. In: Goyal SM, Ridpath JF, editors. Bovine viral diarrhea virus: diagnosis, management and control. Ames (IA): Blackwell Publishing; 2005. p. 105–20.
47. Potgieter LN. Bovine respiratory tract disease caused by bovine viral diarrhea virus. Vet Clin North Am Food Anim Pract 1997;13(3):471–81.

48. Ellis JA, West KH, Cortese VS, et al. Lesions and distribution of viral antigen following an experimental infection of young seronegative calves with virulent bovine virus diarrhea virus-type II. Can J Vet Res 1998;62(3):161–9.
49. Baszler TV, Evermann JF, Kaylor PS, et al. Diagnosis of naturally occurring bovine viral diarrhea virus infections in ruminants using monoclonal antibody-based immunohistochemistry. Vet Pathol 1995;32(6):609–18.
50. Liebler-Tenorio EM, Ridpath JE, Neill JD. Distribution of viral antigen and development of lesions after experimental infection with highly virulent bovine viral diarrhea virus type 2 in calves. Am J Vet Res 2002;63(11):1575–84.
51. Blowey RW, Weaver AD. Alimentary disorders. In: Blowey RW, Weaver AD, editors. Color atlas of diseases and disorders of cattle. 2nd edition. London (UK): Mosby-Elsevier Science; 2003. p. 43–6.
52. Liebler-Tenorio EM, Ridpath JE, Neill JD. Distribution of viral antigen and tissue lesions in persistent and acute infection with the homologous strain of noncytopathic bovine viral diarrhea virus. J Vet Diagn Invest 2004;16(5):388–96.
53. Liebler-Tenorio EM, Ridpath JF, Neill JD. Lesions and tissue distribution of viral antigen in severe acute versus subclinical acute infection with BVDV2. Biologicals 2003;31(2):119–22.
54. Liebler-Tenorio EM, Ridpath JF, Neill JD. Distribution of viral antigen and development of lesions after experimental infection of calves with a BVDV 2 strain of low virulence. J Vet Diagn Invest 2003;15(3):221–32.
55. Ames TR. The causative agent of BVD: its epidemiology and pathogenesis. Vet Med 1986;81:848–69.
56. Potgieter LN, McCracken MD, Hopkins FM, et al. Experimental production of bovine respiratory tract disease with bovine viral diarrhea virus. Am J Vet Res 1984;45(8):1582–5.
57. Potgieter LN, McCracken MD, Hopkins FM, et al. Comparison of the pneumopathogenicity of two strains of bovine viral diarrhea virus. Am J Vet Res 1985;46(1):151–3.
58. Ridpath JF, Fulton RW. Knowledge gaps impacting the development of BVDV control programs in the United States. J Am Vet Med Assoc 2009;235(10):1171–9.
59. Bolin SR, Ridpath JF. Differences in virulence between two noncytopathic bovine viral diarrhea viruses in calves. Am J Vet Res 1992;53(11):2157–63.
60. Carman S, van Dreumel T, Ridpath J, et al. Severe acute bovine viral diarrhea in Ontario, 1993–1995. J Vet Diagn Invest 1998;10(1):27–35.
61. Hamers C, Couvreur B, Dehan P, et al. Differences in experimental virulence of bovine viral diarrhoea viral strains isolated from haemorrhagic syndromes. Vet J 2000;160(3):250–8.
62. Kelling CL, Steffen DJ, Topliff CL, et al. Comparative virulence of isolates of bovine viral diarrhea virus type II in experimentally inoculated six- to nine-month-old calves. Am J Vet Res 2002;63(10):1379–84.
63. Ridpath JF, Neill JD, Frey M, et al. Phylogenetic, antigenic and clinical characterization of type 2 BVDV from North America. Vet Microbiol 2000;77(1–2):145–55.
64. Ridpath JF, Neill JD, Peterhans E. Impact of variation in acute virulence of BVDV1 strains on design of better vaccine efficacy challenge models. Vaccine 2007;25(47):8058–66.
65. Corapi WV, French TW, Dubovi EJ. Severe thrombocytopenia in young calves experimentally infected with noncytopathic bovine viral diarrhea virus. J Virol 1989;63(9):3934–43.
66. Bolin SR, McClurkin AW, Cutlip RC, et al. Severe clinical disease induced in cattle persistently infected with noncytopathic bovine viral diarrhea virus by

superinfection with cytopathic bovine viral diarrhea virus. Am J Vet Res 1985; 46(3):573–6.

67. Chase CC, Elmowalid G, Yousif AA. The immune response to bovine viral diarrhea virus: a constantly changing picture. Vet Clin North Am Food Anim Pract 2004;20(1):95–114.

68. Elvander M, Baule C, Persson M, et al. An experimental study of a concurrent primary infection with bovine respiratory syncytial virus (BRSV) and bovine viral diarrhoea virus (BVDV) in calves. Acta Vet Scand 1998;39(2):251–64.

69. Brodersen BW, Kelling CL. Effect of concurrent experimentally induced bovine respiratory syncytial virus and bovine viral diarrhea virus infection on respiratory tract and enteric diseases in calves. Am J Vet Res 1998;59(11):1423–30.

70. Ridpath JF, Bendfeldt S, Neill JD, et al. Lymphocytopathogenic activity in vitro correlates with high virulence in vivo for BVDV type 2 strains: criteria for a third biotype of BVDV. Virus Res 2006;118(1–2):62–9.

71. Bendfeldt S, Ridpath JF, Neill JD. Activation of cell signaling pathways is dependant on the biotype of bovine viral diarrhea viruses type 2. Virus Res 2007; 126(1–2):96–105.

72. Potgieter LN, McCracken MD, Hopkins FM, et al. Effect of bovine viral diarrhea virus infection on the distribution of infectious bovine rhinotracheitis virus in calves. Am J Vet Res 1984;45(4):687–90.

73. Haines DM, Moline KM, Sargent RA, et al. Immunohistochemical study of *Hemophilus somnus*, *Mycoplasma bovis*, *Mannheimia hemolytica*, and bovine viral diarrhea virus in death losses due to myocarditis in feedlot cattle. Can Vet J 2004;45(3):231–4.

74. Kahrs RF, Scott FW, de Lahunta A. Bovine viral diarrhea-mucosal disease, abortion, and congenital cerebellar hypoplasia in a dairy herd. J Am Vet Med Assoc 1970;156(7):851–7.

75. Ward GM. Bovine viral diarrhea-mucosal disease implicated in a calf with cerebellar hypoplasia and ocular disease. A case report. Cornell Vet 1971;61(2):224–8.

76. Brown TT, De Lahunte A, Scott FW, et al. Virus induced congenital anomalies of the bovine fetus. II. Histopathology of cerebellar degeneration (hypoplasia) induced by the virus of bovine viral diarrhea-mucosal disease. Cornell Vet 1973;63(4):561–78.

77. Scott FW, Kahrs RF, De Lahunte A, et al. Virus induced congenital anomalies of the bovine fetus. I. Cerebellar degeneration (hypoplasia), ocular lesions and fetal mummification following experimental infection with bovine viral diarrhea-mucosal disease virus. Cornell Vet 1973;63(4):536–60.

78. Allen JG. Congenital cerebellar hypoplasia in jersey calves. Aust Vet J 1977; 53(4):173–5.

79. Narita M, Fukunaga N, Inui S. Congenital cerebellar hypoplasia in newborn calves. Natl Inst Anim Health Q (Tokyo) 1979;19(4):114–20.

80. Coetzer JA. [Brain teratology as a result of transplacental virus infection in ruminants]. J S Afr Vet Assoc 1980;51(3):153–7 [in Afrikaans].

81. Riond JL, Cullen JM, Godfrey VL, et al. Bovine viral diarrhea virus-induced cerebellar disease in a calf. J Am Vet Med Assoc 1990;197(12):1631–2.

82. Hewicker-Trautwein M, Liess B, Trautwein G. Brain lesions in calves following transplacental infection with bovine-virus diarrhoea virus. Zentralbl Veterinarmed B 1995;42(2):65–77.

83. Straver PJ, Journee DL, Binkhorst GJ. Neurological disorders, virus persistence and hypomyelination in calves due to intra-uterine infections with bovine virus diarrhoea virus. II. Virology and epizootiology. Vet Q 1983;5(4):156–64.

84. Osburn BI, Castrucci G. Diaplacental infections with ruminant pestiviruses. Arch Virol Suppl 1991;3:71–8.
85. Otter A, Welchman Dde B, Sandvik T, et al. Congenital tremor and hypomyelination associated with bovine viral diarrhoea virus in 23 British cattle herds. Vet Rec 2009;164(25):771–8.
86. Constable PD, Hull BL, Wicks JR, et al. Femoral and tibial fractures in a newborn calf after transplacental infection with bovine viral diarrhoea virus. Vet Rec 1993; 132(15):383–5.
87. Blanchard PC, Ridpath JF, Walker JB, et al. An outbreak of late-term abortions, premature births, and congenital deformities associated with a Bovine viral diarrhea virus 1 subtype b that induces thrombocytopenia. J Vet Diagn Invest 2010; 22(1):128–31.
88. Bielefeldt-Ohmann H. An ocular-cerebellar syndrome caused by congenital viral diarrhea virus-infection. Acta Vet Scand 1984;25:26–49.
89. Bielefeldt-Ohmann H, Bloch B. Electron microscopic studies of bovine viral diarrhea virus in tissues of diseased calves and in cell cultures. Arch Virol 1982;71(1):57–74.
90. Bistner SI, Rubin LF, Saunders LZ. The ocular lesions of bovine viral diarrhea-mucosal disease. Pathol Vet 1970;7(3):275–86.
91. Brown TT, Bistner SI, de Lahunta A, et al. Pathogenetic studies of infection of the bovine fetus with bovine viral diarrhea virus. II. Ocular lesions. Vet Pathol 1975; 12(5–6):394–404.
92. Kahrs RF, Scott FW, de Lahunte A. Congenital cerebella hypoplasia and ocular defects in calves following bovine viral diarrhea-mucosal disease infection in pregnant cattle. J Am Vet Med Assoc 1970;156(10):1443–50.
93. Done JT, Terlecki S, Richardson C, et al. Bovine virus diarrhoea-mucosal disease virus: pathogenicity for the fetal calf following maternal infection. Vet Rec 1980;106(23):473–9.
94. Larsson B, Jacobsson SO, Bengtsson B, et al. Congenital curly haircoat as a symptom of persistent infection with bovine virus diarrhoea virus in calves. Arch Virol Suppl 1991;3:143–8.
95. Wijeratne WV, O'Toole D, Wood L, et al. A genetic, pathological and virological study of congenital hypotrichosis and incisor anodontia in cattle. Vet Rec 1988; 122(7):149–52.
96. Brodersen BW, Kelling CL. Alteration of leukocyte populations in calves concurrently infected with bovine respiratory syncytial virus and bovine viral diarrhea virus. Viral Immunol 1999;12(4):323–34.
97. Lehmkuhl HD, Gough PM. Investigation of causative agents of bovine respiratory tract disease in a beef cow-calf herd with an early weaning program. Am J Vet Res 1977;38(11):1717–20.
98. Liu L, Lehmkuhl HD, Kaeberle ML. Synergistic effects of bovine respiratory syncytial virus and non-cytopathic bovine viral diarrhea virus infection on selected bovine alveolar macrophage functions. Can J Vet Res 1999;63(1):41–8.
99. Edwards S, Wood L, Hewitt-Taylor C, et al. Evidence for an immunocompromising effect of bovine pestivirus on bovid herpesvirus 1 vaccination. Vet Res Commun 1986;10(4):297–302.
100. Castrucci G, Ferrari M, Traldi V, et al. Effects in calves of mixed infections with bovine viral diarrhea virus and several other bovine viruses. Comp Immunol Microbiol Infect Dis 1992;15(4):261–70.
101. Falcone E, Cordioli P, Tarantino M, et al. Experimental infection of calves with bovine viral diarrhoea virus type-2 (BVDV-2) isolated from a contaminated vaccine. Vet Res Commun 2003;27(7):577–89.

102. Aly NM, Shehab GG, Abd el-Rahim IH. Bovine viral diarrhoea, bovine herpes-virus and parainfluenza-3 virus infection in three cattle herds in Egypt in 2000. Rev Sci Tech 2003;22(3):879–92.
103. Shahriar FM, Clark EG, Janzen E, et al. Coinfection with bovine viral diarrhea virus and *Mycoplasma bovis* in feedlot cattle with chronic pneumonia. Can Vet J 2002;43(11):863–8.
104. Haines DM, Martin KM, Clark EG, et al. The immunohistochemical detection of *Mycoplasma bovis* and bovine viral diarrhea virus in tissues of feedlot cattle with chronic, unresponsive respiratory disease and/or arthritis. Can Vet J 2001; 42(11):857–60.

Bovine Respiratory Coronavirus

Linda J. Saif, MS, PhD

KEYWORDS

- Bovine respiratory coronavirus • Shipping fever
- Wild ruminant coronaviruses

Bovine coronaviruses (BCoVs) cause respiratory and enteric infections in cattle and wild ruminants.[1–3] BCoVs belong to the family Coronaviridae in the order Nidovirales and are members of subgroup 2a along with swine hemagglutinating encephalomy-elitis virus (HEV), canine respiratory CoV, and human CoV-OC43 and HKU1. HEV, which causes wasting disease, is an exception;[4] the others cause enteric and/or respi-ratory disease. Recently discovered severe acute respiratory syndrome (SARS)-CoVs, which are associated with respiratory and enteric infections in humans and animals (eg, civet cats, raccoon dogs, bats), belong to a new CoV subgroup 2b.[1,5]

BCoV is a pneumoenteric virus that infects the upper and lower respiratory tract and intestine. BCoV is shed in feces and nasal secretions and infects the lung. BCoV is the cause of 3 distinct clinical syndromes in cattle: calf diarrhea (CD),[1,2] winter dysentery (WD) with hemorrhagic diarrhea in adults,[3,6–12] and respiratory infections in cattle of various ages including the bovine respiratory disease complex (BRDC) or shipping fever of feedlot cattle.[2,13–25] All BCoV isolates examined to date, regardless of clinical origin belong to a single serotype based on virus cross-neutralization tests.[8,14] Although 2 to 3 subtypes of BCoV as determined by biologic properties and antigenic variation identified by neutralization tests or using monoclonal antibodies (MAbs) are recognized, each encompasses viruses from all 3 clinical syndromes.[2,3,8,14,15] Despite genetic differences (point mutations but not deletions) detected in the spike (S) gene between enteric and respiratory isolates, including ones from the same animal,[26–28] in vivo challenge revealed a high level of cross-protection between such isolates.[29,30] No consistent antigenic or genetic markers have been identified to discriminate BCoVs from the different clinical syndromes. Reviews describing the role of BCoV in CD and WD are available.[1,3,7] This article focuses on respiratory BCoV infections including

This work was partially supported by grant R21 AI062763 from the NIAID, NIH. Salaries and research support were provided by state and federal funds provided to the Ohio Agricultural Research and Development Center, The Ohio State University.

Department of Veterinary Preventive Medicine, Food Animal Health Research Program, Ohio Agricultural Research and Development Center, College of Veterinary Medicine, The Ohio State University, 1680 Madison Avenue, Wooster, OH 44691, USA
E-mail address: saif.2@osu.edu

viral characteristics, epidemiology and interspecies transmission, diagnosis, pathogenesis and clinical signs, and immunity and vaccines.

VIRAL CHARACTERISTICS

BCoV is enveloped and pleomorphic, ranging from 65 to 210 nm in diameter, and covered with a double layer of short (hemagglutinin) and long (spike) surface projections (**Fig. 1**).[2] Like other enveloped viruses, BCoV is sensitive to detergents and lipid solvents (eg, ether, chloroform) and is inactivated by conventional disinfectants, formalin, and heat. The large genome consists of single-stranded, positive-sense RNA of 27 to 32 kb encoding 5 major structural proteins. Among these, the 50-kDa nucleocapsid (N) is highly conserved among strains, so it is often the target for viral RNA detection assays.[29] Unique to some group 2 CoVs including BCoV and wild ruminant CoVs, is the presence of a surface hemagglutinin-esterase (HE) glycoprotein (120–140 kDa). The HE acts as a receptor-destroying enzyme (esterase) to reverse hemagglutination. Like other CoVs, BCoV also possesses an outer-surface S glycoprotein (190 kDa). It consists of an S1 subunit that contains the dominant neutralizing epitopes and an S2 subunit that mediates viral membrane fusion. HE and S are important viral proteins that are involved in attachment to host cell receptors and hemagglutination of chicken, rat, mouse, and hamster erythrocytes. MAbs to the HE or S protein prevented BCoV-induced villous atrophy in vivo in intestinal loops of calves, confirming their dual role in in vivo protection.[31] HE and S proteins elicit neutralizing antibodies that can block viral attachment and infectivity, so they are important for immunity and vaccines.

Variation in tissue tropism and host range among CoVs is attributed mainly to changes in the S protein. Researchers have sequenced the partial or full-length S gene of multiple BCoV strains to ascertain the genetic basis of the broad host range of BCoV (see section on Epidemiology) and occurrence of the distinct clinical syndromes. Several groups have compared the S (or S1) or full-length genomic sequences[22,26–28,32–36] of WD or respiratory and enteric BCoV isolates, including isolates from the same animal. The porcine respiratory CoV evolved as an S gene deletion mutant (deletions of 621–681nuceotides) of swine transmissible gastroenteritis virus, acquiring an almost exclusive respiratory tropism.[37] No similar large S gene deletions were detected in respiratory BCoV strains, most of which also possess an

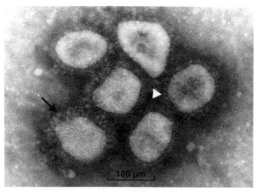

Fig. 1. Immune electron microscopy of tissue culture-adapted respiratory BCoV. Particles reacted with antisera to BCoV showing shorter surface HE (*arrowhead*) and longer spikes (*arrow*) resulting in a dense outer fringe. Bar equals 100 μm.

enteric tropism as revealed by calf challenge studies.[29] Focusing on the hypervariable region (amino acids [aa] 452–593) containing the neutralizing epitope (S1B) of the S1 subunit, 4 groups[22,26,27,36] reported that respiratory strains (or respiratory and enteric isolates from the same feedlot calf) had changes in aa residues 510 and 531 compared with the reference enteric Mebus strain and a WD strain (DBA). One of the polymorphic positions (aa 531) discriminated between enteric (aspartic acid or asparagine) and respiratory (glycine) BCoV strains in 2 studies,[26,36] but not in others.[27,28,34] Therefore, like the antigenic and biologic differences observed among BCoV isolates, variability was not necessarily related to the clinical origin of the isolates.[14,15] BCoV, like other RNA viruses, represents a quasispecies or swarm of viruses;[38] some viruses within a population may be more suitable for replication in respiratory versus intestinal sites, contributing to the sequence differences reported for paired enteric/respiratory isolates from the same host.[28] Zhang and colleagues[28] noted that in the process of cell culture adaptation, an enteric BCoV strain accumulated mutations to resemble the corresponding respiratory BCoV isolate from the same animal. Consequently interpretation of the comparative sequence analysis of enteric and respiratory strains of BCoV may be compromised by lack of complete genome sequences and the laboratory manipulation of field strains (multiple cell culture passage and plaque isolations) before sequencing.

All investigators showed that the greatest aa sequence divergence (42 aa changes at 38 distinct sites)[27] and the most differences by phylogenetic analysis were between the historic reference Mebus enteric BCoV strain (1972) and the more recent BCoV isolates, regardless of their clinical origin. This result demonstrates that BCoVs, like other RNA viruses, are evolving in the field, with recent isolates more similar to contemporary strains than to historic strains. If the genetic divergence affects neutralizing or other key epitopes allowing viruses to escape existing immunity,[36] then vaccines containing more contemporary or broadly cross-reactive BCoV strains may be required to enhance the efficacy of existing or newly developed BCoV vaccines. Sequential sera from cattle with respiratory BCoV infections associated with BRDC pneumonia reacted with higher neutralizing and hemagglutination inhibition (HI) titers to a more contemporary respiratory lung isolate (97TXSF-Lu15-2) than to much older historic enteric BCoV strains, including a derivative of the high cell culture–passaged Mebus 1972 strain (L9-81) and an older wild type strain (LY138-3).[39] However, in a previous report from the same laboratory,[35] an earlier isolate of a respiratory BCoV strain (BRCV-G95) was more similar to the enteric LY-138 strain than to the older Mebus strain L9-81 based on S-specific MAb reactivity. These data concur with the greater phylogenetic and antigenic divergence described between the Mebus cell culture–passaged strain compared with the more recent enteric and respiratory BCoV isolates.[14,15,28,40] In the studies by Lin and colleagues,[39] it is likely that the antigenic variation observed reflects the timeframe differences, independently of the enteric versus respiratory origin of the isolates. Repeating these immunologic assays using more recent enteric BCoV strains is necessary to clarify this issue.

EPIDEMIOLOGY AND INTERSPECIES TRANSMISSION
Respiratory BCoV Infections in Calf Respiratory Disease

BCoV is ubiquitous in cattle worldwide based on BCoV antibody seroprevalence data.[2,3,7] Respiratory BCoV is associated with mild respiratory disease (coughing, rhinitis) or pneumonia in 2- to 6-month-old calves. It is detected in nasal secretions, lung, and often intestine as well as feces (**Table 1**).[2,3,16,24,41–44] Four respiratory

Table 1
Summary of clinical signs and pathogenesis of respiratory BCoV infections

Disease Syndrome	Clinical Signs	Cells Infected	Lesions		Shedding[a]		Ages Affected
			Respiratory	Enteric	Nasal	Fecal	
Calf pneumonia	Cough Rhinitis ± Pneumonia ± Diarrhea Fever/anorexia	Nasal/± lung Tracheal ± Intestinal Epithelial cells	± Pneumonia	± J, I, Colon Villous atrophy	Sporadic 5 d	Sporadic 5 d	2 wk–6 mo
Shipping fever/BRDC	Cough/dyspnea ± Rhinitis ± Pneumonia ± Diarrhea Fever/anorexia	Nasal/tracheal Bronchi/alveoli ± Intestinal Epithelial cells	Interstitial Emphysema Bronchiolitis Alveolitis	± NT	5–10 d (17 d)	4–8 d (17 d)	6 mo–10 mo

In experimental challenge studies, the incubation periods for disease onset and shedding ranged from 3 to 8 days.
Abbreviations: I, ileum; J, jejunum; NT, not tested.
[a] Shedding detected by infectivity or antigen assays; data in parentheses denote shedding detected by reverse transcriptase polymerase chain reaction.

disease outbreaks associated with BCoV infection but without concurrent detection of other common respiratory viruses, bacteria, and mycoplasmas were investigated in dairy and beef cattle in Italy.[41] In 3 of 4 outbreaks, the classic signs of bovine respiratory disease (dyspnea, fever, respiratory distress) were evident in 2- to 3-month-old calves, and BCoV was detected by quantitative reverse transcriptase polymerase chain reaction (qRT-PCR) in nasal samples. In 2 of 4 outbreaks, respiratory disease and enteric disease were present: BCoV was detected simultaneously in nasal and fecal specimens. In 1 of these 2 herds, clinical signs were present in calves, heifers, and lactating dairy cattle. In the second, concurrent infection with a group A bovine rotavirus was detected. Researchers also detected ocular shedding of BCoV in lower titers in one of the herds, suggesting that ocular swabs could be another diagnostic specimen for detection of BCoV. BCoV was isolated in human rectal tumor (HRT)-18 cells from nasal swabs of calves from 3 of the 4 outbreaks.

BCoV seroprevalence studies in 135 Norwegian dairy herds indicated that calves (>150 days old) in herds with BCoV-seropositive calves had an increased risk (hazard ratio = 3.9) of respiratory disease compared with herds with BCoV-seronegative calves.[45] In studies of dairy calves in Ohio from birth to 20 weeks of age, Heckert and colleagues[16,24] documented fecal and nasal shedding of respiratory BCoV, but with diarrhea prominent in the initial infection. Subsequently, repeated or intermittent nasal shedding episodes occurred in the same animal, with or without respiratory disease, but with transient increases in serum antibody titers consistent with reinfection. These findings suggest a lack of long-term mucosal immunity in the upper respiratory tract after natural respiratory BCoV infection, confirming similar observations for human[46] and porcine respiratory CoV infections.[47]

Within a herd, reservoirs for respiratory BCoV infection may be virus cycling in clinically or subclinically infected calves, young adult cattle in which sporadic nasal shedding occurs,[16,24] or clinically or subclinically infected adults.[3,48] Respiratory BCoV is transmitted via fecal-oral and potentially respiratory (aerosol) routes.

Respiratory BCoV Infections Associated with the BRDC in Feedlot Cattle

Respiratory BCoV has been increasingly implicated since 1995 in BRDC associated with respiratory disease and reduced growth performance in feedlot cattle (see **Table 1**).[13,17–21,23,25] Respiratory BCoV was detected from nasal secretions and lungs of cattle with pneumonia and/or from feces.[15,17–21,23,25] In a follow-up study, a high percentage of feedlot cattle (45%) shed BCoV nasally and in feces as determined by enzyme-linked immunosorbent assay (ELISA).[13] Application of nested RT-PCR detected higher respiratory BCoV nasal and fecal shedding rates of 84% and 96%, respectively.[23] Storz and colleagues[20] reported that 25 of 26 Texas feedlot cattle that died had a respiratory BCoV infection. Respiratory BCoV and *Pasteurella* sp were isolated from lungs of the cattle with necrotizing pneumonia.

Some investigators have shown an association between nasal shedding of respiratory BCoV and respiratory disease. In a large feedlot study (n = 1074 cattle), Lathrop and colleagues[17] noted that feedlot calves shedding respiratory BCoV nasally and seroconverting to respiratory BCoV (>4-fold) were 1.6 times more likely to have respiratory disease and 2.2 times more likely to have pulmonary lesions at slaughter than animals that did not shed respiratory BCoV. Similarly, in studies by Hasoksuz and colleagues[23] and Thomas and colleagues,[25] calves shedding respiratory BCoV nasally were 2.7 and 1.5 times, respectively, more likely to have respiratory disease than calves that were not shedding. Nasal shedding of respiratory BCoV or an antibody titer less than 20 increased the risk of requiring treatment for respiratory disease in another report.[49] Intranasal (IN) vaccination of such calves using a commercial, modified, live

BCoV calf vaccine on entry to a feedlot reduced the risk of treatment for BRDC in the latter study.

Respiratory and enteric shedding of respiratory BCoV are common in feedlot cattle with peak shedding at 0 to 4 days after arrival at feedlots. In one study, 3-day pre-arrival specimens were tested, and nasal shedding consistently preceded fecal shedding.[25] Many cattle (61%–74%) shed respiratory BCoV at the buyer-order before shipping to feedlots.[21] A high percentage (91%–95%) of feedlot cattle seroconverted (2–4-fold increased titers) to respiratory BCoV by 3 weeks after arrival.

An important observation from several studies was that cattle arriving with relatively high respiratory BCoV antibody ELISA titers or neutralizing antibodies in serum were less likely to shed respiratory BCoV, seroconvert, or develop BRDC.[13,18,25,50,51] Furthermore, some investigators showed that respiratory BCoV infections had a negative effect on weight gains in feedlot cattle,[13,23] which suggests that respiratory BCoV may affect herd health and performance. Conversely, higher serum antibody titers against respiratory BCoV have been associated with increased weight gains.[25,50]

BCoV Interspecies Transmission and Wildlife Reservoirs

Possible wildlife reservoirs for BCoV have been identified. Captive wild ruminants from the United States including sambar deer (*Cervus unicolor*), white-tailed deer (*Odocoileus virginianus*), waterbuck (*Kobus ellipsiprymnus*), elk (*Cervus elephus*), and more recently, giraffe[52] harbor CoVs that are closely related to BCoV biologically, genetically, and antigenically (cross-neutralizing).[53,54] Bovine-like CoVs have also been identified in water buffalo calves[55] and in alpacas.[56] Deer and waterbuck isolates were from animals with bloody diarrhea resembling WD in cattle. Serologically, 6.6% and 8.7% of sera from white-tailed deer in Ohio and mule deer in Wyoming, respectively, were seropositive for antibodies to BCoV by indirect immunofluorescence tests.[54] Caribous (*Rangifer tarandus*) were also BCoV seropositive.[57] These studies confirm the circulation of CoVs that are antigenically closely related to BCoV in captive and native wild ruminants.

Several CoVs from wild ruminants have recently been fully sequenced to assess their genetic similarity to BCoV.[40,52] The antigenically related giraffe, sambar and white-tailed deer, waterbuck, and sable antelope CoVs share high (99.3%–99.6%) aa sequence identity with enteric and respiratory BCoV strains, supporting their close genetic relatedness. Wild ruminant CoV isolates from sambar and white-tailed deer and waterbuck also infected the upper respiratory and intestinal tracts of gnotobiotic calves and caused diarrhea,[54] affirming experimentally that wild ruminants may serve as a reservoir for CoV strains that are transmissible to calves. The possibility exists that native wild ruminants may transmit bovine-like CoVs to cattle (see later) or vice versa. Few serologic surveys of wild ruminants in native habitats have been done. A particular concern is that such interspecies infections may culminate in more genetically divergent BCoV strains including recombinant strains, increasing the possibility of their transmission to other species. Analysis of CoV genomic sequence data has revealed that porcine HEV and human respiratory CoV OC43 represent CoVs that likely evolved from ancestral BCoV strains.[58]

Many CoVs have restricted host ranges; some such as the BCoV and more recently the SARS-CoV seem to be promiscuous.[5,59] Coronaviruses genetically (>95% nucleotide identity) and/or antigenically similar to BCoV have been detected from respiratory samples of dogs with respiratory disease,[60] and from humans[61] and wild ruminants (see earlier discussion). A human enteric CoV isolate from a child with acute diarrhea (HECoV-4408) was genetically (99% nucleotide identity in the S and HE gene with BCoV) and antigenically closely related to BCoV, suggesting that it is a BCoV variant able to infect humans. A recent report confirmed that the HECoV-4408 strain infects (upper respiratory tract and intestine) and causes diarrhea and intestinal lesions in gnotobiotic calves. This strain induced complete cross-protective immunity against the virulent BCoV-DB2 enteric strain. An enteric BCoV also experimentally infected dogs, causing subclinical infection and seroconversion.[62] Furthermore, the virulent BCoV-DB2 enteric strain caused mild disease (diarrhea) in phylogenetically diverse species such as avian hosts, including baby turkeys but not baby chicks.[63] These data raise intriguing questions of whether dogs or wild birds (such as wild turkeys) can also be a reservoir for bovine-like CoVs transmissible to cattle or wild ruminants, or conversely, if cattle (or ruminants) can transmit CoVs to dogs, wild birds, or poultry. There are few if any seroprevalence surveys for bovine-like CoVs in avian species and only limited data for wild ruminants.[54,57] The reasons for the broad host range of BCoV are unknown but may relate to the presence of a hemagglutinin on BCoV and its possible role in binding to diverse cell types. Experimental evidence for interspecies transmission of bovine-like CoVs between wild ruminants, dogs, birds, and cattle is of concern for open feedlots where wild birds may congregate or cattle may be exposed to dogs, wild ruminants, or their feces.

DIAGNOSIS

BCoV commonly infects the upper respiratory and the intestinal tract with shedding detected in nasal secretions and/or feces.[13,23,43,64] BCoV has also been detected or isolated from lung in animals with respiratory disease. Uncomplicated BCoV infections are characterized as acute infections with a short duration of virus shedding (see **Table 1**). The sensitivity of the assay used to detect BCoV shedding influences the detection rates and the length of time that the virus is detected. Generally, nucleic acid detection assays are among the most sensitive (RT-PCR, nested RT-PCR, real-time qRT-PCR) barring interference by inhibitors common in fecal samples.

The acute transient nature of BCoV infections necessitates sample collection at disease onset or shortly thereafter (see **Table 1**). For BRDC-associated infection, the peak of BCoV nasal (or fecal) shedding is often seen on entry into the feedlot or within the first week of arrival.[13,21,23,25] This pattern of BCoV shedding is likely attributable to the stress of shipping and the transmission of new BCoV strains among mixed source, comingled calves from auction barns.[21,25] For cattle with BRDC, differential diagnosis is needed because multiple respiratory viral and bacterial pathogens contribute to this syndrome and the ensuing fatalities.

To diagnose BCoV from animals with suspected respiratory (or enteric) disease necropsy, samples to be submitted include tissues from the upper respiratory tract (eg, nasal, pharyngeal, tracheal tissues) and lung,[14,20,21] and as available tissues from the distal small intestine and colon.[64] For live animals, ideally, nasal secretions collected using sterile polyester-tipped swabs (1 per nostril) and feces collected in sterile fecal cups (via anal stimulation using sterile gloves) should be transported on ice to the diagnostic lab.[13,15] Also tracheobronchial lavage fluids can be aspirated from live calves with acute respiratory disease. In at least 1 study, they were found to be positive for BCoV antigen by ELISA.[65]

BCoV infections can be diagnosed by detection of virus, viral antigen, or viral RNA in tissues, secretions, or excretions of infected animals. Comprehensive methods used by our laboratory for the isolation and detection of BCoV from nasal secretions, lung homogenates or feces, or titration of BCoV serum or neutralizing antibodies have been published recently[66] and are not reiterated in detail in this article. These methods include procedures for primary virus isolation, propagation, and plaque induction in our cloned line of HRT-18 cell cultures.[15,20,21,23] This cell line is used most successfully and almost universally for isolation of respiratory and enteric BCoV strains and bovine-like CoVs from wild ruminants and dogs. Some BCoV field strains fail to grow in cell culture, so sensitivity for BCoV detection may be low.

For viral antigen detection in respiratory (trachea, lung) or intestinal (ileum, colon) tissues (frozen or paraffin-embedded), immunofluorescent or immunohistochemical staining is performed using hyperimmune antiserum or MAbs to BCoV. Detection of BCoV in nasal secretions or feces is accomplished by immune electron microscopy, which has the advantage of detecting other viruses, but its sensitivity is relatively low.[16,54] BCoV antigens are most commonly detected by ELISA using MAbs to improve assay specificity and sensitivity. Advantages include rapid test results and applicability to large sample numbers. Highly sensitive molecular assays to detect BCoV RNA in nasal secretions, lung lysates, or feces are becoming more widely used. These assays include RT-PCR and the more sensitive nested RT-PCR and real-time qPCR assays.[29,67] Ideally these assays should target conserved regions of the BCoV genome (polymerase or N protein) to detect divergent strains. For feces, controls are needed to detect interference by PCR inhibitors that need to be eliminated or diluted out for assay validity.

Antibodies to BCoV can be quantitated by virus neutralization and HI tests that measure functional neutralizing or hemagglutinating antibodies, respectively, that often correlate with immunity.[14,51] In addition, ELISAs are used to quantitate overall or isotype-specific antibodies (IgM, IgA, IgG1, IgG2) in serum, nasal secretions, or feces, because certain isotypes (ie, IgA, IgG1, IgG2) may be better correlated with mucosal immunity or neutralizing or HI antibodies.[16,24,51,68,69] Because BCoV antibodies are widespread in cattle, paired acute and convalescent serum samples are needed for serologic diagnosis of BCoV infections.

PATHOGENESIS AND CLINICAL SIGNS

Research on respiratory and enteric BCoV infections of cattle has provided important information on BCoV disease pathogenesis, possible potentiators for increased disease severity, and vaccine strategies. Enteric BCoV infections are generally most severe in calves. Respiratory BCoV infections in adults are more severe or even fatal when combined with other factors including stress and transport of animals (shipping fever of cattle) that increase corticosteroid levels, high doses of virus exposure, aerosols, and coinfections with other respiratory pathogens (viruses, bacteria, bacterial lipopolysaccharides). Such variables, by accentuating viral shedding or increasing titers shed may also contribute to virus transmission.

Respiratory BCoV Pathogenesis in Younger Calves and Cattle with WD

Besides causing diarrhea in young calves (1–3 weeks of age) and cows with WD, BCoV is implicated as a cause of mild respiratory disease (coughing, rhinitis) or pneumonia in 2- to 6-month-old calves.[16,24,42–44] Clinical signs include coughing, fever, rhinitis, and inappetence, often with concurrent diarrhea. BCoV has been isolated from nasal and pharyngeal swabs and lung wash of sick calves. Experimental calf challenge studies using calf respiratory BCoV isolates confirmed fecal and nasal shedding (averaging 5 days) and diarrhea, but only variable mild respiratory disease.[42,43] BCoV respiratory infections in the field are likely exacerbated by stress or respiratory coinfections that may include the common bovine respiratory viruses, bacteria, and *Mycoplasma* sp.

In 2 experimental studies of WD in BCoV-seronegative or -seropositive dairy cows, fecal shedding of BCoV was coincident with or preceded diarrhea and persisted for 1 to 4 days. No respiratory disease or fever was evident in the BCoV-seropositive cows, but nasal shedding of BCoV was detected in 1 of 5 cows.[6] BCoV-seronegative cows directly exposed to calves experimentally infected with a WD strain of BCoV developed transient fevers, mild cough, and serous mucopurulent discharge.[10] These data are consistent with field outbreak reports indicating variable signs of respiratory disease in cattle with WD.[7,9] WD isolates of BCoV are antigenically closely related to calf enteric and respiratory isolates, but the various strains, regardless of clinical origin, elicited cross-protection against one another in calf challenge studies.[12,29,30]

A plausible scenario for the pathogenesis of BCoV and its transit to the intestine has been proposed based on the time course of BCoV nasal and fecal shedding in natural and experimental BCoV infections.[16,25,64] Following initial and extensive replication in the nasal mucosa, BCoV may spread to the gastrointestinal tract after the swallowing of large quantities of virus coated in mucous secretions. This initial respiratory amplification of BCoV and its protective coating by mucus may allow larger amounts of this labile, enveloped but infectious virus to transit to the gut after swallowing, resulting in intestinal infection and fecal shedding.

Respiratory BCoV Pathogenesis in Feedlot Calves

The BRDC of feedlot calves is characterized by fever, dyspnea, inflammatory and necrotizing lung lesions leading to bronchopneumonia, weight loss, and death. It is most pronounced during the first weeks after arrival at feedlots and overlaps with a high prevalence of respiratory viral and secondary bacterial coinfections and various environmental or host stress factors during this period. A growing number of reports in the past decade have provided epidemiologic or experimental evidence suggesting that BCoV respiratory infection contributes substantially to the BRDC. Multiple previous studies (see section on Epidemiology) have documented nasal and fecal shedding of BCoV by calves shortly after arrival in feedlots and subsequent seroconversion to BCoV (see **Table 1**). Storz and colleagues[19] showed a progression in development of the BRDC for natural cases, initiated by BCoV respiratory infection (nasal shedding) upon arrival followed by dual infections with BCoV and respiratory bacteria (*Mannheimia hemolytica* and *Pasteurella multocida*). This progression led to pneumonia and deaths in 26 cases, most of which had concurrent high titers of BCoV and bacteria in the lungs. The cattle died within 5 to 36 days after the disease onset. Clinical signs included high fever and severe respiratory distress. Gross lung lesions consisted of subacute exudative and necrotizing lobar pneumonia involving 50%–80% of the lung volume. Histologic lung lesions were characterized as fibrinous, necrotizing lobar pneumonia, but with moderate to severe bronchitis and bronchiolitis. The investigators concluded that these data supported a role for BCoV in the BRDC as defined by Evans' criteria for causation. In this and another study,[20] researchers confirmed the presence of BCoV antigen in respiratory epithelial cells or isolated BCoV from nasal secretions, trachea, bronchi, or lung alveoli and documented the presence of interstitial emphysema, bronchiolitis and alveolitis in concert with bacterial infection (see **Table 1**). Although BRDC is recognized as a multifactorial disease, this evidence supports a role for BCoV in inciting the disease. Multifactorial/multiagent experiments describing interactions between respiratory viruses, bacteria, and stress have highlighted their synergistic effects in the BRDC[70] but no such experiments have been reported for BCoV. Such studies of feedlot age, BCoV-seronegative stressed calves are needed to further elucidate the role of BCoV in the BRDC and the mechanisms involved in predisposing calves to development of fatal pneumonia.

Cofactors that Exacerbate Respiratory BCoV Infections, Disease, or Shedding

Underlying disease or respiratory coinfections, dose and route of infection, and immunosuppression (corticosteroids) are all potential cofactors that can exacerbate the severity of BCoV infections and enhance virus transmission or host susceptibility. The BRDC (shipping fever) is recognized as a multifactorial, polymicrobial respiratory disease complex in young adult feedlot cattle, with several factors exacerbating respiratory disease, including BCoV infections.[13,17–21,23,25,49] The BRDC can be precipitated by several viruses, alone or in combination (BCoV, bovine respiratory syncytial virus, parainfluenza-3 virus, bovine herpesvirus), and viruses capable of mediating immunosuppression (eg, bovine viral diarrhea virus). The shipping of cattle long distances to feedlots and the comingling of cattle from multiple farms creates physical stresses that overwhelm the animal's defense mechanisms and provide close contact for exposure to high concentrations of new pathogens or strains not previously encountered. For the BRDC, various predisposing factors (viruses, stress) allow commensal bacteria of the nasal cavity (eg, *Mannheimia haemolytica*, *Pasteurella* sp, *Mycoplasma* sp) to infect the lungs leading to a fatal fibrinous pneumonia.[17,19–21]

It is also possible that antibiotic treatment of animals coinfected with BCoVs and bacteria, with massive release of bacterial lipopolysaccharides (LPS), could precipitate induction of proinflammatory cytokines, which may further enhance lung damage. Van Reeth and colleagues[71] showed that pigs infected with porcine respiratory CoV followed by a subclinical dose of LPS from *Escherichia coli* within 24 hours developed enhanced fever and more severe respiratory disease compared with each agent alone. The investigators concluded that the effects were likely mediated by the significantly enhanced levels of proinflammatory cytokines induced by the bacterial LPS in synergy with the CoV infection. Thus, there is a need to examine LPS and lung cytokine levels in BCoV-infected feedlot cattle as possible mediators of the severity of BRDC.

Corticosteroids induce immunosuppression and reduce the numbers of CD4 and CD8 T cells and certain cytokine levels.[72–74] A recrudescence of BCoV fecal shedding was observed in 1 of 4 WD-BCoV-infected cows treated with dexamethasone.[6] Similarly, treatment of weaned pigs with dexamethasone before porcine respiratory CoV inoculation led to increased disease severity and reduced T-cell immune responses in the treated pigs.[73,74]

IMMUNITY AND VACCINES

An understanding of the pathogenesis of respiratory BCoV infections including the target organs infected and how virus is disseminated to these organs should assist in development of vaccine strategies. The realization that BCoV infects epithelial cells lining the respiratory and/or intestinal tracts may necessitate development of vaccines effective at both sites of infection to provide optimal protection. In addition, vaccines for mucosal pathogens may fail to induce sterilizing immunity or to prevent respiratory reinfections, as observed for natural or experimental respiratory BCoV infections.[16,29] Consequently, the major focus for vaccine should be to prevent the severe disease-requiring treatments and the weight loss/reduced gain in the infected animals. These objectives may be best accomplished by vaccinating calves on farm before shipping to auction barns or feedlots because BCoV infections occur at the auction barn or shortly after arrival at feedlots necessitating rapid onset of immunity.

Despite its economic impact, no respiratory BCoV vaccines have been developed to prevent BCoV-associated pneumonia in young calves or in the BRDC of feedlot cattle. The correlates of immunity to respiratory BCoV infections remain undefined. Limited data from epidemiologic studies of BCoV infections in cattle suggest that serum antibody titers to BCoV may be a marker for respiratory protection. In multiple studies the BCoV antibody isotype (IgG1, IgG2, IgA), neutralizing and HI antibody titer, and magnitude of antibody titer in serum of naturally infected calves or in cattle on arrival in feedlots were correlated with protection against respiratory disease, pneumonia, or BCoV respiratory shedding.[13,24,25,39,50,51,69] However, whether the serum antibodies are themselves correlates of respiratory protection or only reflect previous enteric or respiratory exposure to BCoV is uncertain and requires additional research. If serum BCoV neutralizing antibodies are indeed a correlate of immunity to respiratory BCoV infection,[51] then parenteral vaccines to boost levels of existing BCoV antibodies may be protective.

Lin and colleagues[51,69] assessed the kinetics of the neutralizing and HI antibody responses to respiratory BCoV in sera of cattle during an epizootic of pneumonia associated with the BRDC. Cattle shedding respiratory BCoV at the start of the epizootic had low levels of neutralizing and HI antibodies, whereas cattle with high levels of antibodies against the HE and S viral glycoproteins remained negative for respiratory BCoV. The neutralizing and HI-BCoV antibody levels in serum were highly correlated. Moreover all the BCoV antibody isotypes measured (IgM, IgG1, and IgG2) were significantly correlated with the levels of neutralizing and HI antibodies. In cattle with fatal respiratory BCoV infections, only IgM antibody responses were detected.

Alternatively, in a recent study, IN vaccination of feedlot calves with a modified live-BCoV calf vaccine on entry to a feedlot reduced the risk of treatment for BRDC in calves.[49] The immune correlates for the BCoV vaccine were not identified, but based on data from IN-modified live infectious bovine rhinotracheitis vaccines, the investigators speculated that locally induced interferon or IgA antibodies could be involved. The data further suggest that IN administration of a BCoV CD strain induces cross-protection against field exposure to a respiratory BCoV. The findings concur with results of experimental challenge studies of calves confirming cross-protection among BCoV strains of distinct clinical origin. Inoculation of gnotobiotic or colostrum-deprived calves with CD, WD, or respiratory BCoV strains led to nasal and fecal CoV shedding followed by complete cross-protection against diarrhea after challenge with a calf diarrhea strain.[29,30] Subclinical nasal and fecal virus shedding (detected only by RT-PCR) in calves challenged with the heterologous BCoV strains[29,30] confirmed field studies documenting subclinical BCoV infections and the potential for subclinically infected animals to be a reservoir for BCoV in infected herds.[16,24] Consequently, the goal is to develop vaccines that are protective against divergent field strains of BCoV, including ones from the distinct clinical syndromes. Inclusion of a mixture of strains representing CD, WD, and respiratory isolates may be an ideal strategy to develop a single broad-spectrum BCoV vaccine effective against BCoV infections associated with each of the clinical syndromes including respiratory disease.

FUTURE RESEARCH

Future areas for research include understanding the basic mechanisms of how BCoVs induce a broad spectrum of respiratory disease (ranging from mild to fatal) and the cofactors and interactions that exacerbate disease or lead to enhanced shedding and transmission. Relatively little is known about the basis of interspecies transmission of BCoVs or why they have broad host ranges. Little is understood about the ecology of bovine-like CoVs present in wildlife reservoirs or their potential to emerge as either public or animal health threats. A lack of basic understanding of the attributes required for effective respiratory BCoV vaccines and the immune correlates of protection remain obstacles to vaccine development.

SUMMARY

- BCoV causes pneumoenteric infections in cattle and wild ruminants. Detection of similar CoV strains among wild ruminants and in dogs, with evidence for experimental interspecies transmission to calves, suggests that these species could harbor CoVs transmissible to cattle or vice versa.
- BCoV is associated with 3 clinically distinct syndromes in cattle: CD, WD in adults, and respiratory disease in cattle of various ages.
- Greater biologic, antigenic, and genetic diversity is evident between contemporary and historic BCoV strains than between enteric and respiratory strains. There are no consistent markers to discriminate between respiratory and enteric BCoVs.
- Existence of a single serotype of BCoV and cross-protection among strains from the different clinical syndromes suggests that a single broadly cross-reactive strain of BCoV may suffice for a vaccine. Alternatively, because of variations among field strains, including ones from the 3 clinical syndromes, a single vaccine composed of CD, WD, and respiratory BCoV isolates may provide a broader spectrum of protection against all 3 syndromes.
- An accumulating body of evidence suggests that BCoV respiratory infections contribute substantially to the BRDC of feedlot cattle.
- Underlying disease or respiratory coinfections, dose and route of infection (fecal/oral or aerosols), and immunosuppression (corticosteroids) related to shipping or immunosuppressive viral coinfections are potential cofactors that could exacerbate the severity of BCoV infections and the BRDC.
- Samples for antemortem diagnosis of BCoV infections include nasal swabs, tracheobronchial aspirates, and feces collected in the acute stage of infection; postmortem tissues include ones from the upper respiratory tract, lung, ileum, and colon. Highly sensitive molecular assays (RT-PCR, nested RT-PCR, qRT-PCR) are being used increasingly to detect BCoV RNA in diagnostic samples including tissue homogenates (lung, and so forth).
- Because most cattle are seropositive to BCoV, in suspect herd outbreaks, collection and testing of paired sera for BCoV antibody tests is essential for diagnosis.
- There are no BCoV vaccines to prevent respiratory BCoV infections in cattle, and the correlates of immunity to respiratory BCoV infections are unknown.
- In multiple studies, the serum BCoV antibody isotype (IgG1, IgG2, IgA), neutralizing and HI antibody titer, and magnitude of antibody titer in serum of cattle on arrival in feedlots were correlated with various parameters of protection against the BRDC. Whether the serum antibodies are correlates of protection or only reflect previous BCoV exposure is uncertain.
- Because BCoV infections commonly occur at or shortly after arrival of cattle to feedlots or at auction barns, use of BCoV vaccines in preconditioning calf programs before shipment of calves would be the most beneficial.

REFERENCES

1. Saif LJ. Coronaviruses of domestic livestock and poultry: interspecies transmission, pathogenesis and immunity. In: Perlman S, Gallagher T, Snijder E, editors. The nidoviruses, vol. 18. Washington, DC: ASM; 2007. p. 279–98.

2. Clark MA. Bovine coronavirus. Br Vet J 1993;149:51–70.

3. Saif LJ, Heckert RA. Enteric coronaviruses. In: Saif LJ, Theil KW, editors. Viral diarrheas of man and animals. Boca Raton (FL): CRC Press; 1990. p. 185–252.

4. Pensaert MB. Hemagglutinating encephalomyelitis virus. In: Straw B, Zimmerman JJ, D'Allaire S, et al, editors. Diseases of swine. 9th edition. Ames (IA): Iowa State Press; 2006. p. 353.

5. Saif LJ. Animal coronaviruses: what can they teach us about the severe acute respiratory syndrome? Rev Sci Tech 2004;23:643–60.

6. Tsunemitsu H, Smith DR, Saif LJ. Experimental inoculation of adult dairy cows with bovine coronavirus and detection of coronavirus in feces by RT-PCR. Arch Virol 1999;144:167–75.

7. Saif LJ. A review of evidence implicating bovine coronavirus in the etiology of winter dysentery in cows: an enigma resolved? Cornell Vet 1990;80:303–11.

8. Tsunemitsu H, Saif LJ. Antigenic and biological comparisons of bovine coronaviruses derived from neonatal calf diarrhea and winter dysentery of adult cattle. Arch Virol 1995;140:1303–11.

9. Cho KO, Halbur PG, Bruna JD, et al. Detection and isolation of coronavirus from feces of three herds of feedlot cattle during outbreaks of winter dysentery-like disease. J Am Vet Med Assoc 2000;217:1191–4.

10. Traven M, Naslund K, Linde N, et al. Experimental reproduction of winter dysentery in lactating cows using BCV – comparison with BCV infection in milk-fed calves. Vet Microbiol 2001;81:127–51.

11. Van Kruiningen HJ, Khairallah LH, Sasseville VG, et al. Calfhood coronavirus enterocolitis: a clue to the etiology of winter dysentery. Vet Pathol 1987;24:564–7.

12. Benfield DA, Saif LJ. Cell culture propagation of a coronavirus isolated from cows with winter dysentery. J Clin Microbiol 1990;28:1454–7.

13. Cho KO, Hoet AE, Loerch SC, et al. Evaluation of concurrent shedding of bovine coronavirus via the respiratory tract and enteric route in feedlot cattle. Am J Vet Res 2001;62:1436–41.

14. Hasoksuz M, Lathrop S, Al-dubaib MA, et al. Antigenic variation among bovine enteric coronaviruses (BECV) and bovine respiratory coronaviruses (BRCV) detected using monoclonal antibodies. Arch Virol 1999;144:2441–7.

15. Hasoksuz M, Lathrop SL, Gadfield KL, et al. Isolation of bovine respiratory coronaviruses from feedlot cattle and comparison of their biological and antigenic properties with bovine enteric coronaviruses. Am J Vet Res 1999;60: 1227–33.

16. Heckert RA, Saif LJ, Hoblet KH, et al. A longitudinal study of bovine coronavirus enteric and respiratory infections in dairy calves in two herds in Ohio. Vet Microbiol 1990;22:187–201.

17. Lathrop SL, Wittum TE, Brock KV, et al. Association between infection of the respiratory tract attributable to bovine coronavirus and health and growth performance of cattle in feedlots. Am J Vet Res 2000;61:1062–6.

18. Lathrop SL, Wittum TE, Loerch SC, et al. Antibody titers against bovine coronavirus and shedding of the virus via the respiratory tract in feedlot cattle. Am J Vet Res 2000;61:1057–61.

19. Storz J, Lin X, Purdy CW, et al. Coronavirus and Pasteurella infections in bovine shipping fever pneumonia and Evans' criteria for causation. J Clin Microbiol 2000; 38:3291–8.

20. Storz J, Purdy CW, Lin X, et al. Isolation of respiratory bovine coronavirus, other cytocidal viruses, and *Pasteurella* spp from cattle involved in two natural outbreaks of shipping fever. J Am Vet Med Assoc 2000;216:1599–604.

21. Storz J, Stine L, Liem A, et al. Coronavirus isolation from nasal swab samples in cattle with signs of respiratory tract disease after shipping. J Am Vet Med Assoc 1996;208:1452–5.
22. Gelinas AM, Sasseville AM, Dea S. Identification of specific variations within the HE, S1, and ORF4 genes of bovine coronaviruses associated with enteric and respiratory diseases in dairy cattle. Adv Exp Med Biol 2001;494:63–7.
23. Hasoksuz M, Hoet AE, Loerch SC, et al. Detection of respiratory and enteric shedding of bovine coronaviruses in cattle in an Ohio feedlot. J Vet Diagn Invest 2002;14:308–13.
24. Heckert RA, Saif LJ, Myers GW, et al. Epidemiologic factors and isotype-specific antibody responses in serum and mucosal secretions of dairy calves with bovine coronavirus respiratory tract and enteric tract infections. Am J Vet Res 1991;52:845–51.
25. Thomas CJ, Hoet AE, Sreevatsan S, et al. Transmission of bovine coronavirus and serologic responses in feedlot calves under field conditions. Am J Vet Res 2006;67:1412–20.
26. Chouljenko VN, Kousoulas KG, Lin X, et al. Nucleotide and predicted amino acid sequences of all genes encoded by the 3' genomic portion (9.5 kb) of respiratory bovine coronaviruses and comparisons among respiratory and enteric coronaviruses. Virus Genes 1998;17:33–42.
27. Hasoksuz M, Sreevatsan S, Cho KO, et al. Molecular analysis of the S1 subunit of the spike glycoprotein of respiratory and enteric bovine coronavirus isolates. Virus Res 2002;84:101–9.
28. Zhang X, Hasoksuz M, Spiro D, et al. Quasispecies of bovine enteric and respiratory coronaviruses based on complete genome sequences and genetic changes after tissue culture adaptation. Virology 2007;363:1–10.
29. Cho KO, Hasoksuz M, Nielsen PR, et al. Cross-protection studies between respiratory and calf diarrhea and winter dysentery coronavirus strains in calves and RT-PCR and nested PCR for their detection. Arch Virol 2001;146:2401–19.
30. El-Kanawati ZR, Tsunemitsu H, Smith DR, et al. Infection and cross-protection studies of winter dysentery and calf diarrhea bovine coronavirus strains in colostrum-deprived and gnotobiotic calves. Am J Vet Res 1996;57:48–53.
31. Deregt D, Gifford GA, Ijaz MK, et al. Monoclonal antibodies to bovine coronavirus glycoproteins E2 and E3: demonstration of in vivo virus-neutralizing activity. J Gen Virol 1989;70(Pt 4):993–8.
32. Jeong JH, Kim GY, Yoon SS. Molecular analysis of S gene of spike glycoprotein of winter dysentery bovine coronavirus circulating in Korea during 2002–2003. Virus Res 2005;108:207–12.
33. Liu L, Hagglund S, Hakhverdyan M, et al. Molecular epidemiology of bovine coronavirus on the basis of comparative analyses of the S gene. J Clin Microbiol 2006;44:957–60.
34. Kanno T, Hatama S, Ishihara R, et al. Molecular analysis of the S glycoprotein gene of bovine coronaviruses isolated in Japan from 1999 to 2006. J Gen Virol 2007;88:1218–24.
35. Zhang X, Herbst W, Kousoulas KG, et al. Comparison of the S genes and the biological properties of respiratory and enteropathogenic bovine coronaviruses. Arch Virol 1994;134:421–6.
36. Yoo D, Deregt D. A single amino acid change within antigenic domain II of the spike protein of bovine coronavirus confers resistance to virus neutralization. Clin Diagn Lab Immunol 2001;8:297–302.

37. Saif LJ, Sestak K. Transmissible gastroenteritis and porcine respiratory coronavirus. In: Straw B, Zimmerman JJ, D'Allaire S, et al, editors. Diseases of swine. 9th edition. Ames (IA): Blackwell Publishing; 2006. p. 489–516.

38. Domingo E, Baranowski E, Ruiz-Jarabo CM, et al. Quasispecies structure and persistence of RNA viruses. Emerg Infect Dis 1998;4:521–7.

39. Lin XQ, O'Reilly KL, Storz J. Antibody responses of cattle with respiratory coronavirus infections during pathogenesis of shipping fever pneumonia are lower with antigens of enteric strains than with those of a respiratory strain. Clin Diagn Lab Immunol 2002;9:1010–3.

40. Alekseev KP, Vlasova AN, Jung K, et al. Bovine-like coronaviruses isolated from four species of captive wild ruminants are homologous to bovine coronaviruses, based on complete genomic sequences. J Virol 2008;82:12422–31.

41. Decaro N, Campolo M, Desario C, et al. Respiratory disease associated with bovine coronavirus infection in cattle herds in Southern Italy. J Vet Diagn Invest 2008;20:28–32.

42. McNulty MS, Bryson DG, Allan GM, et al. Coronavirus infection of the bovine respiratory tract. Vet Microbiol 1984;9:425–34.

43. Reynolds DJ, Debney TG, Hall GA, et al. Studies on the relationship between coronaviruses from the intestinal and respiratory tracts of calves. Arch Virol 1985;85: 71–83.

44. Thomas LH, Gourlay RN, Stott EJ, et al. A search for new microorganisms in calf pneumonia by the inoculation of gnotobiotic calves. Res Vet Sci 1982;33:170–82.

45. Gulliksen SM, Jor E, Lie KI, et al. Respiratory infections in Norwegian dairy calves. J Dairy Sci 2009;92:5139–46.

46. Callow KA, Parry HF, Sergeant M, et al. The time course of the immune response to experimental coronavirus infection of man. Epidemiol Infect 1990;105:435–46.

47. Callebaut P, Cox E, Pensaert M, et al. Induction of milk IgA antibodies by porcine respiratory coronavirus infection. Adv Exp Med Biol 1990;276:421–8.

48. Crouch CF, Acres SD. Prevalence of rotavirus and coronavirus antigens in the feces of normal cows. Can J Comp Med 1984;48:340–2.

49. Plummer PJ, Rohrbach BW, Daugherty RA, et al. Effect of intranasal vaccination against bovine enteric coronavirus on the occurrence of respiratory tract disease in a commercial backgrounding feedlot. J Am Vet Med Assoc 2004; 225:726–31.

50. Martin SW, Nagy E, Shewen PE, et al. The association of titers to bovine coronavirus with treatment for bovine respiratory disease and weight gain in feedlot calves. Can J Vet Res 1998;62:257–61.

51. Lin X, O'Reilly KL, Burrell ML, et al. Infectivity-neutralizing and hemagglutinin-inhibiting antibody responses to respiratory coronavirus infections of cattle in pathogenesis of shipping fever pneumonia. Clin Diagn Lab Immunol 2001;8:357–62.

52. Hasoksuz M, Alekseev K, Vlasova A, et al. Biologic, antigenic, and full-length genomic characterization of a bovine-like coronavirus isolated from a giraffe. J Virol 2007;81:4981–90.

53. Majhdi F, Minocha HC, Kapil S. Isolation and characterization of a coronavirus from elk calves with diarrhea. J Clin Microbiol 1997;35:2937–42.

54. Tsunemitsu H, el-Kanawati ZR, Smith DR, et al. Isolation of coronaviruses antigenically indistinguishable from bovine coronavirus from wild ruminants with diarrhea. J Clin Microbiol 1995;33:3264–9.

55. Decaro N, Martella V, Elia G, et al. Biological and genetic analysis of a bovine-like coronavirus isolated from water buffalo (*Bubalus bubalis*) calves. Virology 2008; 370:213–22.

56. Jin L, Cebra CK, Baker RJ, et al. Analysis of the genome sequence of an alpaca coronavirus. Virology 2007;365:198–203.
57. Elazhary MA, Frechette JL, Silim S, et al. Serological evidence of some bovine viruses in the caribou (*Rangifer tarandus caribou*) in Quebec. J Wildl Dis 1981; 17:609–12.
58. Vijgen L, Keyaerts E, Lemey P, et al. Evolutionary history of the closely related group 2 coronaviruses: porcine hemagglutinating encephalomyelitis virus, bovine coronavirus, and human coronavirus OC43. J Virol 2006;80:7270–4.
59. Saif LJ. Comparative biology of coronaviruses: lessons for SARS. In: Peiris M, Anderson LJ, Osterhaus AD, et al, editors. Severe acute respiratory syndrome. Oxford (UK): Blackwell; 2005. p. 84–99.
60. Erles K, Toomey C, Brooks HW, et al. Detection of a group 2 coronavirus in dogs with canine infectious respiratory disease. Virology 2003;310:216–23.
61. Zhang XM, Herbst W, Kousoulas KG, et al. Biological and genetic characterization of a hemagglutinating coronavirus isolated from a diarrhoeic child. J Med Virol 1994;44:152–61.
62. Kaneshima T, Hohdatsu T, Hagino R, et al. The infectivity and pathogenicity of a group 2 bovine coronavirus in pups. J Vet Med Sci 2007;69:301–3.
63. Ismail MM, Cho KO, Ward LA, et al. Experimental bovine coronavirus in turkey poults and young chickens. Avian Dis 2001;45:157–63.
64. Saif LJ, Redman DR, Moorhead PD, et al. Experimentally induced coronavirus infections in calves: viral replication in the respiratory and intestinal tracts. Am J Vet Res 1986;47:1426–32.
65. Uttenthal A, Jensen NP, Blom JY. Viral aetiology of enzootic pneumonia in Danish dairy herds: diagnostic tools and epidemiology. Vet Rec 1996;139:114–7.
66. Hasoksuz M, Vlasova A, Saif LJ. Detection of group 2a coronaviruses with emphasis on bovine and wild ruminant strains. Virus isolation and detection of antibody, antigen, and nucleic acid. Methods Mol Biol 2008;454:43–59.
67. Decaro N, Elia G, Campolo M, et al. Detection of bovine coronavirus using a TaqMan-based real-time RT-PCR assay. J Virol Methods 2008;151:167–71.
68. Heckert RA, Saif LJ, Mengel JP, et al. Mucosal and systemic antibody responses to bovine coronavirus structural proteins in experimentally challenge-exposed calves fed low or high amounts of colostral antibodies. Am J Vet Res 1991;52:700–8.
69. Lin XQ, O'Reilly KL, Storz J, et al. Antibody responses to respiratory coronavirus infections of cattle during shipping fever pathogenesis. Arch Virol 2000;145: 2335–49.
70. Jakab GJ. Viral-bacterial interactions in pulmonary infection. Adv Vet Sci Comp Med 1982;26:155–71.
71. Van Reeth K, Nauwynck H, Pensaert M. A potential role for tumour necrosis factor-alpha in synergy between porcine respiratory coronavirus and bacterial lipopolysaccharide in the induction of respiratory disease in pigs. J Med Microbiol 2000;49:613–20.
72. Giomarelli P, Scolletta S, Borrelli E, et al. Myocardial and lung injury after cardiopulmonary bypass: role of interleukin (IL)-10. Ann Thorac Surg 2003;76:117–23.
73. Jung K, Alekseev KP, Zhang X, et al. Altered pathogenesis of porcine respiratory coronavirus in pigs due to immunosuppressive effects of dexamethasone: implications for corticosteroid use in treatment of severe acute respiratory syndrome coronavirus. J Virol 2007;81:13681–93.
74. Zhang X, Alekseev K, Jung K, et al. Cytokine responses in porcine respiratory coronavirus-infected pigs treated with corticosteroids as a model for severe acute respiratory syndrome. J Virol 2008;82:4420–8.

Mycoplasma bovis in Respiratory Disease of Feedlot Cattle

Jeff L. Caswell, DVM, DVSc, PhD[a],*, Ken G. Bateman, DVM, MSc[b],
Hugh Y. Cai, DVM, MSc, DVSc[c], Fernanda Castillo-Alcala, DVM, DVSc[d]

KEYWORDS

- Mycoplasma bovis • Pneumonia • Cattle • Beef feedlots
- Arthritis • Mannheimia haemolytica

Mycoplasma bovis has emerged as an important cause of pneumonia, arthritis, and tenosynovitis in feedlot cattle. The role of *M bovis* in pneumonia and otitis media in younger calves, mastitis, keratoconjunctivitis, and decubital abscesses is reviewed elsewhere.[1–4] *Mycoplasma bovis* is best recognized as a cause of chronic pneumonia that often progresses to fatal disease despite prolonged therapy with multiple antibiotics, with characteristic gross pulmonary lesions of caseonecrotic bronchopneumonia in which the cranioventral areas of lung consolidation contain round white nodules of dry friable material. *Mycoplasma bovis* appears to play a role in other forms of acute and chronic pneumonia in feedlot cattle, but its importance in these forms of disease remains uncertain because clinical features are not etiologically specific and the prevalence of infection in clinically healthy cattle is high.

PATHOGENESIS AND VIRULENCE FACTORS

Several important characteristics of mycoplasmal biology are of clinical significance: the small size of their genome confers a reliance on the host animal for several metabolic requirements; the presence of a cell membrane but absence of a cell wall makes mycoplasmas insensitive to β-lactam antibiotics; and because of limited survival in the environment, transmission is considered to be mainly by direct contact with infected

This work was supported by research grants from the Ontario Cattlemen's Association, the Canadian Cattlemen's Association, and the Natural Sciences and Engineering Research Council of Canada. Dr Caswell acted as a paid consultant for Pfizer in 2008.
[a] Department of Pathobiology, University of Guelph, Guelph, Ontario N1G 2W1, Canada
[b] Department of Population Medicine, University of Guelph, Guelph, Ontario N1G 2W1, Canada
[c] Animal Health Laboratory, Laboratory Services Division, University of Guelph, Guelph, Ontario N1G 2W1, Canada
[d] Ross University School of Veterinary Medicine, PO Box 334, Basseterre, St Kitts, West Indies
* Corresponding author.
E-mail address: jcaswell@uoguelph.ca

animals.[5] *Mycoplasma bovis* is not considered to be a significant human pathogen, although there is one case report of its isolation from a person with lobar pneumonia.

Mycoplasma bovis survives for several days in the environment, but this is not regarded as an important source of infection. Young calves can acquire *M bovis* by ingestion of contaminated milk,[1] and this might be a basis for the few calves that are infected with this pathogen on arrival in feedlots. However, most *M bovis* infections in feedlot cattle are thought to be acquired by contact with the nasal secretions of infected calves, and there is limited evidence that stress or transportation enhance the shedding of *M bovis* in nasal secretions.[3,6]

Mycoplasma bovis is capable of adhering to host cells, evading the immune response, and injuring host tissues, and some of the virulence factors responsible for these processes are known. *Mycoplasma bovis* can adhere to bovine tracheobronchial epithelial cells, which presumably facilitates colonization of the lung. However, in contrast to *M hyopneumoniae* and several other pathogenic mycoplasmas, this adhesion does not result in ciliostasis.[7] Adhesion to host cells differs among bacterial strains, and there is limited evidence that it correlates with pathogenicity of the bacterial strain. Adhesion of *M bovis* to host cells is partly mediated by variable surface proteins (VSPs), a family of lipoproteins on the bacterial surface, and unrelated proteins, including pMB67 and p26.[8–10] A complex genetic system determines which of the five VSPs are expressed or not at a given time, and modifies the size and antigenicity of the expressed protein. The resulting patterns of VSPs on the surface of the bacterium presumably allow *M bovis* to adapt to different conditions within the host microenvironment and adhere to different host cell types.[11,12]

Infection elicits a robust immune response, and evasion of the immune defenses is necessary for *M bovis* to chronically colonize the lung and disseminate to the joints. Following natural infection, calves develop *M bovis*-specific IgM and IgG in serum, and higher levels of IgA in nasal and lung fluids.[13] *Mycoplasma bovis*-specific serum IgM is detectable by 7 days and maximal at 14 days after experimental infection, but total *M bovis*-specific serum antibody titres continue to increase for 63 days after infection.[14] The predominance of immunoglobulin G1 over IgG2 isotypes may imply skewing toward a Th2 response, but this finding awaits confirmation.[14] T-cell responses have been documented following experimental infection, particularly of CD8+ T cells but also of CD4+ and γδ T cells, and these T cells express IFN-γ and IL-4.[14] However, the role of the T-cell response, and particularly whether a Th1/Th2 bias affects immunity, remains unknown.

The major antigenic targets of the host antibody response are the VSP proteins, and unrelated proteins, including pMB67 and P48.[11,15,16] It might be expected that high titres to these antigens would result in bacterial killing, for *M bovis*-specific IgG1 and IgG2 are both known to activate complement in vitro. However, the available evidence suggests that this immune response is non-protective. In vitro exposure of *M bovis* to antibodies specific for the VSP antigen expressed by that isolate induces a change in pattern of VSP expression by the bacteria.[17] As a result, changes in the expression, conformation, and antigenicity of the VSP and pMB67 proteins are thought to be one way in which *M bovis* continuously evades the host antibody response.

In addition to alteration of surface antigens, *M bovis* has other mechanisms of evading the host immuno-inflammatory response. *Mycoplasma bovis* can induce apoptosis of lymphocytes, and a C-terminal fragment of VSP-L impairs the in vitro lymphocyte proliferative response to mitogens.[18,19] The bacterium can adhere to neutrophils and inhibit oxidative burst in these cells.[20] Finally, biofilms are produced by some strains of *M bovis* and result in resistance to desiccation in the environment.

Biofilm formation is strain dependant and appears to be associated with VSP expression, and could potentially play a role in evading the immune response and conferring resistance to antimicrobials.[21]

The mechanism by which *M bovis* causes injury to lung tissue is an area of considerable uncertainty. *Mycoplasma bovis* produces hydrogen peroxide during oxidation of nicotinamide adenine dinucleotide and the amount of peroxide produced varies among different bacterial isolates.[22] A similar phenomenon has been well studied in the case of *M mycoides* ssp. mycoides SC (the cause of contagious bovine pleuropneumonia), where the amount of peroxide produced is positively correlated with the cytotoxicity of the strain.[23] However, caution is warranted in extending these findings to *M bovis*, because the enzymes and substrates for peroxide production differ between these two mycoplasmas. Nonetheless, oxidative injury induced by hydrogen peroxide might be one mechanism by which *M bovis* causes injury to host tissues. The production of a polysaccharide toxin was found in one report but not confirmed in another paper, and the absence lipopolysaccharide or other secreted toxins presumably accounts for the chronic indolent clinical appearance of *M bovis* pneumonia that differs from the acute depression and anorexia seen in pneumonia caused by *M haemolytica*.

PATHOLOGIC AND EPIDEMIOLOGIC FINDINGS

Recognition of the prevalence of *M bovis* infection is important to understanding the pathogenesis of the disease and to interpretation of laboratory tests. In general, the prevalence of calf infection prior to arrival in feedlots is low, typically between 0% and 7%. In contrast, infection is much more widespread once cattle have been in the feedlot for about 2 weeks or longer, with a prevalence of 40% to 100% in most studies.[6,24,25] The increased prevalence of infection at this time probably results from spread of infection following comingling of infected and noninfected calves, although stress-associated increases in prevalence of detectable infection may also contribute.[13] Thus, pulmonary and nasal infection with *M bovis* is generally uncommon in pre-weaned beef calves, but becomes common within 2 weeks after arrival in feedlots, and is detectable in most calves later in the feeding period.

M bovis can be recovered from nasal swabs or bronchoalveolar lavage (BAL) fluid of many at-risk but otherwise healthy calves. This fact complicates any attempt to associate infection with a particular form of disease, because the mere presence of *M bovis* within a clinical sample does not indicate that it is causing the observed disease. Instead, observations that would suggest that *M bovis* causes a particular form of pneumonia include: (1) demonstrating the same clinical signs and lesions in experimentally challenged calves, (2) isolation of *M bovis* and failure to isolate other pathogens from naturally occurring cases that had not received antibiotic therapy, (3) finding a different prevalence of infection in calves with and without the disease condition, and (4) associating the concentration or microscopic location of the infectious agent with the characteristic lesion.

Chronic caseonecrotic bronchopneumonia with or without arthritis is the lesion that is most reliably known to be caused by *M bovis*. Most commonly, lesions are distributed in the cranioventral areas of the lung, with relative sparing of the caudal and dorsal aspects of the caudal lobes. Lesions are usually bilateral, and vary greatly in their extent from 20% to 90% of the total lung tissue. The affected areas of lung are red and collapsed or consolidated, but these are features similar to other forms of bronchopneumonia.[26–30] The unique aspect of the lesion is the presence of multiple foci of caseous necrosis within these areas of affected lung. In severe cases, these foci form nodules that are visible from the pleural surface; more mild lesions are only detected when a cut section of lung is examined. Such foci are usually round, coalescing, well demarcated, white, and vary from pinpoint to several centimeters in diameter. The key feature is the friable caseous nature of the lesions; the content is dry and crumbly when manipulated with a knife (**Figs. 1** and **2**).

Histologically, the caseonecrotic foci develop in airways, in alveoli, or in interlobular septa, and consist of eosinophilic material that often contains the ghostlike outlines of necrotic leukocytes. Necrotic and non-necrotic macrophages and fewer neutrophils are present at the periphery, and there is often a capsule of fibrous tissue containing lymphocytes and macrophages. *Mycoplasma bovis* antigen is most abundant at the edge of these necrotic foci, free and within macrophages, and is less copious in the cytoplasm of neutrophils, within edematous alveoli, and infrequently among ciliated tracheobronchial epithelial cells.[26–30]

The typical caseonecrotic foci are readily distinguished from abscesses, which have a fluid purulent center, although caseonecrotic foci may develop into abscesses if there is concurrent infection with *Arcanobacterium pyogenes*. It is usually possible to distinguish the caseonecrotic foci from foci of coagulation necrosis, although this may be more challenging. The *M haemolytica*-associated foci of coagulation necrosis are irregularly shaped, flat, have normal tissue strength, and are red with a thin white rim; whereas the *M bovis*-associated caseous foci are round, bulging, friable, and white. This distinction is important because the caseonecrotic lesions indicate *M bovis* as a cause of the pneumonia, whereas foci of coagulation necrosis are common in pneumonia caused by *Mannheimia haemolytica*. However, as discussed later in this article, there may be transition between these two disease process in some cases and it remains possible that some coagulative foci are caused by *M bovis* infection. Similarly, the contribution of *M bovis* is most certain when numerous large foci of caseous necrosis dominate the landscape of the consolidated cranioventral lung,

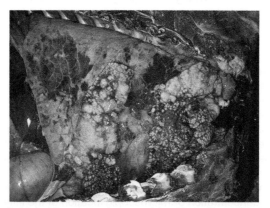

Fig. 1. Caseonecrotic bronchopneumonia caused by *Mycoplasma bovis*. This calf did not receive metaphylactic antibiotic on arrival to the feedlot. It was first treated for respiratory disease at 10 days after arrival in the feedlot, and was euthanized 4 weeks later. Necropsy findings in the lung are shown; the head is at the right and the abdomen at the left. The cranioventral 60% of the lungs are collapsed or consolidated, dark red, and contain numerous white nodules of caseous necrosis. Tracheobronchial and mediastinal lymph nodes were enlarged, and the tendon sheath adjacent to the stifle joint contained similar foci of caseous necrosis. *Mycoplasma bovis*, *Mannheimia haemolytica*, and *Mycoplasma arginini* were isolated in large number from the lungs, *M bovis* was isolated from the joint, and BVDV was not identified by isolation or immunohistochemistry.

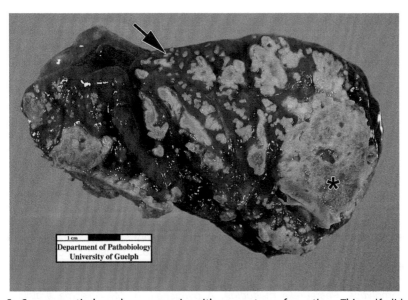

Fig. 2. Caseonecrotic bronchopneumonia with sequestrum formation. This calf did not receive antibiotics on arrival to the feedlot, was treated for pneumonia at 4 days after arrival in the feedlot, received two additional treatments with other antibiotics for pneumonia and lameness, and was euthanized because of intractable lameness at 35 days after arrival. At necropsy, there was bronchopneumonia affecting 50% of the lung, and the photo shows a section of lung tissue containing 2 to 4 mm diameter white foci of caseous necrosis (*arrow*) that coalesce to form a sequestrum (*asterisk*). The scale bar shows 1 cm gradations. Fibrin and cloudy fluid were found in right and left elbow and stifle joints and the right hock joint. *Mycoplasma bovis*, *Mannheimia haemolytica*, and *Mycoplasma arginini* were isolated in large number from the lungs, and *M bovis* and *M arginini* were isolated from the joints. BVDV was not identified by isolation or immunohistochemistry.

but the significance is not as clear when rare foci of caseation are detected within lesions that otherwise resemble those caused by *M haemolytica*.

Variants of these lesions do occur. Caseonecrotic foci can be numerous or few, and uniformly tiny (1 mm) or larger and variable in size (4–20 mm diameter). The lung lesions can be unilateral, although a bilateral distribution is more common. Sequestra develop when the caseous foci enlarge and coalesce, and may involve the entire lobe (see **Fig. 2**). In some cases, the remaining dorso-caudal lung is affected by interstitial pneumonia, with a diffuse or lobular pattern of firm or rubbery texture, reddening, and edema. The caseonecrotic lesions may penetrate the pleural surface and incite fibrinous pleuritis or fibrous pleural adhesions. Arthritis or tenosynovitis is present in 15% to 50% of cases of caseonecrotic bronchopneumonia, may or may not be clinically apparent, and result from hematogenous dissemination of *M bovis* from the lung. Stifle joints are most commonly affected but involvement of other joints is also frequent, as is tenosynovitis and cellulitis along the peroneus tertius and long digital extensor tendons adjacent to the tibia.[30] In contrast to the situation in dairy and veal calves, otitis media as a result of *M bovis* infection appears to be of less importance in feedlot cattle.[26]

The evidence that *M bovis* causes caseonecrotic bronchopneumonia is compelling: *M bovis* can be identified in nearly all lungs with such lesions;[26] *M bovis* antigen is closely associated with the caseonecrotic lesion, being visible at the edge of such foci using immunohistochemistry;[26–28] and the caseonecrotic lesion is seen in calves following experimental infection with M bovis in studies in which infected calves lived for more than 1 month.[31,32] It is less certain whether M bovis is an important cause of bronchopneumonia in which caseonecrotic foci are not present. These lesions are less distinctive pathologically and are historically attributed to M haemolytica, Histophilus somni, or Pasteurella multocida. Nevertheless, M bovis can be the only demonstrable pathogen in some cases of bronchopneumonia that lack caseonecrotic foci,[33] and some descriptions of lesions following experimental infection with M bovis indicate a nonspecific pattern of cranioventral suppurative or catarrhal bronchopneumonia. Thus, M bovis must be regarded as a primary cause of suppurative and catarrhal bronchopneumonia in cattle. However, the proportion of such cases in which M bovis is the initiating or only cause is difficult to assess, because of the high prevalence of M bovis infection in lungs of healthy feedlot cattle, and the fact that most calves dying of pneumonia have received prolonged antibiotic therapy that could obscure the initiating cause. Therefore, the economic importance of M bovis cannot be accurately measured at present, because the clinical signs are not specific, some forms of the lung lesions cannot be easily distinguished from those caused by other bacteria, and effective M bovis-specific preventative or therapeutic strategies are not available.

Most cases of M bovis pneumonia are coinfected with other pathogens, including M haemolytica, Pasteurella multocida, A pyogenes, or Mycoplasma arginini, and less frequently with H somni, Bovine herpesvirus-1, Bovine respiratory syncytial virus (BRSV), or Bovine parainfluenza-3 virus.[26–28,33,34] Bovine viral diarrhea virus (BVDV) infection is common in cattle with caseonecrotic bronchopneumonia.[26,27] Although BVDV is a known predisposing cause of bacterial bronchopneumonia in cattle, it does not seem to preferentially predispose to M bovis pneumonia.[26,35] Mycoplasma bovis infection appears to exacerbate the disease resulting from experimental challenge with M haemolytica, but synergism was not identified with P multocida or BRSV.

In some cases, the caseonecrotic lesions of M bovis infection might evolve out of lesions that were initiated by M haemolytica. This hypothesis is based on the frequent presence of both pathogens in the caseonecrotic lesions, the observation that some foci of coagulation necrosis that contain and are presumably caused by M haemolytica have caseous necrosis and M bovis antigen at their periphery, the similar time of onset of clinical disease in cases with necropsy lesions of either form of pneumonia, and the more chronic appearance of the caseonecrotic foci.[26] Thus, although it is likely that M bovis is the primary or only pathogen in some cases, it is proposed that other cases are initiated by M haemolytica infection, but M bovis may perpetuate these lesions after the M haemolytica infection is eliminated by antibiotic therapy or the developing immune response. This distinction is important because if M bovis is acting as a primary pathogen, then control strategies should specifically target M bovis; whereas if M bovis is a secondary pathogen, then control of M haemolytica and the more well-recognized factors predisposing to shipping fever pneumonia would be a more appropriate intervention.

CLINICAL FEATURES

Feedlot cattle may be pulled to the hospital area for treatment of undifferentiated bovine respiratory disease (UBRD) based on one or more of the following: depression (segregation from the group); lack of rumen fill; persistent cough; excessive nasal discharge; and dyspnea or hyperpnea. It is generally believed that the most sensitive and specific indicators of bronchopneumonia are depression; lack of rumen fill; fever (usually above 40°C/104°F); and absence of signs referable to body systems other than the respiratory tract. Some authors suggest that we should call UBRD undifferentiated fever (UF) because in some situations, in their experience, the necropsy findings in many of the calves that die were attributable to myocarditis, septicemia, pleuritis, or encephalitis caused by *Histophilus somni* infection.[36]

There are few, if any, clinical features that allow differentiation of *M bovis* pneumonia from other causes of pneumonia in feedlot cattle *at first treatment*. *Mycoplasma bovis* pneumonia is only suggested or suspected by chronicity (repeated respiratory treatment failure) or lameness.[37] Often, calves are treated initially as a routine case of UBRD but do not respond or suffer repeated relapses, at which time one begins to suspect involvement of *M bovis*. Many cases of UBRD appear to respond to therapy but develop lameness with or without reappearance of the respiratory component of the disease. The lameness can usually be attributed to swelling and pain in one or more joints, commonly the stifle, hock, carpus or elbow. Other affected joints, such as the hip, may not be evident until necropsy.

Pollock and colleagues[37] described the epidemiology of chronic disease in a Saskatchewan feedlot. Out of 12,039 fall placed calves, 158 (1.3% of the population at risk) were classified as chronically ill and entered a convalescent (chronic) pen. Forty-nine percent were treatment failures for UF, 39% were lame with polyarthritis, and 10% were lame without arthritis. Of those entering the chronic pen, 40% died or were euthanized after an average of 2 weeks and a further weight loss of 48 pounds. The other 60% returned home after a mean of 30 days and a weight gain of 72 pounds. The chronically ill calf population accounted for 40% of all mortality in the feedlot. At necropsy, of the 63 chronically ill calves, 40% had chronic bronchopneumonia and polyarthritis, 21% had polyarthritis only, and 18% had chronic bronchopneumonia. The mean days on feed at the time of death for the chronically ill calves was 51, and for other mortalities it was only 29 days.

In an Ontario mortality study, calves that died of acute fibrinous and suppurative bronchopneumonia or caseonecrotic bronchopneumonia were treated initially at similar times (14 to 15 days) post-arrival, but the calves that had caseonecrotic bronchopneumonia at necropsy lived approximately 2 weeks longer, had more re-treatments, and 52% of them had accompanying arthritis or polyarthritis.[26,38] Many of the death losses caused by chronic pneumonia or arthritis are because of euthanasia and as such, feedlot staff and veterinarians must take an active role to ensure appropriate animal welfare.[37]

Although chronicity and repeated relapses after antimicrobial therapy are hallmarks of cases that have postmortem lesions of caseonecrotic bronchopneumonia,[27,37] it is unknown what proportion of *M bovis* pneumonia cases may recover because they would not be recognizable clinically in the absence of arthritis.

LABORATORY DIAGNOSTIC METHODS

This section considers the laboratory diagnostic techniques for detection of *M bovis*, clinical interpretation of these laboratory data, and methods to measure antimicrobial resistance. Although *M bovis* is more readily isolated in culture than some other pathogenic mycoplasmas, the isolation procedures are specialized and reagents for specific identification of mycoplasmal species are not widely available, so the availability of diagnostic methods varies considerably between laboratories.

Methods to detect *M bovis* in clinical samples include culture to detect viable bacteria, immunohistochemistry to detect bacterial antigen, and PCR-based tests or in situ hybridization to detect bacterial DNA. Isolation in culture is a sensitive method of detecting *M bovis* infection, and is typically performed on lung tissue, nasal swabs, BAL fluid, and joint fluid.[3,39–41] Dacron, calcium alginate, or polyester swabs are preferred over wooden-shaft cotton swabs to avoid inhibition of mycoplasmal growth. Because M bovis grows in association with cells, vigorous swabbing that harvests many cells is recommended, and cultures are best performed on the sediment obtained following centrifugation of fluid specimens. Diagnostic samples should be kept chilled if shipping time is less than 24 hours, or frozen at $-70\,°C$ if longer transport times are needed.

Samples should be inoculated into solid and broth media, such as Hayflick's or other suitable media, and serial dilutions may be needed to overcome the inhibitory effects of antibodies or antibiotics in the samples. Solid medium cultures are incubated at 37°C in 5% to 10% CO_2 and examined daily for M bovis colonies for 10 to 14 days if negative. Broth cultures are incubated at 37 °C for 2 to 3 days then plated on agar and cultured as described earlier. On most media, examination using a stereomicroscope reveals 0.1 to 0.5 mm diameter colonies that have a fried-egg appearance. Although the colony morphology is suggestive, identification of the mycoplasmal species requires additional testing, and must be performed on a pure culture, ideally after three passages of the isolate to ensure its purity. Commonly used methods to specifically identify M bovis include fluorescent antibody test, ELISA, other antibody-based methods, or PCR-based techniques; and such tests must be capable of distinguishing M bovis from the closely related M agalactiae.

Mycoplasma culture has several advantages over other methods to identify M bovis in clinical samples: it is highly sensitive, well established in some laboratories, can isolate multiple mycoplasma species from the same sample, and may reveal unexpected or novel species for which molecular testing is not performed. However, culture techniques are labor intensive, require considerable technical expertise and specialized reagents, and have longer turnaround times than many molecular tests. Further, culture may fail in several situations in which M bovis DNA can still be detected by PCR: samples containing antibodies or antibiotics because they were taken from previously infected or treated animals, samples contaminated with bacteria because of concurrent pulmonary infections or autolysis, samples inadvertently treated with preservatives, or samples from necrotic or autolyzed lesions in which the bacteria may no longer be adequately viable to grow in culture.

Molecular tests to detect M bovis in clinical specimens have been developed in recent years, and include PCR-based amplification of bacterial 16S rDNA followed by melting curve analysis or denaturing gradient gel electrophoresis to distinguish M bovis from M agalactiae, and PCR-based amplification of unique DNA sequences in the uvrC, oppD/F, or DNA polymerase III genes of M bovis. The principle advantages of these tests are the rapid turnaround time, lower cost per test, and compatibility with molecular testing for other pathogens in the diagnostic laboratory. Nevertheless, culture remains as or more sensitive than PCR-based tests, and it is important that this capability is not lost from diagnostic laboratories.

Immunohistochemistry appears to be the most diagnostically specific method to detect M bovis infection, and the test can be performed on formalin-fixed paraffin-embedded tissue sections when no fresh or frozen tissue is available. The major advantage of immunohistochemistry is that M bovis antigen can be localized specifically to areas of necrosis in the lung, and therefore suggests a causal role of M bovis in development of these lesions. A recent study in veal calves found a high correlation between cases with histologically observed necrotizing lesions in the lung, immunohistochemical detection of M bovis antigen at the periphery of these foci, and large numbers of M bovis isolated in culture. In contrast, other cases had other patterns of lung lesions, no M bovis antigen observed by immunohistochemistry, and low numbers of *M bovis* isolated in culture.[42] In situ hybridization, which detects bacterial DNA in histologic sections, has similar advantages of localizing the infection in the context of the histologic lesion, but this method is not widely available in diagnostic laboratories.[43] Thus, although culture is a more sensitive method to detect *M bovis* infection, immunohistochemistry is considered more diagnostically specific.

Finally, because *M bovis* infection elicits a robust antibody response, several effective methods of detecting *M bovis*-specific serum antibody are described. These tests generally detect antibodies to whole bacterial cell lysates or surface antigens, and those available include the passive or indirect hemagglutination test, indirect ELISA, and film inhibition tests. However, most cattle have detectable titres to *M bovis* within 2 to 4 weeks after arrival in feedlots, so serologic testing should not be used to confirm that *M bovis* is the cause of pneumonia in an individual calf or a group.

INTERPRETATION OF LABORATORY DIAGNOSTIC TESTS

Important considerations in interpretation of diagnostic laboratory data for *M bovis* testing include the adequacy of the sample, the high prevalence of healthy infected animals, and the intended purpose of the test. Several studies have shown a poor correlation between nasal swabs and BAL samples with respect to detection of *M bovis* and an increased prevalence of infection in BAL fluid.[44,45] Thus, although nasal or conjunctival swabs are easily obtained and provide information on the infection status of the herd,[46] BAL fluid or samples of lung tissue are probably the only method to reliably determine whether the lung of an individual calf is infected or not. As indicated earlier, cultures of fluid samples are more likely to be positive if sediments rather than supernatants are tested.

Available evidence indicates that many groups of unweaned beef calves have a low prevalence of *M bovis* infection, whereas infection appears to be widespread in most feedlot cattle.[6,24,25] This observation limits the usefulness of culture and serology in making the diagnosis in an individual animal. The diagnosis of *M bovis* pneumonia can be made most reliably at necropsy, if the gross findings are of caseonecrotic bronchopneumonia and *M bovis* antigen is identified within these lesions by immunohistochemistry, or alternatively if *M bovis* infection of the lung is demonstrated by culture or molecular testing in an animal with caseonecrotic lung lesions. Proving a role for *M bovis* in other forms of bronchopneumonia is currently controversial, although a causal role is likely if *M bovis* is the only detectable bacterial pathogen in lung tissue or in BAL samples obtained prior to antibiotic therapy. This approach has limited value as a routine method, because BAL fluid is not readily obtained by most practitioners and because most or all calves with *M bovis* pneumonia receive multiple antibiotic treatments prior to death, so lung tissue from untreated calves with this disease is a rarity. Nevertheless, identifying *M bovis* but not other pathogens in an antibiotic-treated calf with pneumonia is not considered conclusive, because the therapy may well have eliminated the initial cause of the disease. The chronic presence of pneumonia and arthritis suggests *M bovis* as a causative agent. Finally, it is clear that identifying *M bovis* in the lung of a calf with pneumonia does not imply that *M bovis* is the cause of disease, because of the high prevalence of *M bovis* infection in healthy calves and those with other forms of pneumonia.

Conversely, the absence of *M bovis* infection would effectively rule out the disease in an individual animal, particularly if multiple samples of well-preserved specimens from an appropriate site are all negative. Similarly, although serologic tests are of limited value in establishing a positive diagnosis, negative serologic tests are considered valuable in identifying herds that are free of *M bovis* infection.

ANTIMICROBIAL RESISTANCE TESTING

Several methods to test the in vitro antimicrobial susceptibility of M bovis isolates are described, but the disk diffusion methods commonly used for other bacteria are not suitable for M bovis. Suitable methods include the microbroth dilution method, in which detection of bacterial growth is detected by reduction of an indicator dye,[47] and the E test method, in which agar plate cultures of M bovis are exposed to strips that have been impregnated with antibiotics.[48] Such tests are becoming available in some diagnostic laboratories. Important and unresolved issues are the lack of accepted guidelines for establishing breakpoints between susceptible and resistant isolates, an absence of objective information relating in vitro susceptibility to therapeutic efficacy, and geographic differences in patterns of antimicrobial resistance.[49]

PREVENTION AND TREATMENT

Commercial and autogenous vaccines against M bovis have been developed, but although these stimulate antibody production, there is little or no evidence of their efficacy under field conditions. Although there are no published reports of clinical field trials of M bovis vaccines in beef feedlots, the results of one large field trial utilizing an autogenous vaccine have been presented.[50] With more than 5000 calves per treatment group (placebo, vaccinated once, vaccinated twice), no benefit was discernable in any of several relevant morbidity and mortality measurements undertaken.

Because M bovis pneumonia or polyarthritis may develop as a sequel to bacterial bronchopneumonia in some cases (as described earlier), control should be predicated on minimizing the effect of M haemolytica and the more well-recognized factors predisposing to UBRD. Cattle with low antibody titers to BVDV upon arrival and those with rising titers in the first month are more prone to developing UBRD,[51,52] so prevention of persistent BVDV infection in the cow herd, pre-vaccination of calves against BVDV and other viral pathogens prior to entering the feedlot, or vaccination upon arrival at the feedlot should reduce morbidity caused by UBRD. Metaphylactic treatment of high-risk calves with antibiotics is a well-established, beneficial procedure that can reduce UBRD morbidity and case fatality by up to 50%. At the same time, early identification of pneumonia cases, prompt treatment, and timely assessment of the response to therapy is essential. Overconfidence in and reliance on the efficacy of metaphylaxis and long-acting therapeutic antimicrobials can lead to delayed treatment or re-treatment, if clinical signs are not adequately monitored. Housing relapses and keeping chronically ill calves away from calves treated for the first time should avoid the spread of M bovis and BVDV from persistently infected calves. Experienced stockpersons become quite adept at recognizing suspect cases of mucosal disease and such animals should be housed away from other sick animals, examined by veterinarians, and euthanized when a diagnosis is confirmed.

Although there are concerns about extrapolation of in vitro antimicrobial susceptibilities to the live animal, ampicillin, ceftiofur, erythromycin and tilmicosin cannot be recommended as effective for M bovis therapy.[47] Enrofloxacin, florfenicol and spectinomycin have shown excellent in vitro activity against M bovis[47] and would therefore seem to be logical choices for first treatment (in calves that were given metaphylactic antibiotic treatment), relapsing pneumonia cases, and calves with arthritis, which are the cases most likely to involve M bovis. In vitro susceptibility testing of M bovis isolates against tulathromycin shows a high MIC_{50} of 16 μg/mL,[53] but limited evidence in an experimental challenge model of M bovis pneumonia by the same author has shown tulathromycin to be effective against a strain with a similar MIC_{50}.[54] Despite the apparently adequate vitro susceptibilities to these antimicrobials, it must be recognized that the response to therapy may be fair at best because of limited drug distribution into the caseous foci where the *M bovis* bacteria are most numerous.

The assumption that 60% of those cattle entering the chronic pen will survive and reach slaughter[37] presents an obvious management and welfare dilemma: how to maximize the number that recover and minimize the suffering of those that will not? The chronic pen must provide a comfortable, well-bedded environment with good traction underfoot and ready access to feed and water. This facility requires daily assessment by trained staff to euthanize cattle that are unable to adequately rise to feed and drink, and those that develop severe dyspnea that is unlikely to readily respond to therapy. In cold climates, cattle with polyarthritis in certain joints may not be able to tuck their feet under their body in normal sternal posture and are at risk for developing frostbite, so caretakers must be vigilant for this problem.

It is strongly recommended that chronically ill cattle be weighed and examined in a headgate once per week to evaluate progressive changes in their weight, temperature, and clinical signs. Managers and cattle owners often want an experienced veterinarian to participate in this triage exercise. Febrile animals may require further antimicrobial therapy for bronchopneumonia that has developed or relapsed since entering the chronic pen. Positive improvement in other cases may be noted by weight gain within 1 to 2 weeks. Some consider loss of weight and body condition over three consecutive weekly weighings to be justification for euthanasia. It may take, as Pollock and colleagues noted,[37] approximately 1 month before there is adequate improvement in lameness and weight gain to allow cattle to return to their home pen. Occasionally, lameness may not resolve completely, but the animal may be fit for salvage slaughter if body condition is adequate, drug withdrawal times are complete, and the animal can be humanely transported. To summarize, the chronic pen should be triaged on a weekly basis to categorize animals into those that: (1) need further treatment, (2) can return to their home pen, (3) are eligible for salvage slaughter, or (4) must be euthanized because of continued weight loss from intractable pneumonia or lameness. Unfortunately for the animal and the producer, at the time of entry to the chronic pen, our positive and negative predictive value for future euthanasia or return home is somewhere between 50% and 75%. As a result, there is little that we can do except provide an opportunity for convalescence but terminate suffering as needed.

SUMMARY

Mycoplasma bovis has emerged as an important cause of respiratory disease and lameness in beef cattle. Pulmonary infection is uncommon when calves arrive in feedlots, but is widespread after several weeks. Clinical features do not differentiate *M bovis* from other causes of bacterial pneumonia, although chronic respiratory disease, recurrent treatment failure, and lameness caused by arthritis or tenosynovitis are suggestive. *Mycoplasma bovis* causes chronic caseonecrotic bronchopneumonia, characterized by cranioventral pulmonary consolidation with multiple raised white friable foci of caseous necrosis. Although *M bovis* probably causes other forms of bronchopneumonia, its importance in such situations has been difficult to assess. It can act as a primary pathogen, yet many cases are coinfected with other bacteria or viruses, and evidence suggests that *M bovis* colonizes and perpetuates lung lesions that were initiated by other bacteria, such as *M haemolytica*. BVDV appears to predispose to bacterial pneumonia generally rather than to *M bovis* pneumonia in particular. Simply identifying *M bovis* in the lung of a calf with pneumonia does not necessarily indicate that *M bovis* was the cause, and the diagnosis is based on gross, histologic, and immunohistochemical findings. *Mycoplasma bovis* elicits a robust humoral immune response, but the resulting antibodies are not protective because of the variable surface proteins, and vaccines have not yet been shown to prevent disease. *Mycoplasma bovis* infections are responsible for a high proportion of the chronic disease occurring in feedlots, and the welfare of such animals is an important aspect of feedlot health management.

REFERENCES

1. Maunsell FP, Donovan GA. Mycoplasma bovis infections in young calves. Vet Clin North Am Food Anim Pract 2009;25(1):139–77.
2. Foster AP, Naylor RD, Howie NM, et al. Mycoplasma bovis and otitis in dairy calves in the United Kingdom. Vet J 2009;179(3):455–7.
3. Caswell JL, Archambault M. Mycoplasma bovis pneumonia in cattle. Anim Health Res Rev 2007;8(2):161–86.
4. Fox LK, Kirk JH, Britten A. Mycoplasma mastitis: a review of transmission and control. J Vet Med B Infect Dis Vet Public Health 2005;52(4):153–60.
5. Razin S, Yogev D, Naot Y. Molecular biology and pathogenicity of mycoplasmas. Microbiol Mol Biol Rev 1998;62(4):1094–156.
6. Arcangioli MA, Duet A, Meyer G, et al. The role of Mycoplasma bovis in bovine respiratory disease outbreaks in veal calf feedlots. Vet J 2008;177(1):89–93.
7. Howard CJ, Thomas LH, Parsons KR. Comparative pathogenicity of Mycoplasma bovis and Mycoplasma dispar for the respiratory tract of calves. Isr J Med Sci 1987;23(6):621–4.
8. Sachse K, Grajetzki C, Rosengarten R, et al. Mechanisms and factors involved in Mycoplasma bovis adhesion to host cells. Zentralbl Bakteriol 1996;284(1):80–92.
9. Thomas A, Sachse K, Dizier I, et al. Adherence to various host cell lines of Mycoplasma bovis strains differing in pathogenic and cultural features. Vet Microbiol 2003;91(2):101–13.
10. Thomas A, Sachse K, Farnir F, et al. Adherence of Mycoplasma bovis to bovine bronchial epithelial cells. Microb Pathog 2003;34(3):141–8.
11. Sachse K, Helbig JH, Lysnyansky I, et al. Epitope mapping of immunogenic and adhesive structures in repetitive domains of Mycoplasma bovis variable surface lipoproteins. Infect Immun 2000;68(2):680–7.
12. Lysnyansky I, Ron Y, Sachse K, et al. Intrachromosomal recombination within the vsp locus of Mycoplasma bovis generates a chimeric variable surface lipoprotein antigen. Infect Immun 2001;69(6):3703–12.
13. Boothby JT. Dissertation Abstracts International B: Sciences and Engineering. Immunologic responses to Mycoplasma bovis. Ann Arbor: University Microfilms, 1966–1988;44(1):49.
14. Vanden Bush TJ, Rosenbusch RF. Characterization of the immune response to Mycoplasma bovis lung infection. Vet Immunol Immunopathol 2003;94(1):23–33.
15. Behrens A, Poumarat F, Grand DI, et al. A newly identified immunodominant membrane protein (pMB67) involved in Mycoplasma bovis surface antigenic variation. Microbiology (Reading). 1996;142(9):2463–70.
16. Robino P, Alberti A, Pittau M, et al. Genetic and antigenic characterization of the surface lipoprotein P48 of Mycoplasma bovis. Vet Microbiol 2005;109(3):201–9.
17. Le Grand D, Solsona M, Rosengarten R, et al. Adaptive surface antigen variation in Mycoplasma bovis to the host immune response. FEMS Microbiol Lett 1996; 144(2):267–75.

18. Vanden Bush TJ, Rosenbusch RF. Characterization of a lympho-inhibitory peptide produced by Mycoplasma bovis. Biochem Biophys Res Commun 2004;315(2): 336–41.
19. Vanden Bush TJ, Rosenbusch RF. Mycoplasma bovis induces apoptosis of bovine lymphocytes. FEMS Immunol Med Microbiol 2002;32(2):97–103.
20. Thomas CB, Van Ess P, Wolfgram LJ, et al. Adherence to bovine neutrophils and suppression of neutrophil chemiluminescence by Mycoplasma bovis. Vet Immunol Immunopathol 1991;27(4):365–81.
21. McAuliffe L, Ellis RJ, Miles K, et al. Biofilm formation by Mycoplasma species and its role in environmental persistence and survival. Microbiology (Reading). 2006; 152(4):913–22.
22. Khan LA, Miles RJ, Nicholas RAJ. Hydrogen peroxide production by Mycoplasma bovis and Mycoplasma agalactiae and effect of in vitro passage on a Mycoplasma bovis strain producing high levels of H2O2. Vet Res Commun 2005;29(3):181–8.
23. Bischof DF, Janis C, Vilei EM, et al. Cytotoxicity of Mycoplasma mycoides subsp. mycoides small colony type to bovine epithelial cells. Infect Immun 2008;76(1): 263–9.
24. Wiggins MC, Woolums AR, Sanchez S, et al. Prevalence of Mycoplasma bovis in backgrounding and stocker cattle operations. J Am Vet Med Assoc 2007; 230(10):1514–8.
25. Castillo-Alcala F. Molecular characterization of respiratory infection with Mycoplasma bovis in feedlot cattle [D.V.Sc. thesis]. University of Guelph; 2009.
26. Gagea MI, Bateman KG, Shanahan RA, et al. Naturally occurring Mycoplasma bovis-associated pneumonia and polyarthritis in feedlot beef calves. J Vet Diagn Invest 2006;18(1):29–40.
27. Shahriar FM, Clark EG, Janzen E, et al. Coinfection with bovine viral diarrhea virus and Mycoplasma bovis in feedlot cattle with chronic pneumonia. Can Vet J 2002; 43(11):863–8.
28. Khodakaram-Tafti A, Lopez A. Immunohistopathological findings in the lungs of calves naturally infected with Mycoplasma bovis. J Vet Med A Physiol Pathol Clin Med 2004;51(1):10–4.
29. Rodriguez F, Bryson DG, Ball HJ, et al. Pathological and immunohistochemical studies of natural and experimental Mycoplasma bovis pneumonia in calves. J Comp Pathol 1996;115(2):151–62.
30. Clark T. The pathology of chronic pneumonia and polyarthritis syndrome (CPPS) in beef cattle. Proceedings of the International Conference on Bovine Mycoplasmosis, Saskatoon. 2009. Available at: http://www.bovinemycoplasma. ca/documents/07_-_CLARK,_Ted.pdf. Accessed January 22, 2010
31. Thomas LH, Howard CJ, Stott EJ, et al. Mycoplasma bovis infection in gnotobiotic calves and combined infection with respiratory syncytial virus. Vet Pathol 1986; 23(5):571–8.
32. Stipkovits L, Glávits R, Ripley P, et al. Pathological and immunohistochemical studies of pneumonia in calves experimentally induced by Mycoplasma bovis. In: Bergonier D, Berthelot X, Frey J, editors. Mycoplasmas of ruminants: pathogenicity, diagnostics, epidemiology and molecular genetics. Brussels (Belgium): European Commission; 2000. p. 27–30.
33. Byrne WJ, McCormack R, Brice N, et al. Isolation of Mycoplasma bovis from bovine clinical samples in the republic of Ireland. Vet Rec 2001;148(11):331–3.
34. Thomas A, Ball H, Dizier I, et al. Isolation of mycoplasma species from the lower respiratory tract of healthy cattle and cattle with respiratory disease in Belgium. Vet Rec 2002;151(16):472–6.

35. Olaloku N, Schumann F, Campbell J, et al. Prevalence of BVDV in a selected sample of mortalities of feedlot cattle. Government of Saskatchewan, Agrriculture Development Fund research report. Available at: http://www.agriculture.gov.sk.ca/apps/adf/ADFAdminReport/20000066.pdf. Accessed January 22, 2010.
36. Booker CW, Jim GK, Guichon PT, et al. Evaluation of florfenicol for the treatment of undifferentiated fever in feedlot calves in Western Canada. Can Vet J 1997;38(9):555–60.
37. Pollock CM, Campbell JR, Janzen ED. Descriptive epidemiology of chronic disease of calves in a Western Canadian feedlot. Proceedings of the 33rd Meeting of the American Association of Bovine Practitioners. Rapid City (SD) 2000:152–3.
38. Gagea MI, Bateman KG, van Dreumel T, et al. Diseases and pathogens associated with mortality in Ontario beef feedlots. J Vet Diagn Invest 2006;18(1):18–28.
39. Murray PR, Baron EJ. Manual of clinical microbiology. 8th edition. Washington, DC: American Society for Microbiology; 2003.
40. Waites KB. Mycoplasma and ureaplasma. In: Murray PR, Baron EJ, editors, Manual of clinical microbiology: mycoplasmas and obligate intracellular bacteria, vol. 1. 9th edition. Washington, DC: American Society of Microbiology; 2007. p. 1004–20.
41. Nicholas RA, Ayling RD. Mycoplasma bovis: disease, diagnosis, and control. Res Vet Sci 2003;74(2):105–12.
42. Radaelli E, Luini M, Loria GR, et al. Bacteriological, serological, pathological and immunohistochemical studies of Mycoplasma bovis respiratory infection in veal calves and adult cattle at slaughter. Res Vet Sci 2008;85(2):282–90.
43. Jacobsen B, Hermeyer K, Jechlinger W, et al. In situ hybridization for the detection of Mycoplasma bovis in paraffin-embedded lung tissue from experimentally infected calves. J Vet Diagn Invest 2010;22(1):90–3.
44. Thomas A, Dizier I, Trolin A, et al. Comparison of sampling procedures for isolating pulmonary mycoplasmas in cattle. Vet Res Commun 2002;26(5):333–9.
45. Allen JW, Viel L, Bateman KG, et al. The microbial flora of the respiratory tract in feedlot calves: associations between nasopharyngeal and bronchoalveolar lavage cultures. Can J Vet Res 1991;55(4):341–6.
46. Sachse K, Salam HS, Diller R, et al. Use of a novel real-time PCR technique to monitor and quantitate Mycoplasma bovis infection in cattle herds with mastitis and respiratory disease. Vet J 2009. [Epub ahead of print].
47. Rosenbusch RF, Kinyon JM, Apley M, et al. In vitro antimicrobial inhibition profiles of Mycoplasma bovis isolates recovered from various regions of the united states from 2002 to 2003. J Vet Diagn Invest 2005;17(5):436–41.
48. Francoz D, Fortin M, Fecteau G, et al. Determination of Mycoplasma bovis susceptibilities against six antimicrobial agents using the E test method. Vet Microbiol 2005;105(1):57–64.
49. Gerchman I, Levisohn S, Mikula I, et al. In vitro antimicrobial susceptibility of Mycoplasma bovis isolated in israel from local and imported cattle. Vet Microbiol 2009;137(3–4):268–75.
50. Janzen ED, Clark T. Mycoplasma bovis-associated disease. In: Proceedings of the International Conference on Bovine Mycoplasmosis, Saskatoon. 2009. Available at: http://www.bovinemycoplasma.ca/documents/04%20-%20Janzen,%20Eugene.pdf and http://www.bovinemycoplasma.ca/. Accessed April 12, 2010.
51. Martin SW, Nagy E, Armstrong D, et al. The associations of viral and mycoplasmal antibody titers with respiratory disease and weight gain in feedlot calves. Can Vet J 1999;40(8):560–7, 570.

52. Martin SW, Bohac JG. The association between serological titers in infectious bovine rhinotracheitis virus, bovine virus diarrhea virus, parainfluenza-3 virus, respiratory syncytial virus and treatment for respiratory disease in Ontario feedlot calves. Can J Vet Res 1986;50(3):351–8.
53. Godinho KS. Susceptibility testing of tulathromycin: Interpretative breakpoints and susceptibility of field isolates. Vet Microbiol 2008;129(3–4):426–32.
54. Godinho KS, Rae A, Windsor GD, et al. Efficacy of tulathromycin in the treatment of bovine respiratory disease associated with induced Mycoplasma bovis infections in young dairy calves. Vet Ther 2005;6(2):96–112.

Bacterial Pathogens of the Bovine Respiratory Disease Complex

Dee Griffin, DVM, MS[a],*, M.M. Chengappa, DVM, PhD[b],
Jennifer Kuszak, BS, MS[c], D. Scott McVey, DVM, PhD[c]

KEYWORDS

• Bacteria • Pathogens • Bovine respiratory disease complex
• BRDC

The bovine respiratory disease complex (BRDC), also known as shipping fever, is of major economic importance to the North American and the global cattle industries. The United States feedlot industry estimates an annual loss as high as 1 billion dollars due to loss of production, increased labor expenses, drug costs, and death because of bovine respiratory disease (BRD, Hodgins and Shewen).[1,2] Fulton and colleagues[3] estimated that producers lose $40.46/calf for 1 treatment, $58.35/calf for 2 treatments, and $291.93/calf for 3 or more treatments for BRD. BRD is an infectious respiratory disease of cattle with multifactorial causes including *Mannheimia haemolytica*, *Pasteurella multocida*, *Histophilus somni* and *Mycoplasma bovis* as important bacterial pathogens. Pathogenesis involves many factors including stress and possible viral or parasitic infections that often suppress the host immune system, allowing these bacteria to rapidly reproduce in the upper respiratory tract. Regardless of the initiating events, *Mannheimia haemolytica* is considered to be the predominant bacterial pathogen associated with BRD.

The current marketing system in the United States for feeder cattle inherently causes stress on the animals. Most calves are weaned and shipped to a sale barn where they comingle with other cattle of unknown disease and vaccination status. Calves transported over long distances are exposed to additional stressors such as

[a] Great Plains Veterinary Educational Center, School of Veterinary Medicine and Biomedical Sciences, University of Nebraska – Lincoln, PO Box 148, Clay Center, NE 68933-0148, USA
[b] Department of Diagnostic Medicine and Pathobiology, Kansas State University College of Veterinary Medicine, Manhattan, KS 66506, USA
[c] Nebraska Veterinary Diagnostic Center, School of Veterinary Medicine and Biomedical Sciences, University of Nebraska – Lincoln, PO Box 830907, Lincoln, NE 68583-0907, USA
* Corresponding author.
E-mail address: dgriffin@gpvec.unl.edu

Vet Clin Food Anim 26 (2010) 381–394
doi:10.1016/j.cvfa.2010.04.004
0749-0720/10/$ – see front matter © 2010 Elsevier Inc. All rights reserved.

vetfood.theclinics.com

diesel fumes; chilling or overheating, depending on weather conditions; dehydration; starvation; and exhaustion.[4] Once at the feedlot, additional stressors include processing, additional commingling, dusty environments, and introduction to new feed and water. Rice and colleagues[5] note that transportation and cold stressors were found to cause a transient elevation of plasma cortisol levels along with a decrease in serum complement activity in calves acquired through sale barns. These factors may often increase host susceptibility to BRD.

The first line of defense of the innate immune system is the respiratory epithelial surface, which provides mechanical, chemical, and microbiological barriers to prevent infection of BRD-associated pathogens.[6] Nasal passages of healthy and stressed calves contain many opportunistic bacteria including pathogens such as *Mannheimia haemolytica* and other Pasteurellaceae. Stressed calves seem to have a higher density of these bacteria in the nasal passages.[6,7] Bacteria are inhaled via droplets into the lungs[8] and may then adhere to and colonize the epithelial surface. These infected surfaces secrete mucus that coats the surface and prevents adherence of the bacteria. Epithelial cilia of the trachea provide a constant upward movement of the mucus to remove potential pathogens. In the lung, epithelial surfaces are also coated with surfactant proteins A and D[6] as well as defensin peptides. These bactericidal proteins and peptides also adhere to the surface of the pathogens, making them more susceptible to phagocytosis by resident macrophages and neutrophils. Within 4 hours, healthy animals are able to clear 90% of an inhaled administered dose of bacteria.[9]

Coinfection with a virus or bacterium like *Mycoplasma bovis* has been suggested to impair clearance of the infecting bacteria, resulting in lesions in the respiratory track. For example, bovine viral diarrhea virus (BVDV) replicates in and impairs function or destroys alveolar macrophages inducing immunosuppression.[10] The relative virulence of bovine respiratory syncytial virus (BRSV) infection is age and immune status dependent, with most cattle being asymptomatic. Primary infection of the nasal cavity, pharynx, trachea, bronchi, and bronchioli epithelial cells induces loss of cilia or necrosis of bronchial and bronchiolar epithelial cells. Because of the reduced mucociliary clearance, buildup of fluid and cellular debris in the airways and alveoli provides an ideal environment for bacterial colonization. BRSV also depresses phagocytosis and opsonization by alveolar macrophages. Bovine herpes virus-1 (BHV-1) initially infects the epithelial cells of the upper respiratory tract and then spreads to the lower respiratory tract. Necrosis of epithelial cells causing ineffective mucociliary clearance and lesions in the mucosa of the upper respiratory tract exacerbates secondary bacterial infections.[11] Parainfluenza type 3 (PI-3) virus infections are associated with little or no clinical symptoms in cattle, but PI-3 does predispose lung tissue for secondary bacterial infections. Primary infections occur in the epithelial cells in the trachea, bronchi and alveoli, causing necrosis of the ciliated epithelium. This condition results in ineffective mucociliary clearance of fluid, dust, and cellular debris from the airways. Development of clinical disease is associated with stress and exposure to secondary infections by other viral or bacterial pathogens.[12] These factors, individually or in combination, can provide increased opportunity for persistent bacterial infection due to an impaired innate immune responses.[5]

THE BACTERIAL PATHOGENS OF THE BRDC
Mannheimia haemolytica

Mannheimia haemolytica, formally known as *Pasteurella haemolytica*, is a small gram-negative, facultatively anaerobic bacterium usually expressing weak hemolysis on sheep or bovine blood agar plates. It is normally oxidase positive, indole negative, fermentative, nonmotile, and a non–spore-forming rod or coccobacillus.

The genus *Mannheimia* is part of the class α-Proteobacteria, order Pasteurellales, family Pasteurellaceae. In 1999 a new genus, *Mannheimia*, was formed to include trehalose-negative members of the *P haemolytica* subset. *Mannheimia* spp are differentiated from the genus *Pasteurella* by the fermentation of mannitol and the failure to use d-mannose,[13] along with 16S rRNA sequence phylogeny and DNA-DNA hybridization.[14] The *Mannheimia* genus currently contains 5 species: *Mannheimia haemolytica, Mannheimia granulomatis, Mannheimia glucosida, Mannheimia ruminalis,* and *Mannheimia varigena.*[13]

Mannheimia haemolytica is divided into 12 capsular serotypes based on the *P haemolytica* original assignments of A1, A2, A5, A6, A7, A8, A9, A12, A13, A14, A16, and A17.[5] The organism exists as normal flora of the upper respiratory tract in healthy ruminants, mainly in the nasopharynx and tonsillar crypts.[7] A1 and A2 are known to colonize the upper respiratory tract of cattle and sheep, but the predominate serotype isolated from clinically normal cattle is A2.[15] Rice and colleagues (2008) suggest that *Mannheimia haemolytica* maintains a commensal relationship with the host until conditions change as a result of stress or coinfection. Once this commensal relationship is disrupted, the A1 serotype quickly becomes the predominate organism[15] and is responsible for characteristic bronchopneumonia. Hodgins and Shewen[1,2] observed that fibrinous pneumonia could be induced by *Mannheimia haemolytica* alone by using the logarithmic growth phase if delivered directly into the lungs (intratracheal or transthoracic administration) in sufficient numbers ($>5 \times 10^9$ colony-forming units in nonimmune calves), suggesting that *Mannheimia haemolytica* can be a primary pathogen in BRD.

Serotype A1 is isolated most frequently from pneumonic tissue, but A6, A7, A9, A11, and A12 have been isolated from cases of bovine mannheimiosis (previously known as pasteurellosis). Surveys in the United Kingdom and the United States show an increasing prevalence of serotype A6 of up to approximately 30% of serotyped strains associated with bovine mannheimiosis.[15] A1 and A6 are remarkably similar except for differences in capsule structure.[5]

Mannheimia haemolytica has many virulence factors associated with pathogenesis. They include a capsule that is used for adherence and invasion; outer membrane proteins that produce protective immune responses; adhesins used for colonization; neuraminidase that reduces respiratory mucosal viscosity allowing bacteria access to the cell surface[15]; a lipopolysaccharide (LPS) complex that causes hemorrhage, edema, hypoxemia, and acute inflammation, leukotoxin responsible for lysis of ruminant leukocytes and platelets[13]; and a quorum-sensing system that is believed to regulate expression of virulence factors.[16] Because *Mannheimia haemolytica* has the ability to convert from a commensal to a pathogen, control of virulence factor expression and possible undiscovered virulence factors are of significant interest for research.

These virulence factors play an essential role in the ability of *Mannheimia haemolytica* to evade clearance and avoid host defenses while rapidly reproducing in the lower respiratory tract. Leukotoxin seems to be the main virulence factor, which is a 104-kDa protein that is secreted during the logarithmic growth phase.[16] It is a pore-forming cytotoxin of the RTX family that interacts with β_2 integrins of leukocytes.[16] The main functions of β_2 integrins in leukocytes include homing into areas of inflammation, phagocytosis, antigen presentation, and cytotoxicity of foreign substances.[6] CD18 is a common β subunit of β_2 integrins, which studies have shown is used by *Mannheimia haemolytica* leukotoxin as a receptor in ruminant-specific macrophages, neutrophils, and other subsets of leukocytes.[6] There is a concentration-dependent response from bovine leukocytes to leukotoxin. In low concentrations it can induce apoptosis by activating leukocytes to increase calcium uptake while releasing reactive oxygen intermediates, eicosanoids, and cytokines that can intensify local inflammation.[15,16] This helps to explain the severe inflammation observed with fibrinous pleuropneumonia. Leukotoxin in higher concentrations impairs leukocyte function, whereas even greater concentrations will precipitate cell death due to necrosis, directly resulting in lung lesions.[15,16]

Indirect hemagglutination (IHA)[17] has divided the P haemolytica species into 10 serotypes, which were later expanded to 12 serotypes.[18] Further separating of species into biotypes A and T based on fermentation of arabinose and trehalose, in combination with colony morphology, also occurred.[19] Biotype A (serotypes A1, A2, A5-A9, A12-A14, A16, and A17) is now Mannheimia haemolytica, serotype A11 is now Mannheimia glucosida,[13] and biotype T (serotypes T3, T4, T10, and T15) has been reclassified as Bibersteinia trehalosi.[20]

Pulsed-field gel electrophoresis (PFGE) was developed for the separation of large DNA fragments. Schwartz and Cantor[21] developed a technique using an alternating voltage gradient for better resolution of larger molecules. PFGE separates the large DNA fragments by periodically alternating the direction of the electric field, causing the fragments to move in a zigzag fashion through the gel. This system allows for separation of DNA molecules that range in size from less than 20 kb to 10 Mb.[22] PFGE is described as a highly reproducible and discriminatory tool for molecular typing of bacteria as well as other organisms.

Katsuda and colleagues[23,24] used random amplified polymorphic DNA (RAPD) fingerprinting and PFGE to molecularly type 130 isolates of Mannheimia haemolytica serotype A1 from 13 prefectures in Japan. Restriction endonuclease ApaI PFGE profiles formed 6 distinct clusters (A–F). They found the PFGE to be a more discriminative technique for typing Mannheimia haemolytica A1 than the RAPD. Kodjo and colleagues[25] also found PFGE to be more useful in epidemiologic studies then ribotyping (RT) and RAPD for typing Mannheimia haemolytica. Petersen and colleagues[26] used a multilocus sequence typing (MLST) scheme for typing Mannheimia haemolytica, resulting in an unambiguous type scheme that confirmed previous observation of a clonal population.

P multocida

P multocida has 5 capsular serogroups (A–F) and 16 somatic serotypes (1–16).[27–29] The most commonly isolated P multocida in BRD is A:3.[30] P multocida is more commonly identified in respiratory disease affecting younger cattle in syndromes including enzootic neonatal calf pneumonia, and in shipping fever of recently weaned, highly stressed calves.[31] Additional predisposing factors are required for the development of P multocida–associated pneumonia. These factors include immune-modulating stressors such as adverse climate and other environmental conditions, adverse nutritional conditions such as damaged feedstuffs and abrupt ration changes, animal handling and transportation, and the interaction of other infectious agents such as concomitant infections with the other previously listed BRD bacterial pathogens, gastrointestinal bacterial pathogens, and parasites.[27–37]

P multocida is readily isolated from nasal secretions and deep pharyngeal collections in young calves and weaning and feeder cattle.[29,33] The reported isolation rates in clinically normal cattle are between 20% and 60%.[29,36,37] High bacterial recovery rates in clinically normal animals suggest that P multocida is a commensal organism, and recovery in cattle suffering from clinically respiratory disease may not be a true association with a causal relationship. *P multocida* isolation from nasal secretion of calves suffering from clinical respiratory disease is about twice as high as the isolation rate in clinically normal calves.[29,34]

Isolation of *P multocida* as a principle bacterium recovered from pneumonic lungs at necropsy is considered more indicative of a causal relationship.[38–40] Diagnostic microbiologists are more frequently reporting *P multocida* in fatal cases of BRD from feedlots. This finding is contrary to decades of reports implicating *Mannheimia haemolytica* as the principle bacterial pathogen associated with fatal BRD in feedlots. Increased reporting of *P multocida* as a principle bacterial isolate from fatal cases of BRD has lead to questions being raised concerning pathogenic drifts of the bacterium.[29,35,41,42]

An increasing number of cattle have entered the feeding industry as recently weaned calves. This shift in the age for feeder cattle could account for the change in frequency of isolation of *P multocida* compared with the frequency of isolation of *Mannheimia haemolytica* in fatal cases of BRD in feedlots.[4,43–45]

H somni

Like the other BRD bacteria discussed, *H somni* (formerly *Haemophilus somnus*) in calves and feeder cattle is a commensal gram-negative bacterium residing in the nasopharyngeal region but may preferentially colonize the lower respiratory tract.[31,37,46,47] The isolation rate in clinically normal cattle entering feedyards is reported to be as few as 15% to more than 50% of newly received cattle.[37,46] The isolation rate in feeder cattle showing clinical BRD signs is reported to be higher than in clinically normal cattle.[48] The isolation rate is reported to be inversely related to the geometric mean of *H somni* antibody titers for groups of newly received cattle.[47,48] This finding suggests that immunization sufficiently spaced before weaning, commingling, marketing, or transportation stresses might be a key management consideration of minimizing histophilosis.[48,49] The major outer membrane proteins and lipooligosaccharide virulence factors are similar to *Mannheimia haemolytica* but, in addition, a histamine and an exopolysaccharide are produced and play a role in the pathogenesis.[48,50] The immunoglobulin-binding protein has cytotoxic activities, particularly to endothelial cells mediating contraction and allowing for hematogenous spread of the organism.[48]

The bacterium has been associated with several disease manifestations including fibrinopurulent bronchopneumonia as a singular causal pathogen or as a pathogen component of the BRDC, abscessing laryngitis, thromboembolic meningoencephalitis (TEME), polyarthritis-polyserositis, fibrinous pericarditis, and sudden death associated with septicemic-related cardiovascular left ventricular papillary muscle necrosis.[49,51] Abortions and reproductive tract infections have also been reported.[49,51] Generally, the respiratory form is considered the predecessor by weeks to months to the other invasive forms of infection. Clinically, the pneumonia caused by *H somni* is indistinguishable from pneumonia caused by the other BRD bacterial pathogens discussed.[31] Massive fibrin deposition is the most commonly associated observation on gross examination of affected lungs, but similar observations are reported for *P multocida* and *Mannheimia haemolytica*. *H somni*, *P multocida* and *Mannheimia haemolytica* are commonly isolated from the same diseased lung sample.[48] When these similarities are considered along with the commensal nature of the organism, a definitive diagnosis of histophilosis based on gross lesions can be uncertain. Often a BRD-related diagnosis depends on isolating high numbers of the bacterium, but this likelihood can be marginal for samples taken from cattle that have been treated with an antibiotic before an isolation attempt.[48]

Mycoplasma bovis

The role of *Mycoplasma bovis* in BRD of young calves is better understood than it is in stocker and feeder cattle.[31,39,42,47,52–55] The role of *Mycoplasma bovis* can be heavily debated; data defining its relationship in the BRDC are not as clear as they are for the 3 previously mentioned bacterial BRD pathogens. *Mycoplasma bovis* can play a role in enzootic pneumonia with or without associated otitis media, shipping fever, and chronic pneumonia complicated with arthritis or tenosynovitis.[52–54]

Mycoplasma bovis has a trilayered membrane instead of a cell wall. The use of nasal swabs has not been as productive for studying the movement of this bacterium because it is more often found in the deeper respiratory system.[52,55]

Serology using enzyme-linked immunosorbent assays (ELISA) is the practical method used to identify the organism movement. Strain typing requires molecular techniques such as arbitrarily primed polymerase chain reaction (AP-PCR).[52] These techniques have been used mostly to help understand the epidemiology of the organism's movement. The incidence within herds is variable, ranging from absent to more than 90%.[54,56] The prevalence increases as cattle are stressed and comingled. Movement within herds includes dam to offspring. Matched strains between dam and offspring have been identified. The bacterium found in mammary glands is apparently ingested, and aerosolized milk during suckling is the potential route for inoculation of the respiratory tract.[52] After gaining entrance into the respiratory system, *Mycoplasma bovis* can move between the respiratory cells to gain entrance to the blood stream.[52] A bacteremia can be identified within a day of infection and persist for more than a week.[52] The organism can be isolated from other body system tissues after the bacteremia ends.[31,52] This is likely the mechanism for the arthritis most often associated with the respiratory form of mycoplasmosis.[31,52,53]

Mycoplasma bovis can survive in the environment for days to weeks if protected from ultraviolet (UV) radiation. Serology has identified movement of the bacterium within herds and this is most likely animal to animal. When naïve cattle are mixed with *Mycoplasma bovis*–infected cattle the bacterium can be found in some of the naïve cattle within a day, and in most of the naïve cattle within a week.[31,53] Once established in the respiratory tract, *Mycoplasma bovis* may persist for the life of the animal.[52,57] Experimentally infected cattle often stay asymptomatic or develop only mild clinical disease. Severe clinical disease has been reproduced using stress models similar to those used to study the other bacteria most commonly associated with BRD.[31,52] Pneumonia and arthritis are most typically seen 8 to 10 days after inoculation.[52,53] Virulence of *Mycoplasma bovis* is considered to be associated with 5 variable surface lipoproteins (Vsp); VspA, VspB, VspC, VspF, and VspO.[52] A synergistic effect seems to exist between *Mycoplasma bovis* and *Mannheimia haemolytica* because a more severe disease is created when more *Mycoplasma*-infected calves are challenged with *Mannheimia* than when non-*Mycoplasma* calves are challenged.[31,52,53] Other associated BRD causes including stress, commingling, viral infection, and other respiratory bacterial pathogens all play an important role.[30] The same associated BRD components cause some to doubt that *Mycoplasma bovis* has a primary role in many BRD cases.[52,53,58–61]

Lung lesions associated with *Mycoplasma bovis* infection range from mild collapse and consolidated anterior-ventral areas to chronic caseonecrotic bronchopneumonia. The latter appears as nodules of caseous necrosis surrounded by collapsed consolidated lung. Centers of these nodules are not typically liquefied unless the lesion is contaminated with other bacteria. Bronchiectasis may be visible.[52,53]

OTHER BACTERIAL PATHOGENS ASSOCIATED WITH BRD

Other potential bacterial organisms are isolated from bovine pneumonic lung tissues. These include *Arcanobacterium pyogenes*, multiple species of the *Pasteurella* and *Mycoplasma* genera, as well as gram-positive staphylococci and streptococci, and multiple enteric organisms. Occasionally fungal organisms may be recovered. These organisms may be opportunistic pathogens or they may be associated with chronic cases of pneumonia after prolonged antimicrobial therapy. They may also colonize necrotic tissue in cases where animals survive the initial infectious processes. The organisms are also generally considered to be part of the normal upper respiratory tract flora, and isolation may often be coincidental. Isolation of these organisms may not indicate a causal relationship and discretion is required of the clinician.

CLINICAL OBSERVATIONS ASSOCIATED WITH BRD

Clinical signs are typically observed in calves 7 to 10 days after a stressful event (eg, arrival at the feedlot)[4] or as late as 27 days after arrival.[36] Organisms shed from the nasal cavity are a source of infection that is spread through inhalation of droplets containing the bacteria, by direct contact, or by ingesting feed or water supplies contaminated with nasal discharge of infected animals.[13] Identification of sick animals is a major concern of BRD because of the predatory/prey behavior exhibited by animals that perceive animal care personnel as predators and mask early symptoms, delaying or preventing detection and treatment.[36] Symptoms of the illness may range from hardly noticeable to peracute death but may include nasal and ocular discharge, depression, anorexia, fever as high as 42°C, increased respiratory rate, and moist cough, and auscultation reveals moist rales. As the disease progresses, the symptoms become more severe and include respiratory distress, encrusted muzzles, excessive tear production, and dyspnea. Auscultation reveals pleural friction and muffled lung sounds due to consolidation. Calves may exhibit a distressed stance with elbows abducted and neck extended.[1,2,5,13,15,36]

Most respiratory disease cases reported from cattle producers are based on a simple set of observations, and these are generally applied to cattle considered to be at a high risk for developing BRD. Most commonly targeted are stressed or newly received cattle. The observations most commonly targeted are signs that include depression, appetite loss, respiratory character change, and temperate elevation (DART). These clinical signs are not pathognomonic for bacterial pneumonia but these clinical signs have been used for decades to aid in the treatment of BRD.[62] The common and consistent uses of the DART signs as a diagnostic proxy for BRD make case treatment records a useful means of examining incidence rates and various management, environmental, and nutritional causal relationships. However, BRD mortality in groups of cattle is poorly related to the BRD case treatment records.[63–66] The poor correlation between morbidity based on the DART signs and BRD mortality makes it difficult to design interventions directed to specific potential pathogens such as *P multocida* vaccine development. It is even difficult to use antimicrobial minimum inhibitory concentration (MIC) laboratory results from fatal BRD cases in the management of clinical cases based on the DART signs.[35,67–70]

Enzootic calf pneumonia (ECP) is the most common respiratory disease in cattle ascribed to *P multocida*. ECP is most often discussed as a disease of calves, whereas shipping fever, also known as the BRDC or BRD syndrome, is discussed as a disease of older weanling, stocker, or feeder cattle.[30] Differences between ECP and the BRDC are arbitrary, based on age and common management stresses such as marketing and transportation. ECP is most frequently described as a dairy calf disease and generally not considered important in suckling beef calves because the preweaning incidence of respiratory disease is believed to be low; however, this may be an incorrect assumption. Treatment of suckling beef calves is problematic because it is difficult to capture a calf for treatment if it is being guarded by a protective mother. The possibility of injuring the calf while trying to capture it for treatment, or injury to the person trying to treat the calf by the calf's mother, is considerable. Therefore, observations based on case treatment records, as is commonly done with other forms of BRD, are difficult and, thus, an estimate of BRD in suckling calves across the beef industry is impossible. Beef cow-calf operations sometimes complain of BRD in sucking calves, which they refer to as summer pneumonia. P multocida is commonly isolated from specimens collected from live and dead calves.[29,30] Ear infections in newly weaned beef calves, often assumed to be caused by Mycoplasma bovis, frequently yield P multocida as the only isolate.

Passively acquired antibodies to P multocida are reported to be undetectable in calves more than 2 months old.[29] The apparent short half-life of the P multocida passively acquired antibodies makes it difficult to understand how failure of passive transfer could be associated with P multocida BRD in calves more than 2 months old, as described by dairy calf ranch operators and beef cow-calf production units. BRD diagnosis in these situations is generally based on DART signs and, therefore, is only circumstantially related to BRD and cannot be definitively correlated with P multocida.

PATHOLOGY

Acute pleuropneumonia is the major cause of death in animals suffering from BRD. Hodgins and Shewen[1,2] describe lesions as serofibrinous pleuropneumonia. On necropsy, lungs generally have a bilateral consolidation with a firm and heavy texture. Lobules have a marbled appearance, denoting the various stages of the pneumonic process. Sheets of fibrin attached to the parietal and visceral pleura, and possibly the pericardium, are also observed with acute fibrinous or serofibrinous pleuritis. Accumulation of yellow fibrin and edema distends into the infected areas. Large volumes of straw-colored thoracic fluid are occasionally observed, indicating severe exudation. In chronic infections, coagulation necrosis outlined with pale fibrous tissue is observed and becomes progressively thicker over time. Extensive adhesions are formed by organization of fibrin deposits in the pleural and pericardial cavities.[1,2]

Histologic lesions vary with the progression of the disease. Early stages show edema and fibrin deposition with congestion or hemorrhage in the alveoli along with neutrophils and macrophages. In later stages, alveoli contain dark oat-shaped neutrophils with pyknotic, hyperchromatic nuclei indicating cellular toxicity and cell death. Bacteria are observed in foci of necrosis surrounded by fibrous tissue. Chronic lesions often display thrombosis of septal lymphatic vessels.[1]

MANAGEMENT AND THERAPY

Most of the reductions that have occurred with BRD in the past 3 decades have been realized through improved management of cattle and early recognition of sick calves. Improved management practices for dealing with potential stressors and highly susceptible animals may decrease the incidence and severity of BRD infection. It would be ideal for feedlots to purchase fewer stressed or susceptible cattle. Limiting purchase of cattle from sale barns by buying directly from the cow-calf producers would reduce exposure to infected animals. Calves purchased directly, without mixing from other sources, have an expected morbidity of less than 5%[4] compared with animals commingled or acquired from sale barns, which have as high as 69%

expected morbidity within the first few weeks at the feedlot.[5] An added benefit is that this would allow feedlots and cow-calf producers to work together on weaning and vaccination schedules. Transportation time should be minimized and include rest periods with access to feed and water for extended travel. Once on location, calves should be processed within 48 hours and sorted into groups. New animals should not be introduced into established pens. Introduction of any new high-energy ration should be gradual to reduce acidosis, indigestion, and anorexia. Reduction of environmental stressors, such as dust, mud, and feedlot conditions, should be put into place. Long-acting antibiotics given on arrival to cattle that are at high risk of developing BRD have been shown to significantly reduce morbidity and improve rate of gain.[4] However, the common use of antibiotics for disease prevention and growth promotion in domestic animals can potentially lead to the selection of antimicrobial-resistant bacteria. Therefore, rigorous monitoring of antimicrobial susceptibility is imperative for the selection of effective drug treatment of bovine pneumonia.[71]

Treatment of *Mycoplasma bovis* infections has not proven rewarding. The absence of a cell wall in *Mycoplasma* eliminates the consideration of β-lactam antibiotics. The systems and techniques used to evaluate its antibiotic sensitivity have repeatedly found several antibiotics that should be effective. Consistent finding of *Mycoplasma bovis* in the lungs of treated cattle, including lungs from clinically normal cattle collected from packing plants, suggest that the antibiotics used, and the animals' immune systems, were not sufficient to aid the animals to rid themselves of the infection.[52,53,56,57]

ANTIBIOTIC RESISTANCE

Ineffective usage of antimicrobials as prophylaxy, metaphylaxy, or growth-enhancement drugs may result in *Mannheimia haemolytica* exhibiting an increase in resistance to a large number of antibiotics.[15] Exacerbating the issue is the inherent delay of analyzing isolates through a diagnostic laboratory, a high degree of variability among isolates originating from the same animal source, and variation in resistances rates over time.[15] *Mannheimia haemolytica* is frequently found to be resistant to aminoglycosides, β-lactams, sulfonamides, and tetracyclines.[15] Resistance to fluoroquinolones has been observed in recent years.[71]

Antimicrobial resistance is determined by veterinary-specific breakpoints determined by the Veterinary Antimicrobial Susceptibility Testing Subcommittee (CLSI/VASTS). The selected microorganism may still be viable even though growth is inhibited by the antimicrobial agent.[72,73] The subcommittee selects MIC breakpoints and zone-interpretive criteria as defined by susceptible (S), intermediate susceptibility (I), or resistant (R). Veterinary-specific breakpoints are applied to a specific combination of diseases, pathogens, animal species, and antimicrobial regimens. Any change in therapeutic parameters voids the implied clinical outcome, making the predictive values of the breakpoint suspect. These breakpoints are valid only if the laboratory has conducted the susceptibility testing according to CLSI-standardized methods.[72]

The 2 primary approaches to susceptibility testing for veterinary diagnostic laboratories are the serial-dilution method and the disk-diffusion method, also known as the Kirby-Bauer method. Serial dilutions tend to be performed from commercially available plates or panels. These microwell plates contain predetermined concentrations of selected antimicrobials that are precisely inoculated with broth containing a standardized number of bacteria. The presence or absence of observed growth in the wells determines the breakpoint value, which is output as S, I, or R, and may also report the MIC.[72]

In the disk-diffusion or Kirby-Bauer method, a standardized bacterial inoculum is streaked onto an agar plate and antimicrobial-impregnated disks are placed on the inoculated plate. The plate is incubated for 16 to 18 hours and the zones of inhibition are measured and compared with interpretive zone-size criteria. The breakpoint value is reported as S, I, or R, and reports may include extrapolated, estimated MIC values.[72]

As antimicrobial resistance becomes a global issue, greater emphasis needs to be placed on therapies that reduce or minimize the selection of resistant mutants. The mutant prevention concentration (MPC) has been defined by Blondeua,[73] is as "[t]he minimum inhibitory concentration of the most resistant first-step resistant cell present in a high density bacterial population. In other words, the MPC would be an antimicrobial drug concentration threshold that would require an organism to simultaneously possess two concurrent resistance mutations for growth in the presence of the drug." This procedure is carried out to prevent selectively amplifying resistant subpopulations by inhibiting susceptible and first-step–resistant cells with adjusted antimicrobial drug concentrations.[73]

Therapy failure using MIC breakpoints may be caused by many factors; immunocompromised state, prior infection, drug treatment, and acute infection. During such failures, bacterial numbers may not be reduced and selections of resistant organisms resulting from drug concentration are insufficient to block mutant growth. The MPC concept may prevent selection and amplification of resistant subpopulations by increasing drug concentration to prevent mutant growth.[73]

SUMMARY

Pneumonia caused by the bacterial pathogens discussed in this article is the most significant cause of morbidity and mortality of the BRDC. Most of these infectious bacteria are not capable of inducing significant disease without the presence of other predisposing environmental factors, physiologic stressors, or concurrent infections. *Mannheimia haemolytica* is the most common and serious of these bacterial agents and is therefore also the most highly characterized. There are other important bacterial pathogens of BRD, such as *P multocida*, *H somni*, and *Mycoplasma bovis*. Mixed infections with these organisms do occur. These pathogens have unique and common virulence factors but the resulting pneumonic lesions may be similar. Although the amount and quality of research associated with BRD has increased, vaccination and therapeutic practices are not fully successful. A greater understanding of the virulence mechanisms of the infecting bacteria and pathogenesis of pneumonia, as well as the characteristics of the organisms that allow tissue persistence, may lead to improved management, therapeutics, and vaccines.

REFERENCES

1. Hodgins DC, Shewen PE. *Pasteurella* and *Mannheimia* spp. infections. In: Coetzer JAW, Tustin RC, editors. 2nd edition, Infectious disease of livestock, 3. Cape Town (South Africa): Oxford University Press; 2004. p. 1672–6.
2. Fulton RW, Cook BJ, Step DL, et al. Evaluation of health status of calves and impact on feedlot performance: assessment of retained ownership program for postweaning calves. Can J Vet Res 2002;66:173–80.
3. Ames TR. Bovine Respiratory Disease Complex. The Merck Veterinary Manual. 50th edition. Merck and Company. Whitehouse Station (NJ): Merck and Co; 2005. p. 1190–7.
4. Rice JA, Carrasco-Medina L, Hodgins DC, et al. *Mannheimia haemolytica* and bovine respiratory disease. Anim Health Res Rev 2008;8:117–28.

5. Srikumaran S, Kelling CL, Ambagela A. Immune evasion by pathogens of bovine respiratory disease complex. Anim Health Res Rev 2008;8:215–29.
6. Frank GH. Bacteria as etiologic agents in bovine respiratory disease. In: Loan RW, editor. Bovine respiratory disease. College Station (TX): Texas A&M University Press; 1984. p. 347–62.
7. Highlander SK. Molecular genetic analysis of virulence on *Mannheimia (Pasteurella) haemolytica*. Front Biosci 2001;6:D1125–50.
8. Lillie LE, Thomson RG. The pulmonary clearance of bacteria by calves and mice. Can J Comp Med 1972;36:129–37.
9. Potgieter LND. Bovine viral diarrhea and mucosal disease. In: Coetzer JAW, Tustin RC, editors. 2nd edition, Infectious disease of livestock, 2. Cape Town (South Africa): Oxford University Press; 2004. p. 946–69.
10. Babiuk LA, van Drunen Little-van den Hurk S, Tiloo SK. Infectious bovine rhinotracheitis/infectious pustular vulvovaginitis and infectious pustular balanoposthitis. In: Coetzer JAW, Tustin RC, editors. 2nd edition, Infectious disease of livestock, 2. Cape Town (South Africa): Oxford University Press; 2004. p. 875–86.
11. van Vuuren M. Parainfluenza type 3 infections. In: Coetzer JAW, Tustin RC, editors. 2nd edition, Infectious disease of livestock, 2. Cape Town (South Africa): Oxford University Press; 2004. p. 673–6.
12. Songer JG, Post KW. The genera *Mannheimia* and *Pasteurella*. In: Duncan L, editor. Veterinary microbiology: bacterial and fungal agents of animal disease. St. Louis (MO): Elsevier Saunders; 2005. p. 181–90.
13. Gioia J, Qin X, Jiang H, et al. The genome sequence of *Mannheimia haemolytica* A1: insights into virulence, natural competence and Pasteurellaceae phylogeny. J Bacteriol 2006;188:7257–66.
14. Zecchinon L, Fett T, Desmecht D. How *Mannheimia haemolytica* defeats host defense through a kiss of death mechanism. Vet Res 2005;36:133–56.
15. Hodgins DC, Shewen PE. Pneumonic pasteurellosis of cattle. In: Coetzer JAW, Tustin RC, editors. 2nd edition, Infectious disease of livestock, 3. Cape Town (South Africa): Oxford University Press; 2004. p. 1677–84.
16. Czuprynski DJ, Leite F, Sylte M, et al. Complexities of pathogenesis of *Mannheimia haemolytica* and *Haemophilus somnus* infections: challenges and potential opportunities for prevention? Anim Health Res Rev 2004;5:277–82.
17. Biberstein EL, Meyer ME, Kennedy PC. Serological types of *Pasteurella haemolytica*. Cornell Vet 1960;50:283–300.
18. Fodor L, Pénzer A, Varga J. Coagglutination test for serotyping *Pasteurella haemolytica*. J Clin Microbiol 1996;34:393–7.
19. Frank GH, Wessman GE. Rapid plate agglutination procedure for serotyping *Pasteurella haemolytica*. J Clin Microbiol 1978;7:142–5.
20. Blackall RJ, Bojesen AM, Christensen H, et al. Reclassification of [*Pasteurella*] *trehalosi* as *Bibersteninia trehalosi* gen. nov., comb. nov. Int J Syst Bacteriol 2007;57:666–74.
21. Schwartz DC, Cantor CR. Separation of yeast chromosome-sized DNAs by pulsed field gradient gel electrophoresis. Cell 1984;37(1):67–75.
22. Howe J. Appendix: user's guide to the CHEF DR-II pulsed field gel electrophoresis. HDK Lab Manual. 1990.
23. Katsuda K, Kohmoto M, Kawashima K, et al. Molecular typing of *Mannheimia (Pasteurella) haemolytica* serotype A1 isolates from cattle in Japan. Epidemiol Infect 2003;131:939–46.
24. Katsuda K, Kamiyama M, Kohmoto M, et al. Serotyping of *Mannheimia haemolytica* isolates from bovine pneumonia: 1987–2006. Vet J 2007;10:10–6.

25. Kodjo A, Villard L, Bizet C, et al. Pulsed-field gel electrophoresis is more efficient than ribotyping and random amplified polymorph DNA analysis in discrimination of *Pasteurella haemolytica* strains. J Clin Microbiol 1999;37: 380–5.

26. Petersen A, Christensen H, Kodjo A, et al. Development of multilocus sequence typing (MLST) scheme for *Mannheimia haemolytica* and assessment of the population structure of isolates obtained from cattle and sheep. Infect Genet Evol 2009;9:626–32.

27. Boyce JD, Adler B. The capsule is a virulence determinant in the pathogenesis of *Pasteurella multocida* M104 (B:2). Infect Immun 2000;68(6):3463–8.

28. Dabo SM, Confer AW, Quijano-Blas RA. Molecular and immunological characterization of *Pasteurella multocida* serotype A:3 OmpA: evidence of its role in *P. multocida* interaction with extracellular matrix molecules. Microb Pathog 2003;35: 147–57.

29. Dabo SM, Taylor JD, Confer AW. *Pasteurella multocida* and bovine respiratory disease. Anim Health Res Rev 2008;8(2):129–50.

30. Harper M, Boyce J, Adler B. *Pasteurella multocida* pathogenesis: 125 years after Pasteur. FEMS Microbiol Lett 2006;265:1–10.

31. Apley M. Bovine respiratory disease pathogenesis, clinical signs, and treatment in lightweight calves. Vet Clin North Am Food Anim Pract 2006;22(2): 399–411.

32. Aich P, Potter AA, Griebel PJ. Modern approaches to understanding stress and disease susceptibility: a review with special emphasis on respiratory disease. Int J Gen Med 2009;2:19–32.

33. Hunt ML, Adler B, Townsend KM. The molecular biology of *Pasteurella multocida*. Vet Microbiol 2000;72:3–25.

34. Carrol JA, Forsberg NE. Influence of stress and nutrition on cattle immunity. Vet Clin North Am Food Anim Pract 2007;23(1):105–49.

35. Chiase NK, Greene LW, Purdy CW, et al. Effect of transport stress on respiratory disease, serum antioxidant status, and serum concentrations of lipid peroxidation biomarkers in beef cattle. Am J Vet Res 2004;65(6):860–4.

36. Duff GC, Galyean ML. Board-invited review: recent advances in management of highly stressed newly received feeder cattle. J Anim Sci 2007;85:823–40.

37. Angen O, Thomsen J, Larsen LE, et al. Respiratory disease in calves: microbiological investigations on trans-tracheally aspirated bronchoalveolar fluid and acute phase protein response. Vet Micro 2009;137(1–2):165–71.

38. Prado ME, Prado TM, Payton M, et al. Maternally and naturally acquired antibodies to *Mannheimia haemolytica* and *Pasteurella multocida* in beef calves. Vet Immunol Immunopathol 2006;111:301–7.

39. Binder A, Amtsberg G, Dose S, et al. Examination of cattle with respiratory diseases for Mycoplasma and bacterial bronchopneumonia agents. Zentralbl Veterinarmed B 1990;37(6):430–5.

40. Fuller TE, Kennedy MJ, Lowery DE. Identification of *Pasteurella multocida* virulence genes in septicemic mouse model using signature-tagged mutagenesis. Microb Pathog 2000;29:25–38.

41. Loneragan GH, Gould DH, Mason GL, et al. Involvement of microbial respiratory pathogens in acute interstitial pneumonia in feedlot cattle. Am J Vet Res 2001; 62(10):1519–24.

42. Booker CW, Abutarbush SM, Morley PS, et al. Microbiological and histopathological findings in cases of fatal bovine respiratory disease of feedlot cattle in western Canada. Can Vet J 2008;49:473–81.

43. Snowder GD, Van Vleck LD, Cundiff LV, et al. Bovine respiratory disease in feedlot cattle: environmental, genetic and economic factors. J Anim Sci 2006;84: 1999–2008.

44. Macartney JE, Bateman KG, Ribble CS. Comparison of prices paid for feeder calves sold at conventional auctions versus special auctions of vaccinated or conditioned calves in Ontario. J Am Vet Med Assoc 2003;223(5):670–6.

45. Macartney JE, Bateman KG, Ribble CS. Health performance of feeder calves sold at conventional auctions versus special auctions of vaccinated or conditioned calves in Ontario. J Am Vet Med Assoc 2003;223(5):67783.

46. DeRosa DC, Mechor GD, Staats JJ, et al. Comparison of *Pasteurella* spp. simultaneously isolated from nasal and transtracheal swabs from cattle with clinical signs of bovine respiratory disease. J Clin Microbiol 2000;38(1):327–32.

47. Booker CW, Guichon PT, Jim GK, et al. Seroepidemiology of undifferentiated fever in feedlot calves in western Canada. Can Vet J 1999;40:40–8.

48. Corbeil LB. *Histophilus somni* host-parasite relationships. Anim Health Res Rev 2008;8(2):151–60.

49. Booker CM. Histophilosis. The Merck Veterinary Manual. 50th edition. Merck and Company. Whitehouse Station (NJ): Merck and Co; 2005. p. 606–7.

50. Berghaus LJ, Corbeil LB, Berghaus RD, et al. Effects of dual vaccination for bovine respiratory syncytial virus and *Haemophilus somnus* on immune responses. Vaccine 2006;24:6018–27.

51. Orr JP. *Haemophilus somnus* infection: a retrospective analysis of cattle necropsied at the Western College of Veterinary Medicine from 1970–1990. Can Vet J 1992;33:719–22.

52. Caswell JL, Archambault M. *Mycoplasma bovis* pneumonia in cattle. Anim Health Res Rev 2008;8(2):161–86.

53. Maunsell FP, Donovan GA. *Mycoplasma bovis* infections in young calves. Vet Clin North Am Food Anim Pract 2009;25(1):139–77.

54. Byrne WJ, McCormick J, Brice N, et al. Isolation of *Mycoplasma bovis* from bovine clinical samples in the Republic of Ireland. Vet Rec 2001;148(11): 331–3.

55. Khodakaram-Tafti A, Lopez A. Immunohistopathological findings in the lungs of calves naturally infected with *Mycoplasma bovis*. J Vet Med A Physiol Pathol Clin Med 2004;51:10–4.

56. Rosenbusch RF, Kinyon JM, Apley M, et al. In vitro antimicrobial inhibition profiles of *Mycoplasma bovis* isolates recovered from various regions of the United States from 2002 to 2003. J Vet Diagn Invest 2005;17:436–41.

57. Martin SW, Nagy E, Armstrong D, et al. The associations of viral and mycoplasmal antibody titers with respiratory disease and weight gain in feedlot calves. Can Vet J 1999;40:560–70.

58. Shahriar FM, Clark EG, Janzen E, et al. Coinfection with bovine viral diarrhea virus and *Mycoplasma bovis* in feedlot cattle. Can Vet J 2002;43:863–8.

59. Vanden Bush TJ, Rosenbusch RF. Characterization of the immune response to *Mycoplasma bovis* lung infection. Vet Immunol Immunopathol 2003;94: 23–33.

60. Lubbers BV, Apley MD, Coetzee JF, et al. Use of computed tomography to evaluate pathologic changes in the lungs of calves with experimentally induced respiratory tract disease. Am J Vet Res 2007;68(11):1259–64.

61. Woolums AR, Loneragan GH, Hawkins LL, et al. Baseline management practices and animal health data reported by US feedlots responding to a survey regarding acute interstitial pneumonia. Bov Pract 2005;39(2):116–24.

62. Aubry P, Warnick LD, Guard CL, et al. Health and performance of young dairy calves vaccinated with a modified-live *Mannheimia haemolytica* and *Pasteurella multocida* vaccine. J Am Vet Med Assoc 2001;219(12):1739–42.
63. Irsik M. Preparation prevents poor performance. Proceedings maintaining quality production in a dynamic market place. Beef Short Course. University of Florida, Gainesville (FL); 2005. p. 25–31.
64. Seeger JT, Grotelueschen DM, Stokka GL. Comparison of feedlot health, nutritional performance, carcass characteristics and economic value of unweaned beef calves with an unknown health history and weaned beef calves receiving various herd-of-origin health protocols. Bov Pract 2008;42(1):27–39.
65. Richeson JT, Beck PA, Gadberry MS, et al. Effects of on-arrival versus delayed modified live virus vaccination on health, performance, and serum infectious bovine rhinotracheitis titers of newly received beef calves. J Anim Sci 2008;86:999–1005.
66. Richeson JT, Kegley EB, Gadberry MS, et al. Effects of on-arrival versus delayed modified live virus vaccination on health, performance, bovine virus diarrhea virus type I titers, and stress and immune measures of newly received beef calves. J Anim Sci 2009;87(7):2409–18.
67. Smith RA. Feedlot diseases and their control. Proceedings WBC Congress. Quebec (Canada); 2004.
68. McIntosh WMA, Schulz S, Dean W, et al. Feedlot veterinarians' moral and instrumental beliefs regarding antimicrobial use in feedlot cattle. J Community Appl Soc Psychol 2009;19:51–67.
69. Irsik M, Langemeier M, Schroeder T, et al. Estimating the effects of animal health on performance of feedlot cattle. Bov Pract 2006;40(2):65–74.
70. King ME, Salman MD, Wittum TE, et al. Effect of certified health programs on the sale of beef calves marketed through a livestock videotape auction service from 1995 through 2005. J Am Vet Med Assoc 2006;229(9):1389–400.
71. Katsuda K, Kohmoto M, Mikami O, et al. Antimicrobial resistance and genetic characterization of fluoroquinolone-resistant *Mannheimia haemolytica* isolates from cattle with bovine pneumonia. Vet Microbiol 2009;10:10–6.
72. Apley MD. Susceptibility testing for bovine respiratory and enteric disease. Vet Clin North Am Food Anim Pract 2003;19:625–45.
73. Blondeau JM, Borsos S, Hesje C, et al. Comparative killing of bovine isolates of *Mannheimia haemolytica* (MH) by enrofloxacin (ENR), florofenicol (FL), tilmicosin (TIL) and tulathromycin (TUL) using the measured minimum inhibitory (MIC) and mutant prevention concentration (MPC) and maximum serum (Cmax) and tissue (Tmax) drug concentration values. Poster present at International Meeting on Emerging Diseases and Surveillance. Vienna, Austria, February 13–16, 2009.

Bovine Atypical Interstitial Pneumonia

Alan R. Doster, DVM, PhD

KEYWORDS

- Bovine atypical interstitial pneumonia • AIP
- Acute bovine pulmonary edema and emphysema
- Acute bovine pulmonary adenomatosis
- Acute bovine respiratory distress syndrome

Atypical interstitial pneumonia (AIP) of cattle is a term first introduced by Blood[1] to describe a spontaneous respiratory syndrome in cattle characterized by acute pulmonary edema and emphysema. Previous terms used to describe the condition were anatomically descriptive and often colloquial. They included pulmonary adenomatosis, acute alveolar emphysema and edema, bovine pulmonary emphysema, panters, lungers, bovine asthma, pneumoconiosis, and fog fever. Two forms of the disease are recognized; acute and chronic. In acute cases in which cattle succumb to AIP, lungs completely fill the thorax, fail to collapse when the thorax is opened, and are firm on palpation (**Fig. 1**). Diffuse alveolar and interstitial edema and emphysema septa are noted (**Fig. 2**). Involvement of interlobular septa and development of large air-filled bulla are commonly observed. Microscopic lesions include congestion, edema, hyaline membranes, interstitial and interlobular emphysema, alveolar type II epithelial hyperplasia, fibrosis, and cellular infiltration of alveolar septa (**Fig. 3**). In more chronic cases, secondary bacterial involvement often occurs and is typified by cranioventral consolidation and a suppurative inflammatory response that is superimposed on the exudative and proliferative lesions of AIP (**Figs. 4** and **5**).

The term atypical was used to describe the cellular reaction in the lung and the failure of the animal to respond to conventional modes of therapy. Initially, pathogenesis of lesion development was unknown and the reaction in the lung was distinct and unlike that seen in conventional (infectious) forms of pneumonia. Multiple causes were proposed because of the development of AIP under various clinical circumstances. To further clarify the clinical aspects of the disease and correlate them with specific gross and microscopic lesions, Breeze and Carlson[2] suggested that "acute bovine respiratory distress syndrome" be used to describe and distinguish the clinical presentation of acute dyspnea resulting from pulmonary congestion, edema, hyaline membrane

Veterinary Diagnostic Center, School of Veterinary Medicine and Biomedical Sciences, University of Nebraska-Lincoln, East Campus Loop and Fair Streets, Lincoln, NE 68583-0907, USA
E-mail address: adoster@unl.edu

Vet Clin Food Anim 26 (2010) 395–407
doi:10.1016/j.cvfa.2010.03.002
0749-0720/10/$ – see front matter © 2010 Elsevier Inc. All rights reserved.

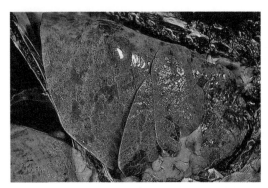

Fig. 1. Lung from heifer with AIP. Lungs completely fill the thoracic cavity. Diffuse pulmonary edema and emphysema are present.

formation, epithelial hyperplasia, and interstitial emphysema, having ruled out other causes of disease such as parasitic bronchitis.

CLINICAL SIGNS

Clinical signs consist of acute respiratory distress and are not specific for any particular cause. Signs usually develop within several days after a change in pasture or diet. Affected cattle are often presented with open-mouth breathing, head and neck extended, and legs abducted (**Fig. 6**). Respirations are shallow, rapid, and often accompanied by a loud expiratory grunt. Temperature is normal or may be slightly increased. Eosinophilia has been recorded in some instances but is not a consistent feature.[1] In extreme cases, subcutaneous crepitation may be evident over the dorsal neck, shoulders, and lumbar areas. Affected animals usually die within 2 to 3 days after initial onset of clinical signs. Morbidity may reach 50%, whereas mortality may range between 30% and 100%. Less severely affected animals may improve without any further consequences other than a slight increase in respiratory rate.

The clinical signs and gross and microscopic lesions of bovine AIP are not diagnostically specific for any particular cause and are similar to those that occur with acute bovine pulmonary edema and emphysema, bovine pulmonary adenomatosis, and other acute respiratory diseases of cattle. To elucidate the cause, the clinical history

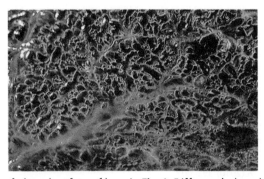

Fig. 2. Closer view of pleural surface of lung in **Fig. 1**. Diffuse subpleural alveolar and interlobular edema and emphysema are evident.

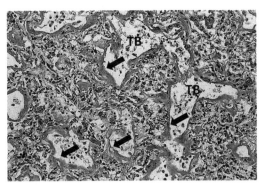

Fig. 3. Photomicrograph of lung from a feedlot steer with AIP. Diffuse necrosis of nonciliated terminal bronchiolar epithelial cells (Clara cells) and type I alveolar epithelial cells has occurred. Thick hyaline membranes line distended alveoli (*arrows*) and the terminal bronchiole (TB).

including husbandry, management practices, and possible exposure to certain toxicants (4-ipomeanol, L-tryptophan, and perilla ketone), and bacterial, viral, or parasitic infections is relevant in formulating an opinion or diagnosis.

PROPOSED CAUSES

Numerous causes have been proposed for AIP. They include exaggerated efforts to expel foreign objects lodged in the respiratory tract, hypersensitivity reactions to various allergens, inhalation of noxious gases, intoxication with pneumonotoxic compounds, and infections with various parasites and viruses.

Bovine AIP has been seen in Europe for more than 200 years and is known colloquially as fog fever. The condition has been associated with the grazing of fog lands, which are pastures that have lush new growth after being cut for haylage or silage. There is no association with fog, smog, or any other atmospheric condition.[2] A similar syndrome is seen in the United States in beef cows more than 2 years of age. It is most commonly associated with the movement of cattle in the early fall from dry summer

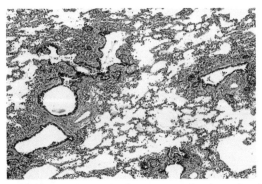

Fig. 4. Photomicrograph of lung from a heifer necropsied 4 days after initiation of clinical signs compatible with AIP. Regeneration of terminal bronchiolar and some alveolar type II cells has occurred. Affected cells are hypertrophied, hyperplastic, and hyperchromatic.

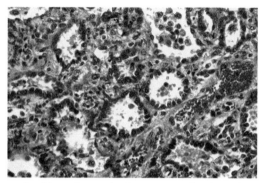

Fig. 5. Photomicrograph of lung from a heifer necropsied 8 days after initiation of clinical signs compatible with AIP. Pulmonary alveoli are lined almost entirely by proliferating type II epithelial cells. Interstitial fibrosis and edema are evident. Alveoli contain degenerate alveolar epithelial cells, macrophages, and few erythrocytes mixed with clumps of fibrin.

grazing to lush green pastures. Grass composition of the pasture does not seem to be as important as the condition that it be lush.[1]

In the United Kingdom, a casual relationship was noted between fog fever and the appearance of immature spiders and gossamer in pastures with affected cattle.[3] It was hypothesized that AIP developed subsequent to grazing of the spider-infested pasture and inhalation of spiders and their gossamer deep into the lung, which resulted in pulmonary irritation and development of violent episodes of coughing in an attempt to expel any foreign material. Ensuing pulmonary damage and respiratory impairment resulted in development of clinical signs and diffuse interstitial pulmonary emphysema. No experimental or further clinical evidence regarding this claim was ever generated.

Sporadic reports of acute pulmonary emphysema and death have been observed in cattle that were exposed to a variety of noxious gases, fumes, or clostridial endotoxins. Silo gas, nitrogen dioxide, chlorine gas, and zinc oxide fumes released from the cutting and welding of galvanized pipe have been associated with development of acute pulmonary edema in exposed cattle.[4–9]

Clostridial endotoxins have been proposed as possible cause of AIP.[10] It was suggested that various clostridial endotoxins damaged pulmonary capillary endothelium,

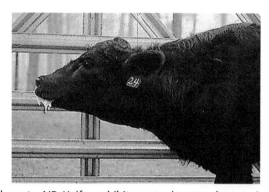

Fig. 6. Heifer with acute AIP. Heifer exhibits acute dyspnea characterized by open-mouth breathing with head and neck in extension and front legs abducted.

which led to development of severe pulmonary edema. Acute dyspnea and emphysema subsequently developed. Experimental evidence is lacking in all instances that propose a noxious gas or clostridia as the cause of AIP.[11]

The acute onset of AIP coupled with gross lesions consisting of severe pulmonary edema and emphysema may mimic the clinical signs and gross lesions seen in an anaphylactic reaction. However, the 2 conditions differ in terms of onset, duration, and microscopic appearance of lesions. Microscopic lesions in bovine anaphylaxis are characterized by pulmonary congestion, edema, intra-alveolar hemorrhage, and interstitial emphysema. Acute necrosis of alveolar and bronchiolar epithelium followed by hypertrophy and hyperplasia are not observed in bovine anaphylaxis, whereas they are characteristic lesions of AIP.[12]

A chronic pulmonary hypersensitivity reaction similar to farmer's lung in humans has been described in cattle and has been incorrectly suggested as a cause of AIP.[13] The condition is seen more commonly in dairy than beef cattle and is believed to be to the result of differences in management and housing practices. The clinical history and microscopic lesions in cattle are similar to those described for extrinsic allergic alveolitis in humans. Pulmonary lesions consist of a multifocal lymphoplasmacytic bronchitis, bronchiolitis, and pneumonia with interstitial fibrosis. Sera from affected humans and cattle often contain antibodies to *Microspora faenia* or other thermophilic fungi found in moldy hay. Cattle dying from AIP do not have significant levels of serum antibodies to any of these fungi, although sera from normal adult cattle fed hay may contain low levels of antibodies to 1 or more of these organisms.[14]

Anaphylaxis resulting from parasitic bronchitis causes severe respiratory disease in cattle and has been suggested as a cause of AIP.[15] Migrating larvae of *Dictylocaulus viviparus*, a lung worm of cattle, can produce an acute pulmonary hypersensitivity reaction accompanied by severe pulmonary edema and emphysema. Eosinophilic alveolitis and bronchitis are characteristic findings in most cases. Microscopic lesions in the lung are similar to those described for other hypersensitivity reactions and are not consistent with pulmonary changes seen with AIP. Definitive diagnosis is made by demonstrating migrating larvae in the lung. It is unlikely that development of AIP can be solely attributed to lungworm infection because the condition has occurred in animals free of *Dictylocaulus* sp infection. Respiratory disease with lesions suggestive of AIP has been reported in cattle infected with migrating larvae of *Ascaris suum* and *Ascaris lumbricoides*.[16,17] The clinical history indicating recent exposure to swine ascarids or ascarid ova and presence of migrating larvae in the lung is diagnostic for this condition.

In summary, experimental and clinical evidence does not support the idea that AIP consistently develops as a sequela to inhalation of foreign materials or poisonous gases, anaphylaxis due to allergens, or parasitic migration even though certain clinical signs and lung lesions may be similar. Careful evaluation of the clinical history, coupled with the appearance of gross and microscopic lesions, will distinguish between the 2 syndromes.

The feeding of moldy sweet potatoes (*Ipomoea batatas*) has been associated with development of acute interstitial pneumonia in cattle.[18-24] The disease was reproduced experimentally by feeding moldy sweet potatoes infected with *Fusarium solani*.[22] 4-Ipomeanol, a 3-substituted furanoterpenoid, was isolated from sweet potatoes damaged by *F solani* and was shown experimentally to be the toxic compound responsible for development of pulmonary lesions typical of AIP in cattle fed the damaged sweet potatoes.[25]

Acute interstitial pneumonia in cattle has been produced by ingestion of leaves and seeds of *Perilla frutescens* (purple mint).[26] The toxic principle is perilla ketone, which is chemically similar in structure to 4-ipomeanol and is activated by pulmonary P450 cytochrome enzymes in the lung, resulting in severe pulmonary damage and development of diffuse pulmonary edema.[27,28]

Acute interstitial pneumonia has been reported in cattle fed various plants of *Brassica* sp including kale, rape, and turnip tops.[29] Specific toxic compounds have not been identified in these plants. AIP has been associated with ingestion of perennial rye grass (*Lolium perenne*) straw infected with the endophyte *Acremonium lolii*. *A lolii* produces toxic compounds including lolitrem-B, which is responsible for the clinical neurologic signs associated with rye grass staggers. Affected animals had gross and microscopic lesions similar to those of cattle with AIP.[30] Experimental feeding of *A lolii*–infected ryegrass straw reproduced typical neurologic signs, but evidence of respiratory disease and pulmonary lesions at necropsy was lacking.

Clinical and experimental evidence indicates that the lung is an important target for chemical injury. Exposure to exogenous compounds capable of causing pulmonary damage may occur through normal respiration or hematogenously via the circulatory system. The lung, like the liver and kidney, contains an active mixed function oxidase (MFO) system. Although it has only 10% to 20% of the metabolic activity of the liver, location and susceptibility make the lung a prime site for bioactivation of certain substances and chemically induced tissue damage.[31] A highly developed MFO system is also found in the nasal mucosa and may cause initial rapid metabolism and activation of xenobiotics inhaled into the respiratory tract.[32]

The monooxygenase activity of the MFO system responsible for metabolism and detoxification of exogenous compounds is located in the smooth endoplasmic reticulum.[33] The greatest activity is associated with the cytochrome P450 enzyme system, which is responsible for electron transport. In the presence of oxygen, the MFO system mediates the oxidation of certain organic substances that form free radicals and electrophils that, in turn, covalently bind cellular proteins and nucleic acids. By covalently binding tissue macromolecules, activated electrophils render them nonfunctional, which ultimately may result in cellular dysfunction and death. Damage as a result of metabolic activation can occur via several mechanisms including peroxidation of lipid membranes, protein thiol depletion, and alteration of intracellular calcium homeostasis.

To mediate toxicity in the host, daughter components generated by metabolic activation are generally more hydrophilic than the parent compound, which promotes their excretion from the body. Certain endogenous substances, particularly sulfur-containing thiols such as glutathione, are capable of binding to MFO-activated compounds and inactivating them, which allows for detoxification and excretion of potential toxicants.[33] Toxicity occurs when there is disturbance of normal cell physiology and depletion of naturally occurring protective enzymes and substances.

Xenobiotic metabolism and bioactivation of certain naturally occurring compounds is not species unique or organ specific. Metabolic activation of certain compounds (eg, 3-methyl indole [3-MI], a metabolite of the amino acid tryptophan; 4-ipomeanol, a product of moldy sweet potatoes; and perilla ketone, a substance found in the purple mint plant) result in development of AIP. Metabolic activation of xenobiotics by nonciliated bronchiolar epithelial cells (Clara cells), type I alveolar epithelial cells, and, to a lesser extent, capillary endothelial cells results in acute necrosis of bronchial and alveolar epithelial cells and capillary endothelial cells.[34] Subsequent to epithelial and endothelial cell damage, acute interstitial edema develops and is followed by alveolar edema and development of dyspnea.

During an experimental study conducted to investigate the effect of amino acid loading on bovine hepatocellular enzymes, high levels of D,L-tryptophan were administered orally to cattle.[35] Several animals developed acute pulmonary edema and emphysema within 24 to 36 hours after administration of the D,L-tryptophan. At necropsy, gross and microscopic lesions were similar to those described for AIP. Further studies showed that the syndrome could only be reproduced with the L-isomer of tryptophan.[36,37] Studies of ruminal degradation products showed that L-tryptophan was metabolized to indolacetic acid (IAA) by ruminal flora that, in turn, was converted to 3-MI by *Lactobacillus* sp in the rumen.[38,39] 3-MI is rapidly absorbed from the rumen into the blood stream. Most of the 3-MI is metabolized by the kidneys and excreted as nonreactive metabolites in the urine. Studies using radiolabeled 3-MI revealed that pulmonary metabolism of 3-MI by the MFO system located in nonciliated terminal bronchiolar (Clara cells) epithelial cells and alveolar type I cells resulted in the formation of a highly electrophilic compound that covalently bonded to cellular proteins and nucleic acids that caused cell necrosis. Intravenous administration of either L-tryptophan or IAA did not produce acute respiratory disease or pulmonary lesions in cattle. These results indicate that further metabolism of both compounds to an intermediate was needed for development of pneumotoxicity.[36,40] However, intravenous 3-MI produced clinical disease similar to that seen with oral doses of L-tryptophan, IAA, or 3-MI. The metabolic basis for pneumonotoxicity by the MFO system was further delineated by pretreating goats with phenobarbital, an inducer of the MFO system.[41] 3-MI toxicity was enhanced in the phenobarbital-pretreated goats compared with 3-MI treated controls. Pretreatment with piperonyl butoxide, an MFO inhibitor, prevented the development of respiratory disease in goats subsequently given 3-MI, and increased the half-life of 3-MI in the blood stream, indicating slowed metabolism.

Clinical field trials were conducted to determine the relationship between consumption of lush forage containing tryptophan and AIP. Cows adapted to foraging dry summer range pastures were suddenly given access to lush green pasture. Analysis of ruminal fluid from cows that developed AIP detected sufficient ruminal concentrations of 3-MI to induce clinical disease. Studies concluded that the composition of ruminal microflora is important in the metabolism of dietary tryptophan contained in lush pastures to 3-MI and development of AIP.[42] A low plane of nutrition brought on by restricted feed intake or the feeding of poor-quality dry forage is believed to alter normal ruminal microflora to one that is capable of converting tryptophan to 3-MI under the appropriate conditions. Tryptophan levels in pastures associated with outbreaks of AIP have not been found to be higher than in pastures in which AIP does not occur.[43] An abrupt dietary change to a more lush forage-based diet results in alteration of the ruminal microflora to one that is capable of metabolism of tryptophan to 3-MI. The level of tryptophan in pasture grasses is not as important as the existence of specific ruminal conditions and the presence of certain organisms such as *Lactobacillus* sp or other microflora capable of metabolizing tryptophan to IAA and 3-MI.[42] Xenobiotic metabolism of ruminal compounds by specific microflora in the rumen, and subsequent bioactivation of these compounds by cytochrome P450 enzymes in Clara cells and type I alveolar epithelial cells, may be the most likely and convincing explanation for the development of AIP in feedlot cattle.[34,44]

The putative compound responsible for causing cellular injury and development of AIP is 3-methyleleindolenine, an electrophilic amine that alkylates and forms stable adducts with cellular macromolecules including proteins and nucleic acids.[45–48] Concentrations of 3-methyleneindolenine in the lungs of feedlot cattle are significantly higher in cattle with AIP and cattle with bronchopneumonia than in healthy pen mates.[49] Metabolism and metabolic activation of 3-MI also produces free radicals that may cause lipid peroxidation of cellular membranes or covalently bind to tissue macromolecules, resulting in cell injury and death.[50,51]

The cause in feedlot cattle is believed to be multifactorial because, unlike pastured cattle, exposure to pasture grasses containing tryptophan is unlikely in most instances. Under most circumstances, feedlot cattle consume highly fermentable rations that often produce continuous subclinical acidosis. Subtle changes in diet, environment, or management practices can produce acidosis that alters the ruminal microflora and causes proliferation of bacteria such as certain *Lactobacillus* sp that are capable of metabolizing tryptophan and IAA to 3-MI.[38,52,53] However, the presence of ruminal acidosis and the increase in the numbers of ruminal *Lactobacillus* sp have not been associated with development of AIP in all instances.[54]

Mortality due to AIP in feedlot cattle has been described to be highest in summer and fall months.[54,55] It is seen almost exclusively on finishing diets containing high concentrations of grain, and frequently occurs near the end of the finishing period. Similarly, occurrence of AIP in pastured cattle is seen most often in the fall, and frequently is associated with a change in pasture or type of dietary forage. In the western United States, changing from a dry summer mountainous pasture to a lush lowland pasture frequently precipitates development of disease. An abrupt change to new pasture growth dominated by legumes or grasses has resulted in outbreaks of AIP 7 to 12 days after the initial dietary change.[1]

According to Blood,[1] all classes, ages, and breeds of cattle are equally affected by AIP, but Monlux and colleagues[56] noted that Hereford cattle appeared to be more susceptible to respiratory disease induced by levels of oral tryptophan. Reports indicate that feedlot heifers are more susceptible than steers.[49,54,57] It was postulated that the high incidence in heifers was due to treatment with melengestrol acetate (MGA), which is used to control estrus. MGA may increase production of prostaglandin H synthetase or induce higher levels of P450 cytochrome enzymes, either of which may accelerate metabolism and conversion of 3-MI to toxic metabolites.[58] However, other studies found no difference in plasma 3-MI adducts among intact or ovariectomized heifers or heifers that were or were not receiving MGA. However, MGA-fed heifers were 3.2 times more likely to be slaughtered early because of the development of AIP than heifers not fed MGA.[54,57]

Based on examination of a limited number of postmortem lung samples from feedlot cattle succumbing to fatal respiratory disease, bovine respiratory syncytial virus (BRSV) infection was proposed as a possible contributing or initiating factor in the pathogenesis of AIP development in feedlot cattle.[59] However, contrary evidence was present in 3 subsequent studies that examined lungs of feedlot cattle purported to exhibit typical clinical signs and to have died of acute interstitial pneumonia.[54,60,61]

Experiments using 3-MI to enhance the infectivity of BRSV in young calves revealed that 3-MI administration followed by inoculation of BRSV did not significantly exacerbate BRSV infection or increase the severity of lung lesions.[62] In contrast, synergism between experimental BRSV infection and administration of 3-MI was observed in calves challenged by aerosolized and intratracheal inoculations of BRSV and immediately given 3-MI orally. Clinical signs of respiratory disease and pulmonary lesions at necropsy were more severe in the BRSV–3-MI challenged calves than sham-inoculated calves or calves given only BRSV or 3-MI.[63] Major differences between the results of the 2 studies were attributed to the use of much younger calves and attenuation of the BRSV through multiple cell culture passages in the initial study. In a subsequent investigational field study, immunity to BRSV in feedlot cattle did not abrogate the potential synergism between BRSV and 3-MI.[64]

A greater incidence of respiratory tract disease due to *Pasteurella multocida* and *Mycoplasma* spp infections have been recorded in cattle dying from AIP compared with normal control pen mates. Inflammation resulting from chronic bacterial infections of the respiratory tract may contribute to development of AIP in some cattle by inducing systemic expression of proinflammatory cytokines that are coupled with the effects of overwhelming bacterial infection and sepsis.[61,65]

4-Ipomenaol and perilla ketone are activated by the P450 MFO system in the lung to form a enedial metabolite capable of causing severe damage to type I cells and Clara cells by binding covalently to nucleic acids and cellular proteins.[66,67] 4-Ipomeanol has been used to intensify the effects of interstitial pneumonia in cattle experimentally induced by parainfluenza type-3 virus and Sendai virus pneumonia in mice.[68,69] Both studies found that administration of 4-ipomeanol enhanced the severity of pulmonary lesions in virus-induced pneumonia, was associated with a higher titer of infectious virus in the lung, and produced a more diffuse distribution of viral antigen in bronchiolar and alveolar epithelium.

THERAPY AND PREVENTION

Conventional therapeutic agents and antagonists of mediators of anaphylaxis are minimally effective in treating AIP. Moderate success has been achieved by attempting to control the ruminal flora by restricting susceptible animals from grazing of lush pastures or reducing intake by prefeeding dry hay before grazing. Such management practices are not always feasible in large-scale operations.[2]

Antibiotics such as tetracycline have been used to alter the composition of ruminal microflora and prevent 3-MI production.[70] Administration of monensin or lasalocid has been shown in vivo to reduce 3-MI production by as much as 90%.[71,72] Oral doses of monensin consisting of 200 mg/head/d reduced conversion of tryptophan to 3-MI and prevented development of AIP. However, for monensin to be effective it must be in the rumen at the time of exposure. Little or no inhibitory effect remains in the rumen 48 hours after withdrawal, so prevention of AIP involves a long-term commitment to preventative therapy.

Mitigation of the effects of 3-MI toxicity and the prevention of AIP in feedlot cattle has been proposed by feeding increased dietary levels of free radical scavengers or their precursors.[73,74] Under laboratory conditions, supplementation with glutathione or one of its precursors, such as cysteine or sulfur, has been effective in reducing cell damage after 3-MI administration in animals and cell cultures.[71,75–77] However, under field conditions, supplementation with feather meal, a source of cysteine, or vitamin E did not influence the rates of death or emergency slaughter due to AIP and had no effect on levels of glutathione in lungs.[78]

SUMMARY

Bovine AIP is a multifaceted disease with several known causes and clinical presentations. Multiple causal agents and management practices have been associated with development of disease. The sporadic incidence and development of disease under a variety of circumstances argues against a common infectious agent, although cases of AIP are often complicated with bacterial, viral, or mycoplasmal organisms. Gross and microscopic lesions represent a basic response of the lung to injury. Metabolic activation of naturally occurring xenobiotic compounds such as 3-MI, perilla ketone, and 4-ipomeanol produce a clinical syndrome that is indistinguishable from naturally occurring AIP that develops on pasture or in the feedlot. Pulmonary injury is mediated by formation and activation of intermediate electrophilic compounds that covalently bind to cellular proteins and nucleic acids and ultimately cause cell death. Clara cells (nonciliated bronchiolar) and type I alveolar epithelial cells are primarily responsible for metabolism and activation of these naturally occurring xenobiotics. Damage to pulmonary epithelial and endothelial cells results in development of pulmonary edema, formation of hyaline membranes, infiltration with inflammatory cells, proliferation of alveolar and bronchiolar epithelial cells, and, if the animal survives, ultimately interstitial fibrosis. Pulmonary emphysema occurs secondary to hypoxia and exaggerated inspiratory efforts. Treatment is usually ineffective after development of clinical signs. Anticipation and correction of an abrupt dietary change, which often precedes development of disease, or the use of preventative measures to avoid development of clinical signs may be the most satisfactory methods of avoiding development of AIP in cattle.

REFERENCES

1. Blood DC. Atypical interstitial pneumonia of cattle. Can Vet J 1962;3(2):40–7.
2. Breeze RG, Carlson JR. Chemical induced lung injury in domestic animals. Adv Vet Sci Comp Med 1982;26:201–31.
3. Begg H, Whiteford WA. Acute interstitial pulmonary emphysema of bovines. Vet Rec 1948;60(12):135.
4. Brightwell AH. "Silo gas" poisoning in cattle. Can Vet J 1972;13(9):224–5.
5. Haynes NB. "Silo filler's disease" in dairy cattle. J Am Vet Med Assoc 1963; 143(6):593–4.
6. Seaton VA. Pulmonary adenomatosis in Iowa cattle. Am J Vet Res 1958;19(72): 600–9.
7. Cutlip RC. Experimental nitrogen dioxide poisoning in cattle. Vet Pathol 1966;3: 474–85.
8. MacDonald DW, Lamoureux MA, Van den Brink M, et al. Chlorine gas poisoning in farm livestock: case report and review. Can Vet J 1971;12(2):33–40.
9. Hilderman E, Taylor PA. Acute pulmonary emphysema in cattle exposed to zinc oxide fumes. Can Vet J 1974;15(6):173–5.
10. Schofield FW. Acute pulmonary emphysema of cattle. J Am Vet Med Assoc 1948; 112(852):254–9.
11. Breeze RG. Respiratory disease in adult cattle. Vet Clin North Am Food Anim Pract 1985;1(2):311–46.
12. Dungworth DL. The pulmonary response of sensitized cattle to aerosol administration of antigen. In: Proceedings of the symposium on acute bovine pulmonary emphysema and related respiratory diseases. University of Wyoming. Laramie (WY): August 23–27, 1965. p. N1–15.
13. Pirie HM, Dawson CO, Breeze RG, et al. A bovine disease similar to farmer's lung: extrinsic allergic alveolitis. Vet Rec 1971;88(14):346–51.
14. Pirie HM, Dawson CO, Breeze RG, et al. Fog fever and precipitins to micro-organisms of mouldy hay. Res Vet Sci 1971;12(6):586–8.
15. Breeze R. Parasitic bronchitis and pneumonia. Vet Clin North Am Food Anim Pract 1985;1(2):277–87.
16. Greenway JA, McCraw BM. Ascaris suum infection in calves. I. Clinical signs. Can J Comp Med 1970;34(3):227–37.
17. Allen GW. Acute atypical bovine pneumonia caused by Ascaris lumbricoides. Can J Comp Med Vet Sci 1962;26(10):241–3.
18. Gibbons WJ. Bovine pulmonary emphysema. Mod Vet Pract 1962;43:34–8.
19. Hansen AA. Potato poisoning. North Am Vet 1928;9:31–4.
20. Monlux W, Fitte J, Kendrick G, et al. Progressive pulmonary adenomatosis in cattle. Southwest Vet 1953;6:267–9.
21. Vickers CL, Carll WT, Bierer BW, et al. Pulmonary adenomatosis in South Carolina cattle. J Am Vet Med Assoc 1960;137(1):507–8.

22. Peckham JC, Mitchell FE, Jones OH, et al. Atypical interstitial pneumonia in cattle fed moldy sweet potatoes. J Am Vet Med Assoc 1972;160(2):169–72.
23. Medeiros RM, Simões SV, Tabosa IM, et al. Bovine atypical interstitial pneumonia associated with the ingestion of damaged sweet potatoes (*Ipomoea batatas*) in northeastern Brazil. Vet Hum Toxicol 2001;43(4):205–7.
24. Hill BD, Wright HF. Acute interstitial pneumonia in cattle associated with consumption of mould-damaged sweet potatoes (*Ipomoea batatas*). Aust Vet J 1992;69(2):36–7.
25. Doster AR, Mitchell FE, Farrell RL, et al. Effects of 4-ipomeanol, a product from mold-damaged sweet potatoes, on the bovine lung. Vet Pathol 1978;15(3):367–75.
26. Wilson BJ, Garst JE, Linnabary RD, et al. Perilla ketone: a potent lung toxin from the mint plant, *Perilla frutescens* Britton. Science 1977;197(4303):573–4.
27. Wilson BJ, Garst JE, Linnabary RD, et al. Pulmonary toxicity of naturally occurring 3-substituted furans. In: Keeler RF, Van Kampen KR, James LF, editors. Effects of poisonous plants on livestock. New York: Academic Press; 1978. p. 311–23.
28. Garst JE, Wilson WC, Kristensen NC, et al. Species susceptibility to the pulmonary toxicity of 3-furyl isoamyl ketone (perilla ketone): in vivo support for involvement of the lung monoxygenase system. J Anim Sci 1985;60(1):248–57.
29. Andrews GA, Kennedy GA. Respiratory diagnostic pathology. Vet Clin North Am Food Anim Pract 1997;13(3):515–47.
30. Pearson EG, Andreasen CB, Blythe LL, et al. Atypical pneumonia associated with ryegrass staggers in calves. J Am Vet Med Assoc 1996;209(6):1137–42.
31. Smith BR, Maguire JH, Ball LM, et al. Pulmonary metabolism of epoxides. Fed Proc 1978;37(11):2480–4.
32. Haschek WM, Witschi HR, Nikula KJ. Respiratory system. In: Haschek WM, Rousseau CG, Wallig MA, editors. Handbook of toxicologic pathology, vol. 2, 2nd edition. San Diego (CA): Academic Press; 2002. p. 3–83.
33. Jeffery EH. Biochemical basis of toxicity. In: Haschek WM, Rousseau CG, Wallig MA, editors. Handbook of toxicologic pathology, vol. 1, 2nd edition. San Diego (CA): Academic Press; 2002. p. 15–37.
34. Bradley BJ, Carlson JR. Ultrastructural pulmonary changes induced by intravenously administered 3-methylindole in goats. Am J Pathol 1980;99(3):551–60.
35. Dickinson EO, Spencer GR, Gorham JR. Experimental induction of an acute respiratory syndrome in cattle resembling bovine pulmonary emphysema. Vet Rec 1967;80(16):487–9.
36. Carlson JR, Yokoyama MT, Dickinson EO. Induction of pulmonary edema and emphysema in cattle and goats with 3-methylindole. Science 1972;176(4032):298–9.
37. Yokoyama MT, Carlson JR, Dickinson EO. Ruminal and plasma concentrations of 3-methylindole associated with tryptophan-induced pulmonary edema and emphysema in cattle. Am J Vet Res 1975;36(9):1349–52.
38. Yokoyama MT, Carlson JR, Holdeman LV. Isolation and characteristics of a skatole-producing *Lactobacillus* sp. from the bovine rumen. Appl Environ Microbiol 1977;34(6):837–42.
39. Carlson JR, Breeze RG. Ruminal metabolism of plant toxins with emphasis on indolic compounds. J Anim Sci 1984;58(4):1040–9.
40. Pirie HM, Breeze RG, Selman IE, et al. Indole-acetic acid, 3-methyl indole and type 2 pneumonocyte hyperplasia in a proliferative alveolitis of cattle. Vet Rec 1976;98(13):259–60.
41. Bray TM, Carlson JR. Role of mixed function oxidase in 3-methylindole-induced acute pulmonary edema in goats. Am J Vet Res 1979;40(9):1268–72.

42. Hammond AC, Bradley BJ, Yokoyama MT. 3-Methylindole and naturally occurring acute bovine pulmonary edema and emphysema. Am J Vet Res 1979;40(10): 1398–401.
43. Mackenzie A, Ford JE, Scott KJ. Pasture levels of tryptophan in relation to outbreaks of fog fever. Res Vet Sci 1975;19(2):227–8.
44. Huang TW, Carlson JR, Bray TM, et al. 3-Methylindole-induced pulmonary injury in goats. Am J Pathol 1977;87(3):647–66.
45. Thornton-Manning J, Appleton ML, Gonzalez FJ, et al. Metabolism of 3-methylindole by vaccinia-expressed P450 enzymes: correlation of 3 methyleneindolenine formation and protein binding. J Pharmacol Exp Ther 1996;276(1):21–9.
46. Skiles GL, Yost GS. Mechanistic studies on the cytochrome P450-catalzyed dehydrogenation of 3-methylindole. Chem Res Toxicol 1996;9(1):291–7.
47. Skordos KW, Skiles GL, Laycock JD, et al. Evidence supporting the formation of 2,3-epoxy3-methylindoline: a reactive intermediate of the pneumotoxin 3-methylindole. Chem Res Toxicol 1998;11(7):741–9.
48. Skordos KW, Laycock JD, Yost GS. Thioether adducts of a new imine reactive intermediate of the pneumontoxin 3-methylindole. Chem Res Toxicol 1998; 11(11):1326–31.
49. Loneragan GH, Gould DH, Mason GL, et al. Association of 3-methyleneindolenine, a toxic metabolite of 3-methylindole, with acute interstitial pneumonia in feedlot cattle. Am J Vet Res 2001;62(10):1525–30.
50. Kubow S, Janzen EG, Bray TM. Spin-trapping of free radicals formed during in vitro and in vivo metabolism of 3-methylindole. J Biol Chem 1984;259(7):4447–51.
51. Bray TM, Emmerson KS. Putative mechanisms of toxicity of 3-methylindole: from free radical to pneumotoxicosis. Annu Rev Pharmacol Toxicol 1994;34:91–115.
52. Yokoyama MT, Carlson JR. Production of skatole and para-cresol by a rumen Lactobacillus sp. Appl Environ Microbiol 1981;41(1):71–6.
53. Honeyfield DC, Carlson JR. Assay for the enzymatic conversion of indoleacetic acid to 3-methylindole in a ruminal Lactobacillus species. Appl Environ Microbiol 1990;56(3):724–9.
54. Ayroud M, Popp JD, VanderKop MA, et al. Characterization of acute interstitial pneumonia in cattle in southern Alberta feedyards. Can Vet J 2000;41(7):547–54.
55. Jensen R, Pierson RE, Braddy PM, et al. Atypical interstitial pneumonia in yearling feedlot cattle. J Am Vet Med Assoc 1976;169(5):507–10.
56. Monlux WS, Cutlip RC, Estes PC. Breed susceptibility to tryptophan-induced pulmonary adenomatosis in cattle. Cornell Vet 1970;60(4):547–51.
57. Stanford K, McAllister TA, Ayroud M, et al. Effect of dietary melengestrol acetate on the incidence of acute interstitial pneumonia in feedlot heifers. Can J Vet Res 2006;70(3):218–25.
58. Popp JD, McAllister TA, Kastelic JP, et al. Effect of melengestrol acetate on development of 3-methylindole-induced pulmonary edema and emphysema in sheep. Can J Vet Res 1998;62(4):268–74.
59. Collins JK, Jensen R, Smith GH, et al. Association of bovine respiratory syncytial virus with atypical interstitial pneumonia in feedlot cattle. Am J Vet Res 1988; 49(7):1045–9.
60. Sorden SD, Kerr RW, Janzen ED. Interstitial pneumonia in feedlot cattle: concurrent lesions and lack of immunohistochemical evidence for bovine respiratory syncytial virus infection. J Vet Diagn Invest 2000;12(6):510–7.
61. Loneragan GH, Gould MS, Mason GL, et al. Involvement of microbial respiratory pathogens in acute interstitial pneumonia in feedlot cattle. Am J Vet Res 2001; 62(10):1519–24.

62. Castleman WL, Lacy S, Slauson DO, et al. Pulmonary lesions induced by 3-meth-ylindole and bovine respiratory syncytial virus in calves. Am J Vet Res 1990; 51(11):1806–13.

63. Bingham HR, Morley PS, Wittum TE. Synergistic effects of concurrent challenge with bovine respiratory syncytial virus and 3-methylindole in calves. Am J Vet Res 1999;60(5):563–70.

64. Bingham HR, Morley PS, Wittum TE. Effects of 3-methylindole production and immunity against bovine respiratory syncytial virus on development of respiratory tract disease and rate of gain of feedlot cattle. Am J Vet Res 2000;61(10): 1309–14.

65. Woolums AR, Mason GL, Hawkins LL, et al. Microbiologic findings in feedlot cattle with acute interstitial pneumonia. Am J Vet Res 2004;65(11):1525–32.

66. Li X, Castleman WL. Ultrastructural morphogenesis of 4-ipomeanol-induced bronchiolitis and interstitial pneumonia in calves. Vet Pathol 1990;27(3):141–9.

67. Chen LJ, DeRose EF, Burka LT. Metabolism of furans in vitro: ipomeanine and 4-ipomeanol. Chem Res Toxicol 2006;19(10):1320–9.

68. Li X, Castleman WL. Effects of 4-ipomeanol on bovine parainfluenza type 3 virus-induced pneumonia in calves. Vet Pathol 1991;28(5):428–37.

69. Durham SK, Babish JG, Castleman WL. 4-Ipomeanol-induced effects on Sendai viral pneumonia in mice. Am J Pathol 1987;126(2):364–75.

70. Hammond AC, Bray TM, Cummins KA, et al. Reduction of ruminal 2-methylindole production and the prevention of tryptophan-induced acute bovine pulmonary edema and emphysema. Am J Vet Res 1978;39(9):1404–6.

71. Carlson JR, Hammond AC, Breeze RG, et al. Effect of monensin on bovine ruminal 3-methylindole production after abrupt change to lush pasture. Am J Vet Res 1983;44(1):118–22.

72. Nocerini MR, Honeyfield DC, Carlson JR, et al. Reduction of 3-methylindole production and prevention of acute bovine pulmonary edema and emphysema with lasalocid. J Anim Sci 1985;60(1):232–8.

73. Kubow S, Bray TM. The effect of lung concentrations of glutathione and vitamin E on the pulmonary toxicity of 3-methylindole. Can J Physiol Pharmacol 1988;66(7): 863–7.

74. Loneragan GH, Morley PS, Wagner JJ, et al. Effects of feeding aspirin and supplemental vitamin E on plasma concentrations of 3-methylindole, 3-methyle-neindolenine-adduct concentrations in blood and pulmonary tissues, lung lesions, and growth performance in feedlot cattle. Am J Vet Res 2002;63(12): 1641–7.

75. Hanafy MS, Bogan JA. Pharmacological modulation of the pneumotoxicity of 3-methylindole. Biochem Pharmacol 1982;31(9):1765–71.

76. Ruangyuttikarn W, Skiles GL, Yost GS. Identification of a cysteinyl adduct of oxidized 3-methylindole from goat lung and human liver microsomal proteins. Chem Res Toxicol 1992;5(5):713–9.

77. Merrill JC, Bray TM. The effect of dietary and sulfur compounds in alleviating 3-methylindole-induced pulmonary toxicity in goats. J Nutr 1983;113(9):1725–31.

78. Sanford K, McAllister TA, Ayroud M, et al. Acute interstitial pneumonia in feedlot cattle: effects of feeding feather meal or vitamin E. Can J Vet Res 2007;71(2): 152–6.

Respiratory Disease Diagnostics of Cattle

Vickie L. Cooper, DVM, MS, PhD[a],*,
Bruce W. Brodersen, DVM, MS, PhD[b]

KEYWORDS

• Diagnostic tests • Diagnostic samples
• Pneumonia • Cattle

It was a dark and stormy night. Bitter winds howled, as snow ripped across the plains blanketing all in its wake with billowing white drifts. Temperatures were frigid. Semitrucks were swept from the road. Interstates were closed. Cattle died. Does it sound a bit melodramatic? Caught your attention?

Although diagnostic testing can provide valuable information when investigating causes of respiratory disease within a group, veterinarians and producers should agree on the diagnostic question, testing goals, and use of results before submitting samples. What processes do the generated data affect? Consulting with a diagnostician and communicating what producer goals are should ensure that appropriate samples are obtained to diagnose or rule in pathogens as well as for the economic use of resources. Evaluating for underlying processes that may be contributing to disease within a group can also be addressed in as expedient a manner as possible.

Cattle appear to be more susceptible to respiratory disease based on anatomic and physiologic factors. It has been hypothesized that cattle have a greater probability of pulmonary exposure to inhaled pathogens because of their greater use of lung capacity for basal breathing compared with other mammalian species.[1] Distinct lobules are separated completely by interlobular septae. Pores of Kohn allow for an alternate route of air exchange between alveoli and are few in the bovine lung.[2] Compartmentalization in the bovine lung may predispose to localized hypoxia in the lung distal to bronchioles or terminal bronchioles especially during times when airways are occluded.[1] Compartmentalization of the bovine lung in combination with the potentially greater exposure of the lung to inhaled pathogens makes bovines a candidate for a relatively greater incidence of pneumonia.

The authors have nothing to disclose.
[a] Department of Veterinary Diagnostic and Production Animal Medicine, Iowa State University, 1600 South 16th Street, Ames, IA 50011, USA
[b] Veterinary Diagnostic Center, School of Veterinary Medicine and Biomedical Sciences, University of Nebraska-Lincoln, 1900 North 42nd Street, Lincoln, NE 68506-0907, USA
* Corresponding author.
E-mail address: vcooper@iastate.edu

It is to be hoped that this article can provide a reference for practicing veterinarians when formulating a diagnostic plan for respiratory disease.

ANIMAL SELECTION

Cattle producers lack the luxury that swine growers or poultry production systems have in terms of ability to sacrifice multiple animals for surveillance of respiratory disease within the population. Antemortem sampling can be a piece of the respiratory disease puzzle in outbreaks. Animals to be selected for antemortem testing should correlate with the herd problem. Animals selected should be in the early stages of the respiratory disease process before treatment. If producers are concerned with animals in chronic stages of disease, which fail to recover or respond to therapy, samples selection should target secondary pathogens. Animals sampled should have signs typical of the process affecting the group. If respiratory disease is the issue, submission of samples from lame, poor doing animals likely leads to inconsistencies in diagnostic testing results. It is important to take diagnostic data in the context in which they are generated, and the tools that are used to generate that data are also important. Bad data or misuse of data can potentially be more harmful than no data at all.

CLINICAL HISTORY

Good clinical histories allow diagnosticians to establish a list of differential diagnoses, select appropriate tests in an economic manner, recommend other testing modalities or sample selection, and evaluate whether samples submitted correspond to the herd problem. Information in regard to affected and unaffected animals within the population can suggest risk factors as well as hone in on underlying agents or deficiencies, which may predispose the group to disease.

Information suggested for provision in a clinical history are

1. Age range of affected animals and ages of animals sampled
2. Age of onset or number of days since arrival (stocker or feedlot operation) and progression in herd
3. Environment or housing or bedding
4. Mortality and morbidity in comparison to past averages for groups. Changes in mortality and morbidity over the course of the problem
5. Duration of illness of affected animals and individuals selected for sampling
6. Duration of problem in the herd
7. Clinical signs and sequence of onset. Changes in signs or severity since onset
8. Treatments and their response. Any treatment given to animals sampled
9. Common factors among affected animals
10. Changes in management, preceding the onset of problem (new feed, new source, feed quality, component quantity)
11. Vaccination history
12. Quarantine and isolation, if any
13. Biosecurity efforts, if any
14. Veterinarian's suspicion of problem's cause
15. Owner's suspicion of problem's cause.[3]

Implementation of electronic correspondence or even something as old-fashioned as invoking the use of a telephone, often expedites the flow of information directly between practitioners and diagnosticians, yielding surprisingly improved results. This is particularly so in regard to test selection.

SELECTING DIAGNOSTIC TESTS

Diagnostic tests are tools. They should be selected based on several criteria including quality of the sample, diagnostic question, producer goals, history, diagnostic laboratory, diagnostician, and economy. Specificity and sensitivity of diagnostic tests are not static figures; they change with time, knowledge drift, sample quality, timing of the disease process, daily stresses, comfort level of technical support staff, and pathogen. These inputs all affect the diagnostic test decision tree that diagnosticians follow on a given case.

NASOPHARYNGEAL AND NASAL SWABS

Nasal swabs have often been used in lieu of doing tracheal wash or bronchoalveolar lavage for antemortem diagnostics. Certainly, for upper respiratory viruses this technique has value. Significance of bacterial isolates or negative test results should be questioned from these samples.

Nasopharyngeal swabs have been used as a noninvasive predictive diagnostic method for natural respiratory infections in calves associated with *Manheimia haemolytica* and *Mycoplasma bovis*. Data demonstrated that *M haemolytica* and *M bovis* isolates from the deep nasopharynx were highly representative of isolates present in the lungs.[4] Evaluation of this method for representative viral entities, which often initiate respiratory disease, was not conducted and would certainly be warranted, particularly in light of recent studies in which 63% of healthy calves were culture positive for bovine bacterial pathogens from bronchoalveolar lavage fluid.[5] This method does hold promise, however, as a repeatable technique to monitor groups of animals through a respiratory disease cycle, if it seems warranted in the clinical setting.

TRACHEAL WASH/BRONCHOALVEOLAR LAVAGE

Tracheal wash and/or bronchoalveolar lavage are antemortem techniques, which can provide samples for a broader diagnostic approach than nasal or nasopharyngeal swabs. Samples can be evaluated by cytologic techniques to establish the inflammatory process and provide differential diagnostics for viral, bacterial, parasitic, and fungal diseases. Samples can be used for both culture as well as polymerase chain reaction. Immunohistochemistry (IHC) for viral and bacterial agents can also be conducted on direct smears or cytospin preparations of the samples, in some instances, for rapid and inexpensive adjunct diagnostics. As noted earlier, bacterial isolates without contextual respiratory disease should be assessed from a clinical perspective. Aseptic technique is required to avoid infection of cutaneous tissues around the tracheal puncture site. Restraint and local anesthesia is required. Sterile saline warmed to body temperature is ideal. Two 60-mL syringes are adequate for a feedlot age animal. For calves or small ruminants, 20- to 30-mL syringe is adequate. Two people are better for this technique than 1. **Fig. 1** indicates appropriate restraint for obtaining tracheal wash and bronchoalveolar lavage samples. **Fig. 2** is an example of the available transtracheal wash kit for large animals. The trochar and cannula system available can be substituted with a 12-gauge needle, assuring that the bevel placement is ventral. In addition, catheters can be replaced with polyethylene tubing (available at hobby stores) that has been cold sterilized and warmed to expand 1 end to slip over a needle hub. Bronchoalveolar lavage can be conducted using nasogastric tubes or commercially available bronchoalveolar lavage tubes, which have an inflatable cuff. These tubes seal off the airway and allow for greater recovery rates of the lavage fluid.

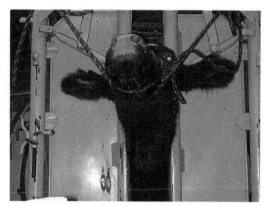

Fig. 1. Correct positioning and restraint for tracheal washes and bronchoalveolar lavage. (*Courtesy of* Karl Kersting, DVM, PhD, Iowa State University, Ames, Iowa.)

POSTMORTEM SAMPLES

Postmortem diagnostic samples should be selected from untreated animals in early phases of the disease. Animals with chronic pneumonia that have been treated with a variety of antimicrobials often provide limited diagnostic laboratory information. This condition should not be interpreted to mean that postmortem on these animals does not provide important information. Degree of involvement, lesions associated with underlying factors, and lesions of the initiating cause of the present pneumonic changes all may be ascertained by evaluation of these animals. They all can provide a wealth of information on what has affected a particular group of cattle. Alternatively, after extensive antimicrobial therapy, bacterial isolates and antimicrobial sensitivity may not provide accurate data for individual organisms or antibiotics.

Submitting live animals to a diagnostic laboratory for a full workup is ideal. If submission of live animals is not possible, submission of samples can be done. Samples that can be submitted are listed in **Table 1**, and it provides an outline for samples needed for a complete diagnostic workup for animals with respiratory disease.

If animals are euthanized, collect blood for submission of serum and in tubes containing anticoagulant before euthanasia. Obtain lung samples for bacterial culture first. Always keep fresh lung samples intended for bacterial culture separate from other tissues to decrease contamination and enhance the probability that pathogens will

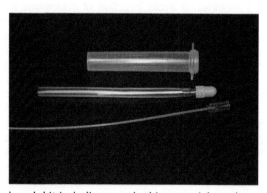

Fig. 2. Transtracheal wash kit including sample shipment vial, trochar, and catheter.

Table 1
Suggested tissues for submission to a diagnostic laboratory for respiratory disease diagnosis

Lung	Formalin fixed, 3 or 4 sections, collected from margins between affected and unaffected areas, and approximately 5 mm thick
Lung	Fresh, 2 pieces of lung approximately 200 g (6 cm × 6 cm × 6 cm)
Serum	3–5 mL (removed from the clot, chilled to 4°C)
Tracheal and mesenteric lymph nodes	Formalin-fixed and fresh
Skin (ear notch)	Formalin-fixed, 1 cm × 1 cm
Ileum	Formalin-fixed, 2–3 cm long
Liver, kidney, and spleen	Fresh, chilled, and formalin-fixed if systemic disease or mineral assessment is warranted

be isolated. Select lung samples for histopathologic examination, IHC and/or fluorescent antibody testing at the junction of affected and less affected tissues. In many cases, IHC or polymerase chain reaction has replaced fluorescent antibody testing as well as virus isolation. This situation is particularly true when tissues have autolyzed during shipment, test specificity is poor, or a 3-week delay for virus isolation results is prohibitive. An advantage of IHC over fluorescent antibody tests is that antigen can be visualized in the proper location or in the proper cell type in tissues. Autolysis reduces the sensitivity and specificity of fluorescent antibody tests. Over fixation of tissues in formalin can be detrimental to IHC test results. Fresh lung samples should be kept and shipped chilled, whereas formalin-fixed tissues can be maintained at room temperature. Chilling slows the fixation process.

SAMPLING TECHNIQUES
Fixatives

Neutral buffered formalin (NBF) at 10% concentration is the most common fixative used in veterinary medicine.

Ten percent NBF can be purchased premixed or prepared from 37% formaldehyde. The formulation for 10% NBF is given in the following list:

- 100 mL of 37% formaldehyde
- 900 mL of distilled water
- 4.0 g of monobasic sodium phosphate
- 6.5 g of dibasic sodium phosphate (anhydrous).

For those in harsher climates, the addition of 1 mL of ethanol to each 9 mL of 10% formalin prevents freezing during cold weather.[3] If 10% NBF is unavailable, 100 proof ethanol can be substituted, with the understanding that tissues must be trimmed to a thickness of approximately 2.5 mm to achieve adequate fixation. If even 100 proof ethanol is not available, samples can be preserved in antifreeze, again with the caveat that samples must be trimmed to approximately 2.5 mm thick to achieve fixation and that once arriving at the diagnostic laboratory, they must be rinsed thoroughly with water, before being placed in 10% NBF and blocked for slide preparation.

Histopathology/IHC

Parenchymal tissue should be trimmed to approximately 5 mm in one dimension and up to 3 to 4 cm in length and width for best fixation in 10% NBF.[3] The optimal ratio of

10% NBF to tissue is 10:1. If specimens are held until fixed, before shipment a smaller volume of formalin can be used to maintain moisture of the specimens, including wrapping formalin-fixed samples in formalin-soaked gauze or quality paper towel. This step reduces issues with leakage as well as total shipping weight.

Plastic leakproof containers with snap or screw top lids, Whirl-Paks (Nasco, Fort Atkinson, WI, USA), or heat-sealed freezer bags are best for shipping formalin.[3] Place the primary container in a second leakproof container or bag to contain spills. Do not tape container tops; if leakage occurs, the result is simply formalin-soaked tape.

Bacteriology

Lung and other parenchymatous organs for culture should be submitted in pieces sizeable enough to be sterilized on surface for sampling of deeper tissue. Samples should be approximately the size of a large lemon and the presence of an intact capsule should be ensured. Submission in sterile well-sealed plastic bags is beneficial. If possible, tissues from untreated animals should be selected. Tissues for culture should be in good condition, collected as soon as possible after death with minimal surface contamination. It is best to keep samples cold and not frozen until reaching the laboratory. Prolonged postmortem interval or gross contamination of samples impedes or precludes isolation of pathogens as well as other testing procedures.

Transtracheal washes, bronchoalveolar lavages, nasopharyngeal swabs, or nasal swabs are best collected from untreated animals within 1 to 2 days of onset of the disease process. These specimens need to be kept chilled and submitted for culture as well as for other techniques listed in the following sections.

Virology

Virus isolation is infrequently used in today's diagnostic laboratories, with the advent of molecular testing techniques and IHC for identification of organisms. Collection of samples for virus isolation follows similar needs of those described for bacterial culture.

Molecular Diagnostics

Molecular diagnostics using polymerase chain reaction and other techniques, including microarray analysis, have replaced more classic diagnostic procedures including virus isolation and culture for *Mycoplasma* spp and other fastidious organisms. Although providing rapid testing with high specificity and sensitivity, results of these tests can be altered by autolysis and bacterial contamination. Samples should be collected as rapidly as possible, free of marked contamination, and kept chilled and submitted to the laboratory.[3]

Parasitology

Nasal discharges may contain embryonated eggs or larvae, and larvae may be found in feces. Coughing may occur in the prepatent period, before adults develop and lay eggs. Lungworms are found in the airways on postmortem examination. Samples can be obtained by collection of discharges in a tube or by nasal washing techniques. Samples should be kept cool and submitted chilled to the diagnostic laboratory.

Examination of feces for lungworm larvae can be conducted (minimum 15 g or 1 tablespoonful required, best submitted chilled in a screw cap tube or double-bagged Whirl-Pak). False-negative results can occur, if the animals are sampled before or after the adult lungworms become patent (egg producing). Furthermore, adult cattle, which are often partially immune, may show disease without the infection ever becoming patent. Thus, laboratory confirmation by demonstration of lungworm larvae in feces is successful in only about 50% of outbreaks in dairy cows.[6]

Serology

Serologic interpretation of respiratory diseases in cattle is extremely difficult. Vaccination procedures and timing of sample collection often distort test results. Close consultation with a diagnostician is recommended to select an adequate population for testing or evaluate value of testing in given situations. Serologic testing is always done on serum and not on plasma. Approximately 0.5 mL of serum should be submitted for each test requested.

Toxicology

Samples of fresh parenchymatous tissues for toxicologic evaluation in diagnostic situations should be frozen to limit changes in toxin levels. Approximately 250 g of tissue should be submitted (approximately a large lemon-sized sample of liver, kidney, or rumen content). Approximately 10 mL of urine, unclotted blood, serum, and ocular fluid is suggested. Situations in which feed is considered a culprit for clinical signs observed, submission of a minimum of 0.5 kg of feed is suggested. Submission in paper or breathable material is recommended, particularly if evaluation of mycotoxins is warranted. An adequate sample of any suspected toxin should be obtained and retained for possible analysis.

To evaluate trace minerals in cattle the best sample is a liver sample compared with serum. A liver biopsy collected by a 12 to 14 gauge biopsy needle is adequate for evaluation of multiple minerals at one time by using inductively coupled plasma analysis. Samples should not be pooled when doing mineral profiles. Pooling effectively averages mineral levels negating the efforts of identifying outliers that exhibit deficits within the population. Animals within affected populations that have not been treated and appear clinically normal are the sample population of choice. A chronic pneumonic calf that has been treated multiple times and has not had adequate or consistent feed intake would have mineral levels altered from abnormal feed intake.

SAMPLE TRANSPORT

At present, shipping of diagnostic specimens is regulated by the federal government. Requirements include a primary watertight container encompassed by sufficient absorbent material to contain spills and enclosed by a secondary solid, watertight packaging (foam box, ice chest, plastic box, or heavy cardboard).

Submitters are often naive in the ways of shippers. As a consequence neatly penned instructions on exteriors of boxes indicating "this side up" or "fragile" are likely barely worth the ink consumed. Think containment and expect that at some point in the package's travel, submission boxes may be upside down, sideways, flying through the air, or dropped.

Formalin-filled containers should be tightly closed and leakproof. Despite the overwhelming number of individuals who put in the effort to seal formalin containers with tape or paraffin wrap, these materials do not impede leakage.

A plastic screw top container or double-bagged Whirl-Paks encompassed by an adequate amount of absorbent material (quality paper towels, commercially available materials, cat litter) works best. Before closing a Whirl-Pak, as much air as possible should be removed. This step avoids damage of the tissues due to jostling of the air-formalin mixture and reduces the possibility of rupture of the Whirl-Pak during shipment.

Fresh specimens should be placed in a larger bag to keep them together and in contact with ice packs. Frozen gel packs are preferred. Crushed ice or ice cubes in bags melt and soak the contents of the box and the box in which the specimens are being shipped. Sufficient numbers of gel packs placed in contact with samples should be used to keep samples cool during shipment.

Include submission forms in a sealed plastic bag to ensure they stay dry during shipment. Label containers with owner name and animal identification. If possible, ship specimens by an overnight courier. Ideally, ship specimens to arrive on a weekday. If delivery on Saturday or on a holiday is anticipated, contact the laboratory.

Communication is frequently the key to receiving and delivering accurate diagnostic data, which can be of greatest use to practitioners and their clients. Keeping things simple and lines of communication open between practitioners and diagnosticians can allow for growth and learning on both sides of the equation.

SUMMARY

Diagnostic sampling and tests can provide valuable information when investigating causes of respiratory disease within a group. Veterinarians and producers should agree on the diagnostic question, testing goals, and use of results before submitting samples. Is the information going to be used? If so, how will it be used? What processes do the generated data affect? Consulting with a diagnostician and communicating what the producer goals are should ensure that appropriate samples are obtained to diagnose or rule in pathogens as well as for the economic use of resources. Evaluating other factors that may be contributing to disease within a group may also be addressed.

ACKNOWLEDGMENTS

Many thanks to Dr Steve Ensley for his input and expertise on toxicology sampling. Thanks as well to Jacqueline Hailey for photography expertise.

REFERENCES

1. Viet HP, Ferrell RL. The anatomy and physiology of the bovine respiratory system relating to pulmonary disease. Cornell Vet 1978;68(4):555–81.
2. Mariassy AT, Plopper CG, Dungworth DL. Characteristics of bovine lung as observed by scanning electron microscopy. Anat Rec 1975;183(1):13–25.
3. Blanchard PC. Sampling techniques for the diagnosis of digestive disease. Vet Clin North Am 2000;16(1):23–36.
4. Godinho KS, Sarasola P, Renoult E, et al. Use of deep nasopharyngeal swabs as a predictive diagnostic method for natural respiratory infections in calves. Vet Rec 2007;160:22–5.
5. Angen O, Thomse J, Larsen LE, et al. Respiratory disease in calves: microbiological investigations on trans-tracheally aspirated bronchoalveolar lavage fluid, and acute phase protein response. Vet Microbiol 2009;137(1–2):165–71.
6. Beggs N. Lungworm infection in organic cattle. Disease surveillance and investigation branch, veterinary science division. Departement of Agriculture and Rural Development 43 Beltany Road, Coneywarren, Omagh, Co. Tyrone BT785NF, Northern Ireland. Internet Communication. Available at: http://www.afbini.gov.uk/adds-cattlelungwormdec05.pdf. Accessed April 15, 2010.

Index

Note: Page numbers of article titles are in **boldface** type.

A

AIP. See Atypical interstitial pneumonia (AIP).
Air surface liquid, in innate immune responses to bovine respiratory disease, 218–219
Airway(s), respiratory, in innate immune responses to bovine respiratory disease, 216
Airway epithelia, in innate immune responses to bovine respiratory disease, 219–220
Anemia(s), bovine pneumonia and, 204–205
Animal husbandry, in bovine respiratory disease management in feedlot cattle, 278–279
Antibody(ies), effect on maternal immunity to respiratory disease in cow/calf
    operations, 230–231
Anti-infective agents, in bovine respiratory disease prevention in stocker cattle, 267–268
Antimicrobial resistance testing, in evaluation of Mycoplasma bovis in respiratory disease
    in feedlot cattle, 374
Antimicrobial therapy, metaphylactic, for bovine respiratory disease in stocker and
    feedlot cattle, **285–301**
    ceftiofur, 291–292
    chlortetracycline, 292–293
    described, 285–286
    florfenicol, 293
    health and feed performance comparison among agents in, 296
    impact on cattle health and performance, 289–290
    implementation/timing of, 287–289
    overview of, 286–287
    oxytetracycline, 293
    sulfamethazine, 292–293
    tilmicosin, 293, 296
    tulathromycin, 296
Aspiration pneumonia, 205–206
Atypical interstitial pneumonia (AIP), bovine, **395–407**
    causes of, 397–403
    clinical signs of, 396–397
    described, 395–396
    prevention of, 403
    treatment of, 403

B

Bacterial bovine pneumonia, 192–200. See also Bovine pneumonia, bacterial.
Bacterial pathogens, of BRDC, **381–394**. See also specific pathogens and Bovine
    respiratory disease complex (BRDC), bacterial pathogens of.
Bacteriology, in bovine respiratory disease diagnostics, 414
BCoVs. See Bovine coronaviruses (BCoVs).

Vet Clin Food Anim 26 (2010) 417–426
doi:10.1016/S0749-0720(10)00025-3
0749-0720/10/$ – see front matter © 2010 Elsevier Inc. All rights reserved.

vetfood.theclinics.com

Printed and bound by CPI Group (UK) Ltd, Croydon, CR0 4YY

03/10/2024

01040457-0008